COMMUNITY NUTRITION

COMMUNITY
NUTRITION

JESSIE CRAIG OBERT, Ph.D., R.D.

Consulting Nutritionist

JOHN WILEY & SONS
New York • Santa Barbara • Chichester • Brisbane • Toronto

*The cover design is a demographic map
showing an areal view of a major city,
focusing in on one community and its
strong nutritional values.*

Library of Congress Cataloging in Publication Data:

Obert, Jessie Craig, 1911–
    Community nutrition.

    Includes bibliographical references and index.
    1. Food relief—United States.   2. Nutrition
policy—United States.   I. Title.

HV696.F6023   362.5   77-13992
ISBN 0-471-65236-9

Printed in the United States of American

10 9 8 7 6 5 4 3 2

To more than eighty nutritionists who worked under my direction in the County of Los Angeles between 1953 and 1976 and who contributed in many ways to my concepts of community nutrition.

PREFACE

This book is intended as a text for the course in community nutrition
and as a handbook for nutritionists, dietitians, home economists, community nurses, health educators, school personnel, physicians, and
others who are interested in developing community nutrition programs.
The community nutritionist is uniquely qualified for this task but, in
many areas where there are no community nutritionists, other health
professionals may assume leadership for community action to solve
nutrition problems. Some of the skills can be performed by aides,
technicians, or volunteers. However, a community nutrition background
is needed to understand how to use the information in diagnosis and
treatment and in the complicated relationships of the community.

Dietitians will find that a knowledge of community nutrition will help
them to provide better care for their discharged patients. They will
understand the problems patients face when they return to home and
community and they will know the community resources that provide
help with specific problems. The book will also help the dietitian who
participates in health planning or community action.

I have given detailed procedures for some of the skills and techniques, but have emphasized the need to develop policy and plan action
on the basis of current circumstance. In some instances I have reported
several points of view without synthesis or recommending a stand on the
question. Such decisions must be made at the time that they are
needed.

My purpose in writing this book is to share the concepts, experiences, and philosophy developed during more than thirty years as a nutritionist, social worker, home economist, and teacher in various organizations. They include the Chicago Welfare Department, Arizona Agricultural Extension, Maricopa County (Arizona) Chapter of the American Red Cross, Ohio State University, University of California at Los Angeles, the school lunch program of Fayette County (Ohio), volunteer service with the Heart Association and Los Angeles county where I served for more than 22 years as Nutrition Program Director and Coordinator.

Many of the examples and program reports are from my experiences in Los Angeles County. Although it is a large county, it includes communities of all sizes and many ethnic groups so that the examples are applicable in other places of different size and characteristics. Some examples are from my participation in programs of voluntary agencies as employee or volunteer, or from programs supported by business or industry.

One of my concepts of community nutrition is that the programs are accomplished by application of a background of subject matter, tools, skills, techniques, and activities to specific communities composed of persons who have common problems. I have tried to show the importance of this background and how it is used.

Significant terms have been specifically defined; I have stated many of them to explain their particular application in community nutrition. References are given at the end of each chapter, sometimes as References Cited, and Additional References, sometimes simply as References, depending on how I used them. Where no references are given, my ideas developed from diffuse sources to which I express my general appreciation.

Some repetition will be found, most of it resulting from the desire to explain a topic in one place and to make each chapter complete.

I have limited the book to programs in the United States. However, the methods, skills, and techniques and much of the subject matter could be applied in other countries.

Jessie Craig Obert

Los Angeles, California
April 2, 1977

ACKNOWLEDGMENTS

I express my appreciation to all who have been my colleagues in community nutrition programs, giving me ideas and in turn using mine. I am especially grateful to four of the many teachers who guided my learning: Margaret E. Lorimer of Park College, Lydia J. Roberts of the University of Chicago, and Mary Brown Patton and Everett C. Shimp of the Ohio State University.

While writing I received much help from persons who supplied class outlines, guides, unpublished materials, examples, and information, or who reviewed portions of the manuscript. Some of them were: Adela Dolney, Esther Eicher, Frances Fischer, Anne Goodwin, Mary M. Hill, Elizabeth Johnson, Rose Ann Langham, Doris Lauber, Wetona Olson, Eileen Peck, Olympia Stapakis, Joyce Vermeersch, and Donna Williams. The Librarians at the University of Southern California and the Los Angeles office staff of Senator Alan Cranston were gracious and helpful on many occasions. My particular thanks go to Virginia Gladney, who reviewed parts of the manuscript and gave me much consultation and encouragement.

J. C. O.

CONTENTS

COMMUNITY NUTRITION

1 THE FIELD

Community nutrition is the field in which the subject matter of nutrition and related science is used by nutritionists to help individuals, families, and communities solve their nutrition problems. Although public health nutrition is community nutrition, it is characterized by having unique responsibilities for health within the area it covers.

Community nutritionists are concerned with the prevention and treatment of nutrition problems that are common to many persons. They identify the problems and causes and arrange appropriate methods of intervention. Community nutritionists perform four basic functions although they work under many titles in a variety of agencies.

CHAPTER

1
INTRODUCTION

Community nutrition is the field of knowledge in which subject matter from a number of areas is applied to the solution of community nutrition problems during the interaction of nutrition personnel and community. The community nutritionist is concerned with all elements that affect nutritional health and the well-being of population groups. Community nutrition differs from other nutrition practice by its attention to people as they relate to the community and are affected by the community. It has a special body of knowledge derived from the nutritional, biological, behavioral, social, and managerial sciences. The body of knowledge supplies information about various topics that is applied in many activities making up the practice of community nutrition.

The areas of learning for the community nutritionist include nutritional science, nutritional needs in both health and disease throughout the life cycle, nutritional care, food science and art, education methods, management, and community organization.

GOALS FOR THE STUDY OF COMMUNITY NUTRITION

Some of the goals for the study of community nutrition are:

1. To acquire the knowledge and to know the skills and tools that constitute the background of the community nutritionist.
2. To understand the community structure for health and to know the

kinds of agencies and organizations that conduct nutrition programs or provide related services.

3. To recognize health and welfare programs that have a nutrition component.

4. To understand the techniques of community organization, management and planning, public education, and professional education.

5. To be able to recognize opportunities for improving food practices.

6. To know sources for leaflets, pamphlets, and other instructional materials suitable for use in community nutrition programs and how to develop new materials.

7. To develop a professional philosophy and value system that will determine the personal approach to community nutrition problems.

HOW TO USE THIS BOOK AS A TEXT

It is expected that the student will have had courses to provide the necessary subject-matter background, including a course in diets in the treatment of disease. This book builds on that background, providing brief subject-matter reviews at various points of use and explaining the application of information in relation to specific skills and activities of community nutrition. Many examples of programs and activities are mentioned in the book. Students should look for other examples in current professional publications and in news stories and advertisements to help them see the application of the tools, skills, techniques, and program methods that are discussed.

Part I, *The Field*, explains the field of community nutrition, reviewing its development and history, the present state, and future trends. In Part II, *The Structure*, there is a description of the community structure and the various organizations and programs that make up the social setting in which the community nutritionist works.

As in other professions the work of the community nutritionist requires certain tools and skills. These are described and explained in Part III, *The Tools and Skills*. Part IV, *The Techniques*, explains the application of community organization, management and planning, professional education, and public education, four broad techniques through which the nutritionist works.

Part V, *The Activities*, describes the body of knowledge necessary for certain activities frequently used in community nutrition. Part VI, *The Practice*, suggests some ways to program with particular attention to conditions and diseases in which nutrition is important for prevention and treatment.

HOW TO USE THIS BOOK AS A RESOURCE

Many persons cooperate in community nutrition programs or assume leadership to solve the nutrition problems of the people they encounter in their regular work. Nutritionists, dietitians, home economists, community nurses, physicians, health educators, and others will find this book a useful reference. It contains suggestions and specific directions on how to carry out many activities, for example, arranging a group educational event in nutrition, and conducting a study of local cultural food practices.

SOLVING THE NEED FOR UP-TO-DATE REFERENCE MATERIALS

The person who uses this book will soon note the absence of tables and charts often included in nutrition texts. This was deliberately done because the community nutritionist needs to keep for constant reference the latest version of such materials. It is suggested that the person who uses this book as a text or reference acquire a pressure binder or large envelope in which these materials can be conveniently filed and easily changed when they become obsolete. Students should make this collection as the materials are covered during the course and have it ready for use in their field work or jobs.

Some materials which should be included are:

Table of Recommended Dietary Allowances (RDA)

Table of United States Recommended Daily Allowances (US RDA's)

Height-weight tables

Growth charts of the Public Health Service

Nutritive Value of Foods

Special food value tables (e.g., cholesterol, folic acid)

USDA Family Food Plans

Various food guides

Recent food prices

Regulations for government food programs that are of particular interest to the individual (e.g., Food Stamp Program, Child Nutrition Programs, Nutrition Programs for the Elderly)

Current poverty guidelines of USDA

The individual user may wish to add others such as a metric conversion table. It is helpful to date each item when acquired and to add the date of publication, price, and source if this information is not printed on the item.

USING CURRENT PUBLICATIONS FOR PROGRAM IDEAS

The student, community nutritionist, and others interested in community nutrition programs should form the habit of reviewing recent journals when starting a new topic or activity. Examples will be found in the publications of many disciplines but most often in the following professional journals:

Journal of the American Dietetic Association
Journal of Home Economics
Journal of Nutrition Education
American Journal of Public Health
Nutrition Today

These journals also carry notice of new publications and films and other teaching materials.

During the course the student should get acquainted with some of the other journals listed in the references. These are in other fields and each will help meet the need for references on particular subjects.

SUMMARY

Community nutrition applies subject matter from nutrition and other fields to the solution of nutrition problems of individuals and families by interaction with the community. The goals for study are to help the student (1) understand the community structure, (2) acquire a background of knowledge, skills, tools, and techniques, and (3) know which methods to use in specific situations. This book will also serve as a reference for professionals and other leaders who conduct community nutrition programs. Some ways to use printed materials and journals have been discussed.

2 COMMUNITY NUTRITION AS A FIELD

Community nutrition was characterized in Chapter 1 as an applied field distinguished by the process of interaction between nutrition personnel and community for the solution of nutrition problems.

A *community nutrition program* is one planned to improve the nutrition of individuals and groups in a *community,* which is a specific group of people who have a common bond such as speaking the same language (as Italian), living under the same government (as a city), or having the same health problem (as high blood pressure).

In this book, *community nutrition program* refers to any nutrition program whether of broad or limited objectives so long as it is characterized by interaction with the community. Community nutrition programs may be conducted by public agencies such as health departments, by voluntary health agencies, such as the Heart Association, by public schools, by colleges and universities, or by other organizations.

PUBLIC HEALTH NUTRITION

Frequently community nutrition and public health nutrition are considered as synonymous terms; however, *community nutrition* is used here in a very broad sense to include all nutrition programs in which there is community interaction. *Public health* has sometimes been defined as health services provided through tax financing and intended for poor people, but its area of responsibility is really the health of the public, that is, of all the people regardless of income or socioeconomic status. In this book, *public health nutrition* will distinguish the nutrition program conducted by an *official agency* such as a state, county, city, or other governmental agency to which has been delegated the official responsibility for the health of persons living in the designated area.

Public health nutrition uses large-scale, organized efforts to solve health problems that affect large numbers of persons for whom group action is necessary or at least more effective than individual efforts. Within a public health jurisdiction, there will be only one public health nutrition program, but it will include a number of activities, each of which is a community nutrition program conducted by public health nutritionists or other members of the agency staff. Some components of a public health nutrition program are planning and coordinating a comprehensive nutrition program for the area served, participating in agency plans for the health care of children and youth, conducting nutrition activities, and providing professional education in the community.

Within the jurisdiction of the public health agency, there may be a number of community nutrition programs conducted independently by other organizations, for example, nutrition education by a local voluntary agency for its service recipients, provision of meals for the elderly, food service and nutrition education in a child care center, and education of teachers and homemakers conducted by the local Dairy Council. By the definition used here, public health nutrition is a community nutrition program, but in the same geographic area there will be other community nutrition programs. Each of these programs will cover a more limited area and scope than the program of the public health agency. Figure 2.1 shows the central role of the public health agency and some of the other programs that may be in the community.

GOALS FOR COMMUNITY NUTRITION PROGRAMS

A community nutrition program should be designed to accomplish specific goals for the population segment that is within its area of responsibility. These goals are:

1. Identification of potential nutrition problems and action for prevention.
2. Identification and correction of existing nutrition problems.
3. Treatment of disease states that have a nutrition component.

These broad goals can cover all community nutrition programs including the public health nutrition program in a large local health

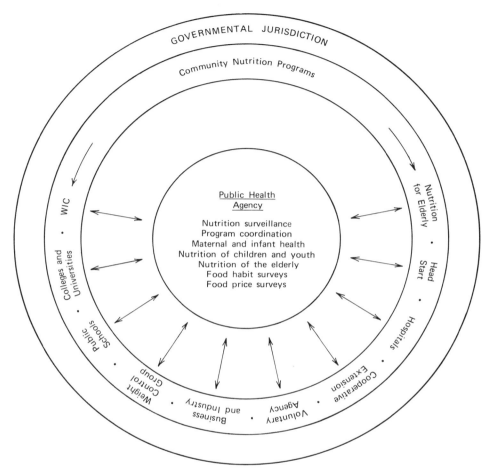

Figure 2.1 Relationship Between the Public Health Nutrition Program and Other Community Nutrition Programs Showing the Central Role of Public Health. (*Source.* Jessie C. Obert, Ph.D., R.D.)

department, the community nutrition program in a small neighborhood agency, and a hospital-oriented community nutrition program.

HISTORY OF COMMUNITY NUTRITION

Community nutrition programs started before the First World War with programs to correct malnutrition in children. Dietitians and home economists conducted a variety of food and nutrition programs in schools, health and welfare agencies and in the United States Agricultural Extension Service. (5) Activities at that time included education about family and child nutrition and supplemental feeding programs with emphasis on teaching people how to take responsibility for their own needs and the needs of those for whose health they were responsible. In 1917 the first nutritionists in state health departments were employed in Massachusetts and New York.

The need for nutrition programs was also recognized in 1917 by one of the founders of the American Public Health Association, who said that past programs had been concerned with food adulteration, that current programs were emphasizing food sanitation and that future programs would be focused on family nutrition. (1) In 1918 Roberts conducted a program in Chicago in which advanced nutrition students held classes in the clinic at Rush Medical College and worked intensively in homes teaching food and health habits, food values and cooking methods. (6)

The continuing concern about child nutrition was evinced by papers on rickets and malnutrition read at the 1921 annual meeting of the American Public Health Association. By this time, nutrition education was conducted in conjunction with school lunch and general health teaching and some nutritionists were employed in public and private health agencies, in Agricultural Extension Service, in the American Red Cross, and in a number of trade associations.

Community nutrition programs during succeeding years related to retarded growth, diseases caused by deficiency of specific nutrients such as rickets, scurvy, and pellagra, and the relationship of nutrition to infectious diseases, especially tuberculosis. These problems continued for several decades until they were corrected by the application of nutritional knowledge such as use of cod liver oil to prevent rickets or by new medication for disease control as in the case of tuberculosis. One of the topics in all the programs was wise use of food money to purchase good nutrition. Attention to food-money management was intensified during the economic depression of the early 1930's, when nutritionists were employed in some welfare agencies to advise on food rations and food orders and to determine minimum adequate allowances for family food and therapeutic diets.

In the 1940's, World War II stimulated a new interest in nutrition with recommendations for programs to maintain good nutrition in the United States. A landmark in nutrition occurred in 1941 with the first issue of the Recommended Dietary Allowances. (4) The "Basic Seven," a new food plan that divided foods into seven groups, was developed and widely used as a teaching device. Bread enrichment was mandated in the United States as a mass effort to increase the consumption of nutrients that were low in the diets of many people. Considerable attention was given to the nutrition of industrial workers and of children in day nurseries. Enactment of the National School Lunch Act in 1946 gave rise to many related community nutrition programs.

A few years later, increasing numbers of older persons resulted in more nutrition programs to improve the nutrition of this age group. These included surveys to identify problems, educational programs, home-delivered meals, and upgrading of food in boarding and nursing homes.

The identification of genetic metabolic diseases and the need for nutrition education for their treatment brought new dimensions as did new programs for health of children and adolescents.

Additional community nutrition activities were developed during the 1960's with emphasis on the problems of hunger and malnutrition. Many activities were funded as part of the Federal poverty programs, including extensive ones to improve the health care of mothers and children with some programs designed to prevent mental retardation. These projects usually had a community component as well as patient counseling by nutritionists.

Further impetus to all nutrition programs was provided in 1968 by the publication *Hunger USA* (3) and the television program "Hunger in America" (2), each presenting a picture of food and nutrition problems of poverty groups. The White House Conference on Food, Nutrition and Health in December 1969 (7) brought together 3000 participants from public, business, and professions who discussed the interrelated problems of nutrition, hunger, and poverty. The panels and task forces presented statements and recommendations about nutritional status, groups with special needs, national food policies, food distribution, mass feeding, agriculture, the food industry, and other topics. The Conference gave impetus to many changes in existing nutrition programs and to new programs concerned with mothers and infants, mental retardation, older people, coronary prevention, alcohol and drug addicts, and food distribution.

In recent years, there has been an increase in the number of community nutritionists, especially in programs for maternal and infant care, older persons, child development, coronary prevention, alcohol and drug addicts, and food distribution. These nutritionists often have a dual role in the community and the clinic.

PRESENT TRENDS

The changes taking place in community nutrition have been brought about by changes in the entire community health field and in emphasis of nutrition programs and nutritional care. Public health programs used to be concerned mainly with disease prevention and health promotion, but considerable emphasis is now placed on therapy and rehabilitation and community nutrition programs are often concerned with treatment of disease as well as with prevention.

Traditionally, most nutritionists were meticulous in establishing the point that they did not participate in diagnosis or prescription, leaving these matters entirely to the physician. Now the role perception includes working from the physician's diagnosis to decide what dietary regime will achieve the medical objective, and instructing on activity and other nutrition-related health practices. Nutritionists also function as project or program directors in a variety of programs in which there is no immediate medical component. In some situations, the nutritionist works with groups of well individuals advising on diet, activity and other health matters which affect nutrition.

SUMMARY

Community nutrition includes any program characterized by interaction with the community. Public health nutrition is the nutrition program in an official governmental agency responsible for health in a specific geographic area, characterized by large-scale efforts to solve the problems of many persons. There may be many community nutrition programs in one public health jurisdiction.

The goals of community nutrition are defined as identifying potential and existing problems, and preventing or treating them, and the treatment of disease by nutrition.

A brief history of community nutrition has been related and present trends described.

REFERENCES CITED

1. Fifty Years of Progress: 1917–1967. *Am. J. Public Health,* 58 1/68 138.
2. Hunger in America, CBS Television Program, 1969.
3. *Hunger, U.S.A.: A Report by the Citizens' Board of Inquiry into Hunger and Malnutrition in the United States.* New Community Press, Washington DC, 1968.
4. Mitchell, Helen, Recommended Dietary Allowances Up To Date, *J. Am. Diet. Assoc.,* 64 2/74 149.
5. Peck, Eileen B., The Public Health Nutritionist-Dietitian: An Historical Perspective. *J. Am. Diet. Assoc.,* 64 6/74 643.
6. Roberts, Lydia J., *Nutrition Work with Children,* University of Chicago Press, Chicago, rev. 1935, p. 320.

7. *White House Conference on Food, Nutrition and Health,* Final Report. Government Printing Office, Washington DC, 1970.

ADDITIONAL REFERENCES

Curran, William J., A Bicentennial Review, *Am. J. Public Health 66* 1/76 93.

Miller, C. Arden, Societal Change and Public Health, *Am. J. Public Health,* 66 1/76 56.

Pollock, H., Hunger U.S.A.: a critical review, *Am. J. Clin. Nutr.,* 22 1969 480.

3 NUTRITION PROBLEMS IN THE UNITED STATES

The goals of all community nutrition programs are to identify potential nutrition problems and prevent them from developing, to identify and correct existing problems, and to treat diseases that have a nutrition component. This chapter will provide an overview of nutrition problems that are targets for intervention in community nutrition programs.

A nutrition program for a specific community should be planned to attack the existing and potential nutrition problems as identified by evidence from that particular community. *Existing problems* are conditions which are already present, for example, 15 percent of the adult women age 40 to 60 in this city are 20 percent or more overweight. *Potential problems* are existing factors likely to lead to undesirable conditions later, for example, that most of the children in the community consume a diet high in saturated fat and sugar.

There are three sources of information about existing and potential nutrition problems in the United States or in a specific community: (1) data on nutritional status, (2) data on the prevalence and consequences of nutrition-related diseases, and (3) information about practices and conditions which contribute to nutrition problems.

Any community nutrition program should be based on these kinds of evidence for the specific community; however, the nutritionist should be informed about pertinent information already available from other sources. This will stimulate ideas about how to obtain relevant data for the specific community and help the nutritionist in organizing the community to develop evaluation methods that will measure progress.

Before anyone can attempt to identify nutrition problems in a community there must be a definition of what constitutes a problem. A *nutrition problem* is any situation or factor that has an adverse effect on the nutrition of an individual or a group or a population so that it must be changed before nutrition can be improved. There are difficulties with this definition, such as whether or not obesity is a nutritional problem when the obese individual is content to be obese, and whether or not saturated fat constitutes a risk factor in coronary heart disease when some professional nutritionists hold other views. A nutrition problem in any specific community needs to be defined by that community in relation to its own situation.

NUTRITIONAL STATUS SURVEYS

Although there have been many studies of small or limited population groups in the United States, it was not until the late 1960's that surveys were conducted to determine the nutritional status of large population groups. Since then information about nutritional status in the United States has been supplied by several surveys made by the Federal government. Results from such studies do not necessarily apply precisely to a specific community, but they provide background for developing a plan to identify and describe local problems.

Methods Used to Determine Nutritional Status

Nutritional status is the physical health of a person as it results from consumption and utilization of food in the body. The nutritional status of an individual is determined by the kind and amount of nutrients supplied to the body and how completely they are used to meet body needs. A survey of nutritional status should show the relationship between food and nutrients ingested, their use in the body, and general health.

Nutritional status·is assessed by anthropometric, clinical and biochemical methods. Dietary studies provide clues that can be used in evaluating other data and in anticipating future problems. (5, 19, 20)

Body Measurements (Anthropometry). Height and weight are used to identify overweight, underweight, and retarded growth. Many studies have used skinfolds, that is, caliper measurements of thickness of a fold of tissue, usually from the upper arm, below the shoulder blade or from the upper abdomen. Measurements used for infants include recumbent height, head circumference, chest circumference, and triceps skinfold.

Clinical Examination. A careful physical examination by a physician, nutritionist, or other specially trained health worker can identify signs that may indicate malnutrition. A clinical finding should be confirmed by laboratory tests. Generally the conditions during the survey are compared with the conditions observed in healthy individuals in other surveys.

Some of the significant clinical signs are hair that is thin, dry, dull or easily plucked; nails that are brittle, ridged, or spoon-shaped; skin pigmentation, dryness or flakiness; pale eye membranes; redness and swelling of mouth, and gums that are soft or bleed easily. Screening for dental caries and other diseases of teeth and gums is a part of the clinical assessment, since dental problems are directly and indirectly related to diet. Measuring blood pressure is usually part of the examination for adults and also for children as early as two years.

Laboratory Tests. These measures provide a precise, objective method of determining levels of nutrients in blood or urine that indicate the status of the body in respect to specific nutrients. (5) The purpose of these measurements is to disclose deficiencies at an early stage or in a marginal state when clinical signs are not yet apparent, as well as to identify disease. The most frequently used tests are determination of hemoglobin or hematocrit to identify iron deficiency anemia, and urinalysis to evaluate protein and sugar. Blood tests are used for trace elements, vitamins, proteins and lipids. Extensive tests are used in research studies or when other signs indicate that problems exist. Bone X-rays are sometimes used to identify retarded growth.

Dietary Studies. Information about food consumed and intake of nutrients helps identify the cause of malnutrition and serves as a basis for recommending dietary changes. (5) The methods most often used to secure this information are (1) a record of the food intake kept by the individual or parent, (2) a recall made by parent or child or taken in an interview, and (3) a diet history taken by a specially-trained interviewer. The number of servings or amounts of foods are compared with standards for amounts of foods in the different food groups. Sometimes calculations are made of the nutrient intakes for comparison with the recommended dietary allowances. Dietary deficiencies shown by these methods should be correlated with the body measurements and biochemical tests. In some types of surveys, dietary studies are made by determining the quantities of all foods used by a family group or household. Dietary data do not diagnose malnutrition or assess nutritional status but supplement other findings and indicate appropriate remedial measures. An extreme shortage of calories or nutrients suggests that biochemical or anthropometric signs of deficiency may appear at a later date.

Preschool Children in the United States

This national study was conducted in 1968–70 by the Children's Hospital Research Foundation under a grant from the United States Department of Health, Education, and Welfare. (12) The purpose was to obtain information on the nutritional status of a sample of preschool children of all income levels. The survey included dietary studies, clinical evaluations, dental examinations, and laboratory tests along with detailed socioeconomic information.

Dietary interviews were conducted with 3441 children aged one to five years. Clinical examinations and biochemical tests were made on about two-thirds of these children.

The dietary data were evaluated by special standards established for the study. The values for protein, vitamin A, vitamin C, thiamin, and riboflavin were set near established minimum requirements, while those for iron and calcium were set at values believed by the researchers also to represent minimum requirements. These values were used with the dietary data to estimate the proportion of children who had inadequate intakes of energy and the selected nutrients.

Clinical examinations showed a few signs of malnutrition, mostly among the poor. There was more dental caries among the poor and the blacks. The anthropometric examination showed that in these age groups black children were heavier and taller than white. Children who had lower dietary intakes, lower biochemical values, and who were small for their age were characterized as showing evidence of nutritional risk.

The major nutrition problem was insufficient food among the poor children with lower than average dietary intakes. Protein intakes were similar for all children and were judged adequate to meet the needs. Ascorbic acid intakes of many children in the low income group were less than 15 milligrams per day, the standard used. Many children used vitamin supplements, although the practice was less common among poor children. The amount of vitamin supplements tended to decrease with age.

Blood protein levels were higher in black children than in white. Serum albumin levels were high even in the lower income groups with levels of white children consistently higher than those of black. There were more low hemoglobin levels among the black children than among the white. The mean hemoglobin values were lowest among the poor, increasing with income and age, and were lower among blacks than among whites. Vitamin A levels were considerably higher in blacks.

The authors suggested that improving socioeconomic status and expanding food programs might be of more value in alleviating the problems than bread and cereal enrichment programs or nutrition education.

Ten-State Nutrition Survey

In 1967 Congress directed the Department of Health, Education and Welfare to determine the extent and location of malnutrition and related health problems in the United States. (29) This Survey, originally called the National Nutrition Survey, was conducted between 1968 and 1970. Emphasis was placed on information about low income families so that the statistical sample of about 40,000 persons was drawn from areas shown by the 1960 census to have the lowest average income. The sample included some higher income families who lived in the selected areas. The population sampled did not necessarily represent all low income people in a state.

The ten states selected for the study were: California, Kentucky, Louisiana, Massachusetts, Michigan, New York, South Carolina, Texas, Washington and West Virginia. Nutritional status was evaluated for the participants by data from physical examinations, anthropometric measurements, dental examinations, and hematocrit and hemoglobin determinations. Selected smaller groups—infants and young children, adolescents, pregnant and lactating women, and persons over 60 years of age—were given more detailed biochemical tests and individual dietary evaluation.

The study group was mainly white but included also blacks and Spanish-Americans (Mexican-American and Puerto Rican). The data were treated to show effects of economic factors on nutritional status.

The results (29) indicated:

1. There was malnutrition or danger of it in a considerable proportion of the survey population, especially among low income persons, more common among blacks and Spanish-Americans than among whites.

2. In all ethnic groups there were more signs of malnutrition, especially growth retardation, in low income areas than in higher income areas, but there was evidence that social, cultural and geographic differences also had an effect on nutrition.

3. There was more evidence of unsatisfactory nutritional status among adolescents, age 10 to 16 years, than in other age groups.

4. Obesity was prevalent among adult females, especially black women, and among children and adolescents.

5. Poor dental health and low levels of dental care were common.

6. Low levels of hemoglobin indicated widespread iron deficiency anemia. Many households had low intakes of iron.

7. Although pregnant and lactating women appeared to have adequate dietary protein, a high proportion had low serum albumin levels.

8. Young people in all groups had a high incidence of low vitamin A levels, with the greatest number among Mexican-Americans in Texas.

9. There was some evidence of vitamin C deficiency, mostly among males and older persons.

10. There was evidence of poor riboflavin status among blacks and young people of all ethnic groups.

Health and Nutrition Examination Survey (HANES)

HANES is a major part of the National Health Survey, a continuing program to obtain information on the health of the American people, initiated by the Congress in 1956 as a regular program of the Public Health Service. (22). The National Health Survey has supplied information on prevalence of diseases, their relationship to age and sex, and information about patients in hospitals and nursing homes. Information for the Survey has been collected from available records, from questions asked of people and from health examinations.

The Health and Nutrition Examination Surveys of 1971–72 were specially designed to determine the nutritional status of a statistical sample of the U.S. population between the ages of 1 and 74. This was the first nutrition survey in this country of a true sample of the civilian non-institutionalized population covering most of its lifespan. It was established to provide an ongoing nutritional surveillance system under which nutritional status can be measured and changes monitored.

The system is also designed to study the adequacy of dietary intakes and utilization of nutrients. Dietary intakes in the 1971–72 survey were obtained by interviews using the 24-hour recall method, with additional questions about food consumption during the preceding three months.

The evaluation of nutritional status was based on clinical examinations, biochemical tests, and anthropometric measurements. Special attention in the examinations was concentrated on chronic diseases and conditions in persons age 25 to 74.

The preliminary findings based (22) on 10,126 persons, about half of the total study group, show:

1. Low transferrin saturation values, especially in children age 1 to 5 years; anemia in older groups as shown by low hemoglobin and hematocrit values, more among blacks than among whites and more at low income levels.

2. Low serum vitamin A values especially among blacks, and among lower income groups.

3. Low serum protein values among all age groups and among whites at all income levels.

4. More evidence of low intakes of iron than of other nutrients. The only group that met the standards for iron intakes was that of males between 18 and 44, however, many black males failed to have adequate intakes.

5. Vitamin A and vitamin C intakes below the standard in 73 percent of the lower income white women, age 18–44, and in higher income black girls, age 12–17.

6. Significant differences in heights, weights, and skinfolds between children from poverty and higher income groups in favor of those from higher income groups.

7. High prevalence of obesity, especially among women, with the percentage in various groups ranging from 18.9 percent for white women age 20 to 44 years to 32.4 percent for black women age 45 to 74 years.

Nutrition Canada 1971–73

A review of this study is included because of the pertinence of the data due to the close geographical location and similarity of lifestyle and eating patterns of Canadians and residents of the United States.

Canada conducted a survey of a random sample of almost 15,000 persons and about 1000 selected women in the third trimester of pregnancy. (14) Selected groups of Eskimos and Indians were also included. The data were interpreted by classifying each of the biochemical and clinical parameters as high, medium and low, and the nutrient intakes into similar categories. Some of the findings were:

1. Overweight, as assessed by the *ponderal index* (ratio of height in inches to cubic root of weight in pounds) was found in 40 percent of adults age 20 to 39 and 60 percent of adults over age 40.

2. Caloric intakes of women were lower than for men, resulting in over-all lower intakes of protein, vitamins (except vitamin C) and minerals.

3. Serum cholesterol values for 10 percent of the men and more than 14 percent of the women were at risk. This may be explained by the early death of men with high cholesterol values or by an increase in risk among women because of current lifestyle.

4. Iron deficiency affects many Canadians of both sexes and all ages, as judged by transferrin saturation. Dietary intakes of iron were generally low.

5. Amounts of dietary calcium and vitamin D were low in diets of many infants, children, and adolescents.

6. There was no consistent effect of season, income, or kind of community on nutritional status. Problems were the same in low income families as in families with higher incomes.

USDA HOUSEHOLD FOOD CONSUMPTION SURVEYS

The United States Department of Agriculture has made five nationwide surveys of food consumption, the latest in 1965–66. (18) Data were collected in the spring of 1965 on the total household food consumption and food intakes of individuals in 7500 households representing all parts of the United States. The total food consumption in 2500 households was also determined for the three other seasons during 1965 and 1966.

Values of seven nutrients—protein, calcium, iron, vitamin A value, thiamine, riboflavin and ascorbic acid—were calculated for each household and individual. A diet was rated good if the calculated values for the seven nutrients equaled or exceeded the total recommended daily allowances for all household members. If the calculated values were less than two-thirds of the allowances for one or more nutrients the diet was rated poor. Diets between poor and good were rated fair. The results showed that:

1. One-half of the households had diets that rated good, while one-fifth rated poor. The percentage of good diets had decreased from 60 percent in 1955 to 50 percent, while the percentage of poor diets had increased from 15 percent to 21 percent.

2. Other differences between the low income (under $3000) and higher income ($7000 to $10,000) groups were noted: 36 percent of the low income group and 9 percent of the higher income group had poor

diets. The use of foods from the milk group, meat group and vegetable-fruit group was lower and the use of bread and cereals was higher among the low income group than among those with higher incomes.

3. There had been changes in consumption of specific foods between 1955 and 1965. The amounts of foods from the milk group decreased, the main change being in a lower use of fresh fluid milk, with less evaporated milk being used while the amount of non-fat dry milk had more than doubled and the use of cheese and frozen milk desserts had increased. The amounts of fresh vegetables and fruits had decreased, but the amount spent for these items had increased because of the higher cost of canned and frozen forms. A shift away from home baking was apparent as the amount of flour had decreased, and there was an increase in bakery products other than bread. There was also an overall increase in the use of breakfast cereals, primarily in the ready-to-eat kind. Small decreases in fats and oils and in sugars and sweets were noted.

It appears from these studies that there had been a deterioration in quality of household food consumption since the previous study. While the significance of these findings is unknown at the present time, they show the kind of information that may be revealed in such studies and suggest ways that the nutritionist may use the data. It is probable that the next studies will show decreases in eggs, meats, and saturated fats, and increases in sugar, polyunsaturated oils, fish, and poultry.

Gortner (6) has reviewed some changes that have taken place since early in the century, noting a change in source of protein, with half of it at that time from animal sources and about half from grain products. Recent studies showed 70 percent of protein was from animal sources. There has been a decrease in use of eggs. The amount of pork fat and milk fat decreased but there was an increase in beef fat, shortening, margarine, and oils.

There had also been changes in crude fiber, another dietary component of particular recent interest but still of unknown significance. Fiber may mean crude fiber, or all materials that affect fecal bulk, or carbohydrates that cannot be used by the body. The consumption of crude fiber was down from 6.1 grams in 1900–1913 to 4.3 in 1974. (6)

There have been efforts to relate fiber to certain costly diseases that affect older persons in the United States. These include (1) diverticular disease, which causes disability in 5 to 10 percent of the over-sixty population, (2) cancer of the colon and rectum, which causes 50,000 deaths per year, and (3) gallstones (cholelithiasis). The annual economic loss in mortality, morbidity, and direct cost from these diseases was estimated at $5 or $6 billion in 1974. (1) However, Hegsted (8) points out that the role of dietary fiber cannot really be evaluated until agreement has been reached on how to define fiber and how to correlate it with disease.

NUTRITION-RELATED DISEASES AND CONDITIONS

Food consumption and nutrition appear to play an important role in the development and treatment of certain diseases, so that the nutritionist needs to be well-informed about the relationship of nutrition to each as a basis for planning prevention and treatment.

Obesity

There are no precise statistics on the extent of obesity in the United States, but it occurs at all ages in both males and females, and at all economic levels. Estimates vary with method of determining body fat and with the standard used. The commonly used methods are based on weight and height or on skinfolds or other measurements.

It has been estimated (30) that 10 percent of adolescents are seriously overweight and that 25 to 45 percent of adults over 30 are overweight. (22) The prevalence is especially high among women, the percentage ranging from 18.9 percent for white women, age 20 to 44 years, to 32.4 percent for black women age 45 to 74 years. (30) While there are many associated and predisposing factors, the true cause of obesity is consuming more calories than are required for basal needs and individual activity.

Obesity is a significant public health concern because it is associated with cardiovascular disease, diabetes, other chronic diseases, prenatal hazards and other health problems. (Figure 3.1) The death rate among overweight men, age 20 to 64 was 50 percent higher than the expected rate, ranging from 31 percent for age 50 to 64 to 80 percent for age 20 to 29. The economic costs of obesity include reduced work efficiency, decreased productivity, increased hazard of disease, and likelihood of early death.

Considerable obesity among infants is reported by pediatricians and nutritionists, and the plethora of requests for help with weight control diets indicates that many individuals consider it a personal problem. An epidemiological study of obesity and disease in 73,532 obesity-prone women showed a correlation between degree of obesity and incidence of diabetes, high-blood pressure, and gallbladder disease. (13)

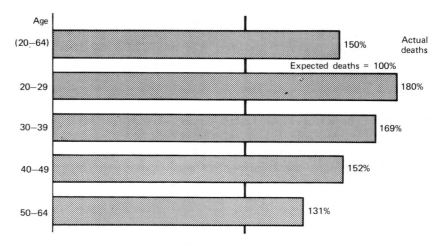

Figure 3.1   Marked Increase of Mortality in Overweight Men. (From: *An Evaluation of Research in the United States on Human Nutrition, Report No. 2, Benefits from Nutrition Research.* U. S. Department of Agriculture, Washington, D. C., 1971, 78.)

Cardiovascular Diseases

These diseases are of significance in community nutrition programs because current methods of prevention include changes in the American lifestyle to maintain normal weight, to keep blood lipids within the normal ranges, and to increase activity. The two cardiovascular diseases that need special attention in nutrition programs are hypertension and atherosclerosis. (4)

In the United States in 1973, cardiovascular diseases accounted for 54 percent of all deaths, more than any other one cause. Atherosclerosis contributes to almost 900,000 deaths annually. It has been estimated that over 23 million people in the United States have hypertension and almost 4 million have coronary heart disease. The economic cost of cardiovascular diseases in the United States has been estimated at almost $23 billion annually. (3)

Atherosclerosis is a disease in which the linings of the arteries are thickened and partly blocked by a build-up of fatty deposits narrowing the inside channel. Though it is significant mainly in adults, it is believed to start early in life so that preventive measures should begin in infancy. The major danger from atherosclerosis is that an artery may be blocked, causing a heart attack or stroke. *Coronary heart disease* is blockage of the coronary artery that causes a heart attack; *cerebral thrombosis,* one form of stroke, occurs when the blocked artery is in the brain. (4) A significant point about heart attacks is the high incidence in young and middle age adults, especially males. Obesity is an important contributing factor, as shown in Figures 3.2 and 3.3.

Hypertension is the medical term for abnormally high blood pressure. (3) The term *high blood pressure* is now being used in public education because of the tendency for people to assume that "tension" implies a disease of the nerves. Blood pressure is measured in millimeters (mm) of mercury and stated as the *systolic* reading (highest reading, taken at the time the heart pumps), over the *diastolic* reading (lowest reading, taken between heart beats), for example, 130 over 75, written 130/75. The normal range for systolic pressure is 100 to 140 mm of mercury. Diastolic pressure is considered as more significant than systolic and should be in the range of 70 to 90 mm of mercury. A reading of 140/90 is considered at the high borderline of normal for all ages, including children.

Diabetes

Diabetes is a disease that occurs when metabolism of carbohydrate is incomplete due to insufficient production of insulin. It is believed to be an inherited disease.

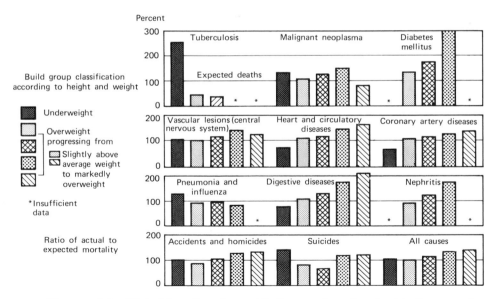

Figure 3.2 High Mortality from All Causes Associated with Increase in Weight: Men, Ages 15–69. (From *An Evaluation of Research in the United States on Human Nutrition, Report No. 2, Benefits from Nutrition Research,* U. S. Department of Agriculture, Washington, D. C., 1971, 79.)

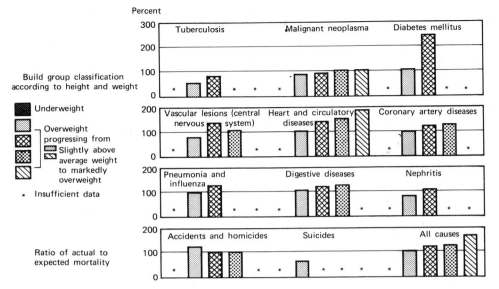

Figure 3.3 High Mortality from All Causes Associated with Increase in Weight: Women, Ages 15–69. (From *An Evaluation of Research in the United States on Human Nutrition, Report No. 2, Benefits from Nutrition Research,* U. S. Department of Agriculture, Washington, D. C., 1971, 80.)

In 1974 diabetes was reported to be in fifth place in the United States as a cause of death from disease. The American Diabetes Association (2) estimates that 10 million people may have it, with one-third undiagnosed because the individual has none of the common symptoms, which include excessive thirst and urination, constant hunger, weight loss, slow healing, and others. It has been estimated that proper nutritional care could reduce the number of cases of diabetes by 50 percent.

A special study by Tokuhata in Pennsylvania reported (17) that in a 12-month period 2640 deaths were officially reported as caused by diabetes but that diabetes was recorded as a contributory cause in an additional 7531 deaths, while about 20,000 residents had actually been diagnosed as having diabetes. Tokuhata suggests that if the same figures apply to the national population, the diabetes problem is much greater than currently reported. He points out that in the Pennsylvania study 58 percent of the complications associated with diabetes were in the major cardiovascular diseases.

Cancer

Cancer is a group of diseases characterized by uncontrolled growth that invades other body systems. It may occur in various body organs or in the nonsolid parts. There has recently been increased evidence from epidemiological studies that nutrition plays an important part in the development of cancer. The evidence was reviewed by Wynder (33), who postulates that one-half of all cancers in women and one-third in men are related to nutritional factors.

There is evidence that a number of nutritional deficiencies (iron, iodine, riboflavin, vitamin A, and pyridoxine) may be implicated in human cancers of the stomach, cervix, and thyroid. (33) Suspicion is attached to excessive intake of specific nutrients in the development of cancer of the colon, pancreas, breast, ovary, and prostate, while obesity is believed to be a factor in cancer of the endometrium and kidney in women. The evidence from both epidemiological and experimental data suggests a relationship to a high intake of fats and possibly to certain types of fat.

There appear to be three ways in which nutrition may influence the development of cancer. (1) Nutrients, food additives, or contaminants may act directly as carcinogens, or may initiate, promote, or accelerate the carcinogenic process. (2) Dietary deficiencies may cause malfunction of the body processes, thereby initiating cancer production. (3) Excesses of either calories or nutrients may likewise lead to metabolic abnormalities that promote cancers. Dietary deficiencies are believed to be the most important of these three avenues because they may produce cell defects that can promote cancer development. (32,33)

Considerable concern has been expressed in the media over the carcinogenic effect of nitrosamines. (16) In a review, Issenberg (10) points out that these compounds are formed from naturally-occurring amines and nitrites and that evaluation of risk will be difficult until more data are available on their environmental occurrence. He believes that it will be impossible to eliminate these compounds from the environment, so work must be directed toward establishing safe levels.

Dental Caries

Dental caries is the most widespread problem in the United States related to both poor nutrition and nature of the food intake. Failure of nutrition during gestation and early life interferes with tooth development, and nutrition throughout life affects the health of both teeth and supporting structures. The kind of food eaten has a direct effect on teeth throughout life, since refined carbohydrates contribute to tooth decay while other foods, especially raw fruits and vegetables, have beneficial effects through a detersive action.

Data from the National Nutrition Survey show that 96 percent of the people over 10 years of age had ten teeth decayed, filled, or missing

(DMF), and that 18 percent reported pain on biting or chewing food. (15)

Figures from the USDHEW for 1963 to 1965 showed that 24 million children ages 6 to 11 had an average per child of 1.4 decayed, 0.4 non-functioning, and 1.2 filled primary teeth. (21) Youths in the 12 to 17 age group had an estimated average of 6.2 DMF teeth, ranging from 4.0 for 12-year-olds to 8.7 for 17-year-olds. White and black males had lower levels than did all races and ages of females. (24)

One of every four adults had no teeth in one or both jaws, while there was an average of 20.4 DMF teeth per person. Half of the people, age 65 to 74 were edentulous. (28)

The economic cost of dental problems in the United States is shown by a total expenditure for FY 1975 of $7.5 billion, with an average per capita expenditure of $34.62. (25)

QUALITY AND SAFETY OF THE FOOD SUPPLY

Concern for the safety of food has existed since early days. In the United States, responsibility for food safety has long been shared by government and the individual. Threats to the safety of the supply come mainly from biological and chemical pollution of food and water.

The greatest problem is food poisoning with from 2 million to 20 million cases a year, caused mainly by microbiological contamination of food. (26) Much is due to poor food handling practices during preparation in home, commercial establishments, institutions, and other places where food is processed. Home canning causes a few cases of poisoning each year.

The major dangers of chemical pollutants are that they may be carcinogenic (cancer-producing), mutagenic (causing a sudden variation in inherited characteristics), or teratogenic (causing malformation of a fetus). (33) They must be controlled by identifying the presence of toxic substances in food, water and air, and by establishing safe levels for humans. Unsafe substances or amounts should be removed from the environment or neutralized to remove harmful effects. Sometimes the danger in a particular chemical comes from interactions with other substances rather than from the chemical itself.

A particular danger occurs when pesticides and other synthetic compounds get into the food chain during the processing of food and water. (26) These dangers arise because of greater production of food and manufactured goods, technological developments, increasing populations, and the increased size of cities and industries.

Harmful chemicals may also enter food by direct contamination, or during processing, or from packaging materials. Further research is needed to establish safe levels, and to determine the long-term effects of low levels of chemicals in foods. (27)

CONTRIBUTING FACTORS

There are a number of practices and conditions that contribute to the existing nutrition-related problems that have been reported.

Poverty is a social and political problem leading to poor diet, poor housing and inadequate medical care. It must be attacked by social and political action. Food prices and income have a strong impact on food selection, perhaps more than knowledge about proper diet. Miller discusses the need for social reform as the essential avenue for improved health, pointing out that most persons inherit the life circumstances that lead to poor health from the social and economic conditions into which they are born and that many are powerless to change these conditions. (11) The problems of migrant workers, one of the poorest groups, are shown by an infant mortality rate 25 percent above the national average, and mortality rates for tuberculosis and other infectious diseases of two and one-half times the national rate. (23) These problems can only be solved by public health actions of government agencies.

Indifference to the principles of good nutrition and good health is found among all social groups and at all income levels and leads to poor diets, overeating, underactivity and other causes of malnutrition; for example, obesity is due to a combination of physical inactivity and overeating. For most individuals, the nutritional processes occur with little attention, and in healthy individuals there are seldom any obvious symptoms that suggest nutrition problems. Hence there is a lack of concern about nutritional health.

Ignorance of what constitutes healthful living such as the components of good nutrition and good health is another problem; however, Hegsted has suggested (7) that "emphasis on the essential nutrients may be irrelevant to the primary nutritional problems in the U.S." because the real problems may lie in the high consumption of animal products and highly processed foods and the low consumption of fruits and vegetables, a diet that is inefficient and expensive, and perhaps nutritionally unsound.

Thus it can be seen that poverty, indifference, and ignorance account for many nutrition problems. An inadequate amount of food occurs mainly among the poor, causing low intakes of nutrients and calories that lead to undernutrition. The same factors account for excessive calorie intake leading to obesity, and for the high consumption of saturated fats and cholesterol, which are suspect in the etiology of heart disease and cancer. Indifference and ignorance about diet and dental hygiene are involved in development of dental caries.

Misinformation and *faddism* are other causes of eating a poor diet. Misinformation in food and nutrition is incorrect information or information presented in such a way as to guide or lead someone into taking the wrong action. (9) A common example is the presentation of the nutrient content of a specific food so that it appears that these nutrients cannot otherwise be obtained. Misinformation is widespread among members of the general public and occurs among some professionals, but there is little objective data on the extent or even the nature of the problem. It occurs partly because eating is an everyday occurrence for all persons, so everyone knows something about food.

Food faddism is an excessive emphasis on a food or diet over a period of time. It results in fad diets that come and go and recur under different names a few months or years later. They are usually based on misinformation or on the hope of miraculous results. *Quackery* is pretending to be an authority when there is no qualifying background. *Food quacks* are always with us promoting a dietary regimen, a book, or a product on the basis of facts, half-facts, or misinformation. Many food quacks have large vocal followings and are disruptive to community nutrition programs.

The problems of misinformation, faddism, and quackery are that an individual may be led into eating an unbalanced or inadequate diet, into delaying medical care while seeking a cure through food, or into spending an undue proportion of income for food supplements or special foods. Misinformation and faddism present great challenges to the community nutritionist since many people would rather look for a miracle than follow the principles of good health.

DISCUSSION

It is evident that there are many nutrition problems that have different causes; thus their solution needs various kinds of intervention from many sources. Academic institutions must conduct research to identify the relationships of nutrition to disease, to find ways to use nutrition in disease prevention, and to develop more efficient ways of changing food habits. Governments at all levels must plan and provide better health care systems so that individuals can obtain effective preventive care and treatment. Government must determine safe levels of chemicals used in foods and see that these levels are not exeeded. Government must arrange for programs such as the distribution of food, providing it free or at low cost for persons on inadequate incomes. The food industry must take the initiative to solve the problems related to food manufacture and distribution so that safe, nutritious foods are available. Community nutritionists along with others in the field must assume leadership for the accomplishment of these activities, and cooperate to this end by bringing about changes in lifestyle and also legislation that will attack the problems.

SUMMARY

A nutrition problem is any situation or factor that has an adverse effect on nutrition, but each community must define the term further in its own environment. A number of methods are used for assessing nutritional status. They include anthropometric measurements, clinical examinations, laboratory tests, and dietary studies.

Nutrition problems in the United States have been identified by several surveys. All three surveys showed a higher incidence of nutrition problems among the poor. In the preschool survey there was evidence of insufficient food; the researchers suggested that improved socioeconomic status and expanded food programs offered the best ways to alleviate the problems observed.

The ten-state survey showed more nutrition problems among adolescents than in other age groups. The major overall problems were obesity, dental caries, and anemia along with low intakes of iron and vitamins A and C.

HANES showed evidence of anemia, low serum vitamin A, and low serum protein. Low intakes of iron were common, with most sex-age groups having inadequate intakes. Growth retardation was found among children from the poverty groups, and a high prevalence of obesity was noted among women.

The food consumption surveys of 1965–66 indicated that there had been a decrease in the number of "good" diets from 60 percent in the 1955 survey to 50 percent in the 1965–66 survey, and that higher income families had more good diets than lower income families. Changes in food consumption of specific food groups included lower amounts of milk, fresh fruits, and vegetables, and a decrease in flour with an increase in bakery products other than bread. The consumption of crude fiber had decreased from the early years of the century, but the relationship of this finding to cancer or other diseases has not been established.

The nutrition problems of obesity, cardiovascular disease, diabetes, cancer, and dental caries are related to excessive intakes of saturated fat, sweets, or both.

Other factors such as poverty, misinformation, indifference, ignorance, and safety of the food supply also contribute to nutrition problems in the community.

REFERENCES CITED

1. Almy, Thomas P., The Role of Fiber in the Diet, in Winick, Myron, ed., *Nutrition and Aging,* John Wiley & Sons, New York, 1976, 155.
2. American Diabetes Association, *Annual Report: 1974—The Year of Momentum,* American Diabetes Association, New York, 6.
3. American Heart Association, *Heart and Blood Vessels,* 1975, American Heart Association, New York.
4. American Heart Association, *Heart Facts,* American Heart Association, New York, 1976.
5. Christakis, George, ed., Nutritional Assessment In Health Programs, *Am. J. Pub. Health,* 63 11/73, Supplement.
6. Gortner, Willis A., Nutrition in the United States, 1900 to 1974, Symposium on Nutrition and Cancer, Atlantic City, 4/15/75, *Fed. Proc.,* 35 5/1/76 1309.
7. Hegsted, D. Mark, Food and Nutrition Policy—Now and in the Future, *J. Am. Diet. Assoc.,* 64 4/74 367.
8. Hegsted, D. Mark, Summary of the Conference on Nutrition in the Causation of Cancer, Key Biscayne FL., May 19–22, 1975, *Cancer Research,* 35 11/75, Part 2, 3541.
9. Huenemann, Ruth L., Combatting Food Misinformation and Quackery, *J. Am. Diet. Assoc.,* 47 10/65 263.
10. Issenberg, Phillip, Nitrite, Nitrosamines, and Cancer, *Fed. Proc.,* 35 5/1/76 1322.
11. Miller, C. Arden, Issues of Health Policy: Local Government and the Public's Health, *Am. J. Pub. Health,* 65 12/75 1330.
12. Owen, George M., Kathryn M. Kram, Philip J. Garry, Jay E. Lowe, and A. Harold Lubin, A Study of Nutritional Status of Preschool Children in the United States, 1968–1970, *Pediatrics,* 53 4/74, Part II, 597.
13. Rimm, Alfred A., Linda H. Werner, Barbara Van Yserloo, Ronald A. Bernstein, Relationship of Obesity and Disease in 73,532 Weight Conscious Women, *Public Health Reports,* 90 1-2/75 44.
14. Sabry, Z. I., E. Campbell, J. A. Campbell and A. L. Forbes, Nutrition Canada—A National Nutrition Survey, *Nutr. Rev.,* 32 4/74 105.
15. Schaefer, Arnold E., and Ogden C. Johnson, Are We Well Fed? The Search for the Answer, *Nutr. Today,* 4 Spring 1969 7.
16. Shapley, Deborah, Nitrosamines: Scientists on the Trail of Prime Suspect in Urban Cancer, *Science,* 191 1/23/76 268.
17. Tokuhata, George K., Diabetes Mellitus—An Underestimated Health Problem, *Pennsylvania's Health,* Winter 1973 18.

18. U.S. Dept. of Agriculture, *Dietary Levels of Households in the United States,* Report No. 6, Spring, 1965, Government Printing Office, Washington DC, 1969.

19. U.S. Dept. of Health, Education, and Welfare, *First Health and Nutrition Examination Survey, United States, 1971–72: Anthropometric and Clinical Findings,* DHEW Pub. No. (HRA) 75-1229, U.S. Dept. of Health, Education, and Welfare, Rockville MD.

20. U.S. Dept. of Health, Education, and Welfare, *First Health and Nutrition Examination Survey, United States, 1971–72: Dietary Intake and Biochemical Findings,* DHEW Pub. No. (HRA) 74-1219-1, Dept. of Health, Education, and Welfare, Rockville MD.

21. U.S. Dept. of Health, Education, and Welfare, *Decayed, Missing, and Filled Teeth Among Children—United States,* Vital and Health Statistics, Series 11-No. 106, DHEW Pub. No. (HSM) 72-1003, Washington DC, . 8/71.

22. U.S. Dept. of Health, Education and Welfare, *Preliminary Findings of the First Health and Nutrition Examination Survey, United States, 1971–72.* DHEW Pub. No. (HRA) 74-1219-1, Rockville MD.

23. U.S. Dept. of Health, Education and Welfare, *Promoting Community Health,* DHEW Pub. No. (HSA) 75-5016, 1975, 12.

24. U.S. Dept. of Health, Education, and Welfare, *Decayed, Missing, and Filled Teeth Among Youths, 12–17 Years,* Series 11, No. 144, DHEW Pub. No. (HRA) 75-1626, Rockville MD., 10/74.

25. U.S. Dept. of Health, Education, and Welfare, *Forward Plan for Health 1977–1981,* Aug. 1975 19.

26. Ibid., 106.

27. Ibid., 112.

28. U.S. Dept. of Health, Education, and Welfare, *Selected Dental Findings in Adults by Age, Race, and Sex—United States 1960–62,* PHS Pub. No. 1000-Series 11, No. 7, Washington DC, 2/65.

29. U.S. Dept. of Health, Education and Welfare, *Ten-State Nutrition Survey, 1968–1970, Highlights,* Pub. No. (HSM) 72-8134, Government Printing Office, Washington DC, 1972.

30. Weir, C. Edith, *Benefits from Human Nutrition Research,* Human Nutrition Report No. 2, U.S. Department of Agriculture, Washington DC, Aug. 1971, 74.

31. Ibid., 6.

32. Wynder, Ernst L., Introductory Remarks, Conference on Nutrition in the Causation of Cancer, Key Biscayne, FL., May 19–22, 1975, *Cancer Research,* 35 11/75, Part 2, 3238.

33. Wynder, Ernst L., Nutrition and Cancer, *Fed. Proc.,* 35 5/1/76 1309.

ADDITIONAL REFERENCES

Marx, Jean L., Drinking Water: Another Source of Carcinogens, *Science,* 186 11/29/74 809.

Mayer, Jean, *Overweight,* Prentice-Hall, Inc., Englewood Cliffs NJ, 1968, 26.

National Academy of Sciences, Food Protection Committee, *Evaluating the Safety of Food Chemicals,* Washington DC, 1970.

Rimm, Ilonna J., and Alfred A. Rimm, Association Between Sociological Status and Obesity in 59,556 Women, *Preventive Medicine,* 3 1974 543.

Robinson, Corinne H., *Normal and Therapeutic Nutrition,* 14th ed., The Macmillan Co., New York, 1972, 510.

Shubik, Philippe, Potential Carcinogenicity of Food Additives and Contaminants, *Cancer Research,* 35 11/75 3475.

4 BACKGROUND FOR COMMUNITY NUTRITION

Prevention of diseases and conditions by some nutritional means is a major part of community nutrition programs. Prevention occurs at three levels. (9) *Primary prevention* is a direct attack on the cause of a disease, such as providing food through the school lunch to prevent hunger and malnutrition. It may also be accomplished by altering some factor in lifestyle to prevent development of a disease, as reduction in intake of saturated fat to prevent atherosclerosis. A third way of primary prevention is to control a substance believed to be injurious, as the action by the Food and Drug Administration banning certain red dyes in food.

Secondary prevention is action to identify a disease before symptoms appear while intervention can still change the course of the disease. An example is a screening program for detection of high blood pressure in apparently healthy individuals, followed by treatment to prevent heart disease or stroke. The community nutritionist may participate in secondary prevention by identifying food and nutrition practices such as inadequate diet, or excessive intake of calories or salt, which may play a part in the etiology of high blood pressure. Some nutritionists take blood pressures of individuals seen in their regular programs and refer those with high blood pressure to their physicians for care.

Tertiary prevention occurs when an individual has a disease but treatment prevents or minimizes damage to future health, as when diet and medication are used in treatment of diabetes.

IMPORTANCE OF PREVENTION

The importance of prevention has been emphasized by many public health leaders who believe that further significant improvements in the health status of the population in this country will come from more effective prevention rather than from extension of the present medical care system. (17) It appears that medicine has reached its limits in prolonging life until new major advances are made in the prevention and treatment of the diseases that are the major causes of death; in the meantime, further improvements in health are dependent on correcting the living practices that have a role in those diseases. A better design for living includes food as the most important factor in enhancing the quality of life and in prolonging healthy, productive living.

Community nutrition must take the leadership for prevention, in the apparently healthy population, of diseases in which food consumption and nutrition play an important part. The medical community, voluntary agencies, and others are concerned about various aspects of prevention, but their concern is primarily with high risk groups such as persons at risk of diabetes or stroke.

Progress toward this new approach will require a joint effort by the individual and the community to attack social problems that affect the quality of life and health. These include unemployment, poor housing, and lack of recreational facilities. The community health system includes all activities supported by both public and private resources for the maintenance of health and the quality of life. One of the problems is that people do not know how to use the resources that are already available for health protection and disease prevention.

Often the nutrition problems of the individual arise in the larger health problems of the community. The community nutritionist must assume leadership in diagnosing, assessing, and correcting community health problems, considering both medical and psychosocial needs in the preventive and therapeutic aspects of nutritional care. The nutritionist uses a health-oriented and people-oriented way of looking at the nutrition problems of the community, being specifically concerned with people as individuals, families, household units, and communities. The methods and techniques of a community nutrition program vary, but the *sine qua non* is interaction with the community, and provision of nutrition services through public education, professional education, and nutritional care. The community nutritionist uses many methods, pioneers and stimulates change, seeks new approaches and accepts change, using different, appropriate methods to attack various problems.

In the past, the main nutrition problem was getting food, storing it, and preventing food-borne illness. Today, community nutrition helps others plan for the best nutritional care in both health and disease, whether at home, at school, in a public eating place, in a congregate eating situation, or in a group-living facility. The community nutritionist teaches people what to eat and how to purchase, prepare and serve food for health and enjoyment; and is concerned that there is enough money to purchase an adequate diet for each individual, and that the persons responsible for the personal food intake of others know the importance of food, the requirements of a proper diet, and the techniques of getting people to eat it.

Cornely has discussed the need for education for the prevention of the most prevalent diseases, namely, heart disease, hypertension, diabetes, arthritis and cancer. These diseases are the result of many environmental, physiological, social, and psychological factors acting over a long period of time, so that their prevention depends on changes in living that in turn are dependent on personal responsibility for health. (3) A pertinent philosophic question is whether the individual should have the privilege of following health habits that will almost certainly lead to a drain on social resources. (4) Thus far the prevailing philosophy seems to be that the individual does have such a privilege. This is of significance to the nutritionist because it includes nutritional practices such as too much food and too little exercise.

There is a whole range of health and illness with which community nutrition is concerned. It includes the well, the worried well, the early sick, the acutely ill, and the chronically ill; however, the primary purposes of community nutrition should be to *prevent* disease and to maintain and promote good health. In many agencies, treatment of disease is likely to crowd out the preventive activities that contribute the most to these primary goals. Health professionals frequently talk about optimal care and about maintaining the highest level of health and well-being; however, some health authorities believe there is a need to abandon the unrealistic goal of providing high quality health care for every citizen and replace it with the realistic one of providing a level possible of achievement. (3)

BASIC KNOWLEDGE

The basic knowledge of the community nutritionist comes from a number of fields—nutritional science, biological and physical sciences, food science and art, behavioral sciences, social sciences, and managerial science.

The community nutritionist does not do research in the classic sense of scholarly, carefully controlled, exhaustive, critical investigation or experimentation for the purpose of discovering and interpreting new facts of wide significance. The nutritionist does make surveys and studies to obtain information for use in program planning, and developing methods and materials. The community nutritionist must be able to evaluate published reports of research, studies and surveys, and decide whether the findings should be used in the nutrition program. It is important that the nutritionist be able to decide when to adopt new research findings, and when to use new tools and techniques.

As a member of the health team, the nutritionist assumes responsibility for nutrition-related information and procedures. In the past, the nutritionist's role was mainly concerned with public education, but now nutritionists are learning new skills and assuming additional responsibilities to increase the contribution of good nutrition in preventive health care and treatment of disease states. Just as the nurse has learned to assume many tasks formerly performed by the physician (e.g., giving primary care to the prenatal patient), the nutritionist should assume the responsibility for nutritional assessment, nutritional care, and monitoring nutritional status. To perform these functions, the nutritionist will need to master subject matter about child growth and development, nutrition management in pregnancy, and the process of aging.

Nutritional Science

This subject matter that is learned in nutrition courses includes (1) the function and interrelationships of nutrients, (2) the processes of digestion, absorption, metabolism, and excretion, (3) the changing needs in nutrition throughout the life cycle, and (4) the role of nutrition in the disease states that are of major significance in community health, especially atherosclerosis, hypertension, diabetes, cancer, iron deficiency anemia, dental caries, malnutrition (obesity and retarded growth) and nutritional disorders of pregnancy. This information is used to make nutrition a part of a regimen for healthful living because it is a key factor in promotion of health and the prevention and control of many diseases. Attention to nutrition also reduces the occurrence of acute episodes with their resulting need for medical care and hospitalization.

Child Growth and Development. The nutritionist needs a background in physical growth and mental and emotional development to be able to advise nurses, parents, and teachers about food behavior at various ages and about development of good food habits in infants, children, and youth. The nutritionist must interpret to parents the importance and advantages of good food habits to the health of their children. Parents must also understand the effects of their children's starting to school and participating in school feeding programs. They need help in reinforcement of good nutrition practices and correction of poor ones during elementary and secondary school years.

Pregnancy. Nutrition during pregnancy is one of the most important factors in determining the course and outcome of pregnancy for both mother and infant. A good diet that provides adequate amounts of calories and essential nutrients is necessary for the support of the maternal body tissues and for the growth and development of the fetus. The nutritionist needs to know the changes that take place in the mother's body during pregnancy and the stages in development of the fetus.

The relationship of nutrition to toxemias, weight gain, premature birth, low birth weight, and other complications must also be considered in nutrition management. The nutritionist must also understand how to deal with the additional burden of pregnancy in the teenage girl. Good health practices should be promoted, too, with nonpregnant teenage girls to instill desirable food practices and to bring them to pregnancy in a good nutritional state.

Aging. Food, one of the major sources of enjoyment and social satisfaction for older persons, is also one of the most important factors in maintaining health. Physical problems such as poor eyesight, and poor teeth or ill-fitting dentures, or decreased mobility, may make it difficult for older persons to go to market or to prepare their own food. Activity and exercise should be encouraged when possible to avoid bone loss and help the individual continue in an active life.

Lack of ability to chew food makes it difficult for the older person to eat some foods, especially those containing fiber. Many older persons are not milk-drinkers, therefore ingesting inadequate calcium and riboflavin. Economic and social problems such as loneliness, low income, inadequate facilities, and lack of transportation also interfere with adequate food and good nutrition for the elderly and ill. The nutritionist must understand the effect of these problems and be able to help the older person plan for good nutrition.

Food Science and Art

Food science provides our knowledge about food composition and structure, which determine its nutrient content and the ways it can be prepared and used. Food art shows how to make nutritious foods appealing to the eye and the taste, resulting in the consumption of an adequate diet. Home economists, using this science and art, have developed ways to prepare many variations of basic dishes that appeal to every taste and provide day-to-day variety making for palatable and attractive meals. They have also adapted recipes to low, medium, and liberal budgets and made them easy for any cook to follow. The nutritionist uses this information to convey the need for a variety of foods to supply all necessary nutrients, to motivate people to consume this kind of diet, to apply the information to individual and family food practices, and to do this within available resources of energy, time, and money.

Food science and art also teach the basis for food planning, purchasing, storage, and preparation, and the methods for performing these tasks to give maximum palatability and nutrient content consistent with available resources. Many homemakers, food managers, and cooks can plan and prepare meals that fit the above criteria for their particular clientele. The community nutritionist must be able to apply these principles in helping persons with various cultural food practices, at every economic level, in situations with widely varied resources, and with different food likes and dislikes.

Behavioral Sciences

Much of the success of the community nutritionist's work depends on changing the practices of both professionals and the public. The nutritionist must be able to persuade professionals that in the course of their regular work they can conduct nutrition education and promote community changes that affect nutrition. Many of the concepts and methods of psychology and anthropology are used in nutrition education, which must teach the basis of good nutrition and also motivate action to achieve it. Every nutritionist needs to know the social, cultural, and psychological basis of food habits as a background for effecting changes in food practices.

Managerial Science

The community nutritionist performs some managerial tasks, so must be able to use the basic principles of the field. In a small program, the responsibility may include only the nutritionist's own time and limited resources of facilities and materials. In a large program, the responsibility includes other persons and extensive facilities, equipment, and supplies. The nutritionist needs to know how to manage available resources—large or small—for the greatest return at the lowest cost.

BASIC CONCEPTS

Community nutrition may be considered a specific academic discipline based on the various sciences listed in the preceeding discussions. A particular body of knowledge is needed to provide the background for the work. This special body of knowledge includes community structure, tools and skills, techniques, and information about a variety of other topics. The uniqueness of the field lies in how the knowledge is used. Some of the basic concepts are:

1. The community nutritionist understands the function of agencies and organizations which conduct or influence nutrition programs and knows how to work with them for good nutritional care.
2. The community nutritionist identifies problems, determines goals, and surveys resources before planning a program.
3. Community nutrition practice is based on application of the techniques of program management, professional education, public education, and community organization with individuals, families, and communities.
4. Specific knowledge, techniques, skills, and tools are used in conducting community programs.
5. The same principles and methods are used in all community nutrition programs, regardless of size, with adaptations for the specific program.

Discussion

Community nutrition programs may be based in various government agencies, voluntary health agencies, out-patient clinics and hospitals, and other organizations that have health care as their primary function; or in schools, social agencies, public recreation departments, and businesses that have other primary functions but are also concerned about health.

The focus of community nutrition is on the home or household unit or other setting where some functions of the home are conducted. Today's "household unit" must include the household composed of one or two adults, one parent and child or children, and the commune as well as the more conventional family of two parents and children. There are also many alternates that provide the food which used to be provided in the home. They include the school, the public eating place, the congregate living or feeding environment, and other places where food practices are determined, where children learn their food habits, and where adults and families put theirs into practice. The home or alternate is also the place where changes in food practices become a reality. Most community nutritionists have a high commitment to give attention to the food practices of the entire household unit, because what each member eats is intimately related to the food of other household members, and to the control of the home situation and the ability to follow a medical plan for one member.

Not all nutrition activities that take place outside the home are community nutrition. Overall planning for nutritional care in a community will include hospitals and extended care facilities so that continuity of care can be achieved as an individual moves from one to another. However, the actual care in the facility is not community nutrition. Individual and group patient instruction in a hospital or clinic may involve the community, as when the diet counselor works with the community in solving the problems of a specific population group such as the obese.

Community nutrition includes using appropriate resources in services that provide good nutrition or that teach people how to provide it for themselves, and applying these services for individuals and groups in the community. Figure 4.1 shows the process and the relationships.

Community nutrition is based on the premise that nutrition problems can best be solved by attention to the nutritional care of people as groups in the community environment. The community nutritionist must know how to use nutrition as a preventive measure in a community characterized by having a majority of well people and a minority of sick. The community nutritionist works with both to help them achieve the benefits of good nutrition for prevention of future ill health and for treatment for the smaller number of sick persons who are part of that community and who in turn constitute a smaller community sharing a common disease problem.

Improvement of health involves changing the way people think, feel, and behave. This requires a change in the values that determine health habits and in how people use available resources, so that more time and money are devoted to achieving health and less for other things. One of the basic needs in achieving and maintaining health is a regimen that includes proper food and sufficient activity throughout a lifetime based on a belief that good health is one of life's most precious possessions.

The nutritionist must believe that community nutrition programs can contribute in an important way to the solution of current health problems. A nutrition program is justified only by the contributions it makes to the social and economic development of a group, a community or a nation. Nutrition, as a part of health, should be promoted not for its own sake but to achieve productivity, efficiency and happiness. This presentation with the tangible benefits clearly in evidence will facili-

Subject Matter Input	*Change into Usable Form*	*Resulting Program Action*
Nutritional science	Nutrition scientists identify function of nutrients in body and recommend amounts for daily ingestion.	Nutritionists use these amounts as the basis for planning dietaries.
Food technology	Food scientists determine nutrients in foods and develop food composition tables.	Nutritionists use tables to develop food guides and patterns to show foods to eat each day.
Medical knowledge	Nutritional scientists identify action of nutrients in disease.	Dietitians develop therapeutic diets for treatment of various disease states.
Behavioral science	Behavioral scientists develop methods of inducing changes in food practices.	Nutritionists apply methods to change food practices of individuals and groups.
Community organization	Social scientists develop methods of correcting the causes of social problems by community action.	Community nutritionists use the methods of community action to alleviate the problems of hunger and malnutrition.

Figure 4.1   How Subject Matter Is Used in Community Nutrition.

tate acceptance by the public, by program administrators, and by government.

Community nutrition programs, whether concerned with prevention or treatment, have often been considered only as nutrition education, but nutrition education is only one method of education for the public and it should be recognized that there are other obstacles to effecting change besides lack of information and motivation. It is the job of the community nutritionist to find ways to solve these problems. It is, for example, futile to teach people to eat a good diet when the amount of money available for food is too small to buy a good diet, or to teach the consumption of enriched breads when they are not available. It may be more productive to attack these problems by referral to a social agency for monetary help, or to develop the content of an enrichment law and persuade a legislator to sponsor it.

BASIC TASKS

The activities of the community nutritionist may be classified under six basic tasks. Each community nutritionist will perform these basic tasks but the scope and nature of the activities depend on the specific program. Examples will be given of a nutritionist serving as a program director in a large health agency, a nutritionist in a small child care program, and a nutritionist in a dental care program.

Acting as Program Manager

Most community nutritionists will be responsible for a program or part of a program, sometimes encompassing only their own activities and sometimes the work of a staff. The nutritionist-director of a large program may have a staff of ten nutritionists, a home economist, ten nutrition aides, two secretaries, and a clerk. Management includes planning the program, employing, training and supervising the staff, delegating responsibilities, arranging for record-keeping, and evaluating the program. The nutritionist in the child care program plans the nutrition component of the program, hires a cook and a nutrition aide, and trains and supervises both, oversees record-keeping of meals served, food costs, and food consumption. The nutritionist in a dental clinic, whose main work is counseling individuals and mothers referred by the dentist, manages the available resources that consist of instructional materials, a room for individual and group instruction, and the time available for individual and group counseling.

Providing Education for Professionals and Paraprofessionals

The nutritionist-director hires, orients, trains, and supervises the nutritionists and the home economist, directs them in selecting, hiring, training, and supervising the nutrition aides, and teaches the supervisor of the clerical staff the duties of the particular office. The child care nutritionist provides inservice education for teachers so they can develop good nutrition practices in the children and help parents with their children's food problems. The dental clinic nutritionist works with dentist and dental hygienists to coordinate their nutrition teaching with that of the nutritionist.

Conducting Education for the Public

The nutritionist-director delegates the responsibility for most of this work to nutritionists and other staff, directing them in conducting the various activities through which public education is accomplished. The child care nutritionist actually carries out much of this work but also motivates teachers, the nurse, and the cook to participate and teaches them how to do so. The dental clinic nutritionist works directly with patients and parents, individually and in groups to establish good nutrition practices.

Representing the Nutrition Program in Agency and Community

This function includes acting as promoter and advocate and as a channel of communication between agency and community. It is one of the prime responsibilities of the nutritionist-director who participates in agency planning and in health planning for the community. The child care nutritionist represents nutrition on the agency staff and interacts with other community agencies on mutual concerns. The dental clinic nutritionist may have community involvement with the schools to see that the good practices instituted in the dental clinic are continued and reinforced by the school.

Keeping Informed of Nutrition Research and Programs

All nutritionists need to review current literature and new books, attend lectures and seminars, and utilize other sources of information about current research, subject matter, and program reports. The depth of information depends on the position. The dental clinic nutritionist and child care nutritionist need to know their respective fields in depth. The nutritionist-director must maintain a minimum level of nutrition subject matter in many fields and develop extensive knowledge of administration, management, and program methods.

Making a Nutritional Care Plan for the Specific Community

The community nutritionist serves as a link between the individuals with nutrition problems (the public) and the persons who can do something about them. In planning for the nutritional care of the community, the nutritionist helps the community identify the problems, find the available resources, and decide how each problem can best be attacked. The nutritionist-director in the large agency participates in the general health planning for the community. The nutritionist for the child care agency participates with the agency director in planning for the health of the children. The nutritionist in the dental health clinic leads clinic patients in planning for dental health.

FOCUS FOR COMMUNITY NUTRITION

Community nutrition as a specialty differs in some important aspects from community medicine and community nursing where practice has most often originated with illness or disease. Community nutrition practice has most often originated from problems concerned with food and eating as illustrated by reports from teachers of many children coming to school without breakfast, or of local weight control groups asking for lectures on reducing diets. Until recently, most nutritionists have not had access to statistics on nutritional status from their own programs or from national surveys that could be used to identify the health hazards of poor nutrition. Statistics from nutritional surveys have made it possible for nutritionists to point out the importance of nutritional care as part of the total health program, especially as a preventive health measure.

The lack of statistics to show the prevalence and cost of malnutrition and the value of preventive nutrition programs made it difficult to compete with other health programs for funds. Most of the money in health agencies has been allocated for the prevention of specific diseases, such as heart disease, diabetes, and venereal disease where the problem and cost were readily identified. The major nutritional intervention was in disease treatment by dietitians in hospitals and clinics. Cornely emphasized this in an address before members of the American Dietetic Association in 1971 when he pointed out that 9000 of the 23,000 members were hospital dietitians while only 800 were community nutritionists and suggested need for a greater emphasis on preventive nutrition and greater numbers of community nutritionists. (3)

Community nutrition differs from community medicine and community nursing because it concerns food and eating, which are intimately entwined in everyday living for all persons and are both a foundation for good health and a cause of poor health. Perhaps because of the parallel to medicine and nursing it is easier to identify *clinical dietetics* as the treatment of disease through attention to the nutritional care of the individual than to identify *community nutrition* as a focus on health protection and prevention with individuals and families in the community. Both the community nutritionist and the clinical dietitian use the same base of information about food, nutrition, social sciences, and behavioral sciences. Both practice nutrition as a learned profession

Scientific subject matter
Academic discipline
Application of concepts from many sources
Paramount need for primary care
Primary focus on prevention
Prevention of health problems
Concern for community problems
Difficult and time-consuming process necessary to develop working relationship
  with community
Expertise in adapting methods to lifestyle and environment
Work with individuals and population groups
Identification and solution of health problems
Conflict between institutional and community goals
Delivery of health care
Therapeutic intervention

Figure 4.2 Concepts and Terms from Community Medicine and Community Nursing that Apply to Community Nutrition (1,5).

based on the same body of knowledge. The difference in the two fields is in the place and method of application.

Some of the concepts and terms used in describing community medicine and community nursing that are pertinent also to community nutrition are listed in Figure 4.2.

Scope of Program

The difference between a limited community nutrition program and a broad public health nutrition program has been discussed. The extent of each is determined by the purposes and policies of the sponsoring agency and by available personnel, funds, and other resources. Many community nutrition programs proceed independently of other programs in the area. These programs may be sponsored by different agencies but some may have similar objectives. Some kinds of programs with examples are shown in Figure 4.3.

Each of these community nutrition programs is sponsored by a different agency and operates independently although several are concerned with similar objectives. Under these circumstances duplication of effort may occur, and coordination of all programs is important. Responsibility for leadership for coordination may be assumed by the public health nutritionist or, if there is none, by a coordinating body or council. This kind of group serves as a medium of communication between the persons involved in the various programs and provides a

Kind of Program	Examples
1. Planning for nutritional care of individuals or groups.	a. Developing a plan as a component of comprehensive health planning for the community.
2. Identification and treatment of nutrition problems.	a. Screening and treatment of pre-school children to identify nutrition problems. b. Evaluating food records of older persons and conducting nutrition education for nutritional improvement.
3. Action to improve the underlying causes of nutrition problems.	a. Conducting public education on the nutritional risk factors in prevention of coronary heart disease. b. Providing congregate meals and home-delivered meals for the elderly.
4. Education of the general public for improvement of the nutrition of individuals.	a. Advising weight control groups which motivate and educate for weight loss and monitoring their progress. b. Conducting home-based education by nutrition aides on meal planning, food purchasing and food preparation.
5. Education for professionals who conduct or influence nutrition activities.	a. Planning physician education on new knowledge or nutrition in pregnancy. b. Training of home economists who volunteer to teach nutrition classes for the general public.

Figure 4.3   Kinds of Community Nutrition Programs with Examples.

forum in which relationships and overlapping may be considered so that the total contribution to nutritional improvement may be enhanced.

Community nutrition programs may proceed along three lines:

1. Identifying the needs and resources of each community, matching them as appropriate and developing new resources for unmet needs. The identification of needs makes it possible to plan programs for the solution of specific problems rather than to conduct the same

programs that have always been conducted, or those that have been successful in other places. The identification of resources makes it possible to provide more and better services.

2. Interesting professionals from other fields in strengthening their background and techniques so they can deal competently with the food and nutrition problems of their clients. The nutritionist arranges for inservice education as needed through classes, consultation, or other methods. Many nurses, teachers, health educators and home economists are in positions where they can conduct nutrition education or other activities to meet specific problems. It is important that they have accurate information and confidence in their ability to help with nutrition problems.

3. Educating and motivating people to assume responsibility for their own nutritional care and that of others who are dependent on them. Many people consistently disregard the rules of healthful living for diet, weight control, activity, dental care, sleep, and so forth. Public education may be used to improve attitudes, impart information, and effect changes in practices.

Community Medicine

Haynes defines community medicine as collecting scientific information about community health problems and applying it to the solution of those problems. (6) He has described some of the problems encountered when representatives of a medical center and a community tried to define goals for the community health program. There were conflicts between the goals of the center and those of the professionals and community. The major problems seemed to be that building a community health care system requires a great deal of time over a long period and that it was very difficult and time-consuming for the medical center and the community to reach a consensus because of the many ethnic, economic, and social issues that had to be resolved. Haynes believes that though the community may know what it does *not* want, it frequently does not know what it *does* want, so is open to considering alternatives that are the function of the professionals to formulate.

Tapp and Deuschle consider community medicine as the academic discipline that deals with identifying and solving the health problems of communities or population groups. (15) In their perception, community medicine is characterized by a focus on groups or communities as well as on individuals, and by concern not only about the usual medical skills but about how medical care is delivered, and about preventive medicine and the public health.

Fulmer mentions the need for the health professional to recognize the interactions between patient and family and between home and community with community medicine as the result of interaction among population, health status, environment, and health services systems. (5)

Community Nursing

Community health nursing is defined by Tinkham and Voorhis as the field of nursing that has the family and the community as patients, with most activities taking place in the community rather than in the hospital. (16) The uniqueness of community nursing is seen by Archer and Fleshman to lie in a knowledge of community processes with expertise in helping people by promoting health and providing medical care, and adapting methods and treatment to the lifestyles and environments of the populations involved. (1) Other authors believe that an important part of the field is helping the community identify its health problems and priorities, find the available resources, and devise acceptable solutions. (14) The identifying characteristics of community nursing are emphasis on the health of the entire community and emphasis on the community's helping to solve its own problems.

Archer and Fleshman named five functional categories for community nursing; three that are particularly pertinent to community nutrition will be discussed. (1)

Involvement with Systems. This means working with agencies, organizations, governmental bodies, committees, or groups of other practitioners to find ways to provide services and meet nutrition needs.

A specific example in community nutrition is participating in a community on a committee of a voluntary health agency that plans a seminar on screening and treatment of hypertension. The committee consists of a physician, nutritionist, dietitian, nurse, health educator, and a pharmacist. The seminar includes speakers on methods of screening to identify problems and ways to counsel patients about the kind of treatment needed and its importance.

Working with Population Groups. This includes providing broad services to meet the needs of specific groups, such as mothers and children, by health promotion, disease prevention, treatment and rehabilitation. An example is that of a pregnant women who attends a clinic for high-risk maternity patients where care includes attention to various family problems that may interfere with her ability to follow the recommended health regimen. The nutritionist may refer the family for an emergency food supply, explain the benefits of food stamps, and advise the woman how to plan meals that meet the nutritional needs of various family members and conform to their cultural food practices, their home facilities, and their budget.

Working in a Diagnostic Specialty. An example is working with clients who have a chronic condition such as hypertension. A middle-aged single woman with a dangerously elevated blood pressure may need extensive counseling so she can follow the medical order for sodium restriction and weight loss. She may also be referred to a weight control group, given information and encouragement on ways to increase activity, and suggestions about nutritionally adequate, low calorie meals that are acceptable to her lifestyle.

NUTRITIONIST POSITIONS

Many job titles are used for community nutrition positions to conform with agency policies and community practice. Titles often found are *nutritionist, public health nutritionist, nutrition consultant,* and *nutrition specialist.* Various levels may be designated by numerals such as Nutritionist I and Nutritionist II or by titles such as principal, supervising, or senior nutritionist. (7, 8, 11, 13, 18)

Despite the variation in job titles, most community nutrition positions can be divided into four classes according to function. These are (1) *nutrition counselor* for individuals and groups, (2) *staff nutritionist,* who conducts nutrition activities under a nutrition program manager, (3) *nutrition program manager,* who is responsible for a community program and (4) *nutritionist in group food service.* Many positions combine several of these functions as in a program with one nutritionist who plans and manages the program and counsels the patients.

Any of these positions may appear in government programs, voluntary agencies, business, industry, hospitals, clinics, or health management organizations. Many positions are one of a kind. Some positions are for limited periods of time because of the funding or type of program. Some nutritionists have gone to work in WIC programs funded for only one year at a time. One nutritionist was consultant to a state legislative committee knowing that the position might terminate with the next election. One migrant program was funded only for a nine-month period. One-of-a-kind positions include the legislative consultant just mentioned, the nutritionist in a voluntary agency whose duties combine nutrition and other program activities, and a combination nutritionist-health educator in a small rural health department.

The *nutrition counselor* teaches individuals or groups, usually under general or specific supervision of a public health nutritionist. The nutrition counselor teaches patients about normal or modified diets in home, health center or outpatient clinic and provides consultation to other health professionals on individual diets, or participates in conferences about the patients. An important function of the nutrition counselor is fitting the modified diet into the family food practices. Community involvement occurs when the nutrition counselor helps the client solve problems by making a referral to an appropriate community resource.

The position of nutrition counselor may be filled by graduates of a coordinated internship or in some cases by a person with a bachelor's degree in food and nutrition including a course in diet and disease. Appropriate positions for the graduate lacking a background of nutrition in disease conditions may be found in education or food service programs for normal nutrition of individuals and families.

Other personnel with limited nutrition background may participate in counseling on nutrition or related matters under the direction of the nutritionist. These include the home economist, nurse, nutrition technician and nutrition aide. Regardless of the method used, whether individual counseling, small group counseling, or a larger group method, education on modified diet for a treatment program should have input from both a physician and a registered dietitian or similarly qualified nutritionist. Counseling on complicated therapeutic diets should be done by a person with training in clinical dietetics and counseling.

The *staff nutritionist* conducts part of a program directed by another nutritionist participating in such duties as patient care, studies or surveys to identify needs or resources, program planning, evaluation, selection and preparation of teaching and resource materials, professional education, and providing guidance to individuals about available resources.

The *nutrition program manager* usually designates a person responsible for a program with staff, but any nutritionist who works alone is actually a program manager and is responsible for planning and carrying out the program. In either case, the responsibility and process include managing the resources of money, personnel, and facilities for the most effective program.

The *nutritionist in group food service* is responsible for nutritional care and food service in a group care setting. (11) Special competencies in administration and diet therapy are needed in this program depending on the kind of meals served by the facility. Graduation from a coordinated internship provides a good background for a beginning position to work under supervision of a nutritionist or dietitian responsible for the program. There are some positions with minimal need for management skills, such as a child care setting where a simple meal is served to a small group and nutrition education is conducted for normal individual and family nutrition, or a food service and education program for a small group of elderly persons. These may be filled by a person with a more limited background. (8)

Beginning Positions in Community Nutrition

The positions available for the bachelor's degree nutritionist will depend on the current situation, the kind of positions open at the time, and the number of available nutritionists. Most positions are funded by governmental agencies; the kind and number of positions vary with the state and area. Positions with community implications are also found in voluntary agencies, in business, and in other organizations with a health component. (8)

The best entering position (11) for the bachelor's degree nutritionist is a staff position under the supervision of an experienced nutritionist with graduate education. Most of the more responsible positions require a year of graduate study in community nutrition and at least one year's experience.

In actual practice and in some settings, technical supervision may not be available and the beginning nutritionist may work under the administrative supervision of a program director with a background in administration, medicine, health education, nursing or education. Where there is no technical supervision, the nutritionist has an important responsibility to assure the technical quality of the nutrition component of the program that starts with the application for the position. Often the appointing administrator is not well informed about appropriate qualifications for a specific nutrition position. Sometimes an applicant can supply this information, but in any case the applicant should accept a position only if qualified.

RELATED POSITIONS

There are several related positions that may require or permit participation in nutritional care as part of a nutrition team. The *home economist* who has a good background in foods and nutrition as well as in other aspects of home economics may work in nutrition programs supplementing the nutritionist's work in the areas of home and family management as they interfere with ability to follow a nutritional care regimen. Food budgeting, marketing, food preparation and other aspects of household management are the special province of the home economist, who may also train and supervise nutrition aides. (2)

A *nutrition technician* is a relatively new position for a "technically skilled person who has successfully completed an associate degree program that meets the educational standards established by The American Dietetic Association" for a *dietetic technician* and who has had additional courses and experience to qualify for work in a community health setting. The technician works under the supervision of a community nutritionist, assisting with individual and group education and in other appropriate ways. (10, 12)

A *nutrition aide* is usually a member of the same cultural group with whom the work is done, often from the same neighborhood, and is particularly helpful in finding ways to modify the practices of the cultural group. (11) Inservice training by a nutritionist or home economist prepares this person for a helping role in the nutrition program. The work may include preparing illustrative materials, showing films, helping a patient complete a food record, conducting a food demonstration, or teaching individuals or groups in specific limited ways.

JOB SATISFACTION IN COMMUNITY NUTRITION

The way the community nutritionist derives job satisfaction varies in different programs. Sometimes it comes from seeing progress in continuing work with the same individuals, as in conducting a weight control group. Sometimes it comes from long-term interaction with other professionals in the same agency and in other community organizations. In another program, satisfaction may come from one contact, for example, from providing consultation to a professional about a specific program.

Community nutrition is an interesting, exciting field that has good potential for the future because of current and projected national plans for health and nutrition and increasing information and interest on the part of the general public. Opportunities for work occur in many organizations and programs.

Community nutrition involves working with people from many walks of life and many cultural groups. Because of the universal importance of food, with implications for health and for social and economic affairs, various community nutrition programs can offer the opportunity to work with people in a variety of situations, such as the following:

1. Individuals, both well and sick, for the purpose of changing practices that affect nutrition of well persons of all ages who live in

the community along with those who attend ambulatory care clinics for care of many diseases.

2. Professionals and paraprofessionals from the fields of health, business, education, politics and the media.

The community nutritionist engages in many activities for public education, professional education, and nutritional care serving as a link between the individual with a problem and the persons who can do something about it. Some examples are teaching cooks from day care centers about meal planning, presenting a workshop on food misinformation for elementary school teachers, teaching nutrition to mothers and preschoolers individually or in groups, participating in a symposium on prevention of coronary heart disease, preparing a diet manual for patients of an alcoholism center, participating in a television program on nutritionally adequate lunches, and advising a local food editor about food additives. Some activities are conducted regularly, such as counseling in a weekly diabetic clinic; many others are done once a year or even more rarely, such as conducting a training course for leaders in local weight control groups.

The actual work performed in any specific program depends on its scope and structure. In a program of limited scope such as a meal service for older persons, the nutritionist deals with one meal and one age group; in a public health agency the activities may include many of those mentioned. However, similar methods and techniques are used for all programs regardless of size and nature and are affected mainly by the degree of responsibility for the program.

The work of the community nutritionist is challenging because of the variety, because it changes as health care changes, because there is always a new program, a new group, or a new problem, and because of the opportunity to participate in the process of change by influencing significant action in legislation, health planning, and other areas.

SUMMARY

Prevention of diseases and conditions in which nutrition is an important factor may be at primary, secondary, or tertiary level. The community nutritionist may participate in nutritional care at all three levels. Prevention of diseases that are the major causes of morbidity and mortality is important because it appears that treatment has reached its limit. Further improvements in health will be dependent on correcting living practices that are contributing factors in the etiology of these diseases. Often, nutrition problems are due to socioeconomic and environmental factors such as inadequate income and poor health rather than dietary causes. When this is true, nutrition education is futile since the causes are not under control of the individual. Then the nutrition problems must be attacked in some other way.

The community nutritionist applies basic knowledge from many subjects to the solution of community nutrition problems. Though these subjects are used in other fields, the uniqueness of the community nutrition field lies in how the knowledge is used. Community nutrition has specific basic concepts, tasks, and focus that have been presented and discussed.

Many titles are used for different positions in community nutrition, but the kinds of jobs can be described by four functions: nutrition counselor, staff nutritionist, nutrition program manager, and nutritionist in group food service. Related positions include home economist, nutrition technician, and nutrition aide.

Job satisfaction in community nutrition comes from the variety of activities with professionals, paraprofessionals, community leaders, and public. There are always new programs, new groups, and new problems, and the opportunity to influence change for better nutrition and health.

REFERENCES CITED

1. Archer, Sarah E., and Ruth P. Fleshman, Community Health Nursing: A Typology of Practice, *Nursing Outlook,* 23 6/75 358, 361.
2. Barney, Helen S., and Mary C. Egan, Home Economists as Members of Health Teams, *J. Home Econ.,* 60 6/68 42
3. Cornely, Paul B., Community Concern for Total Health Care, *J. Am. Diet. Assoc.,* 60 2/72 107.
4. Curran, William J., A Bicentennial Review, *Am. J. Public Health,* 66 1/76 93.
5. Fulmer, Hugh S., An Approach to the Teaching of Epidemiology, appendix in Kane, Robert L., ed., *The Challenges of Community Medicine,* Springer Publishing Co., New York, 1974, 336.
6. Haynes, M. Alfred, A New Medical Center, in Ginzberg, Eli and Alice H. Yohalem, ed. *The University Medical Center and the Metropolis,* Josiah Macy Jr. Foundation, New York, 1974, 44.
7. Huenemann, Ruth L., and Eileen B. Peck, Who Is a Public Health Nutritionist?, *J. Am. Diet. Assoc.,* 58 4/71 327.
8. Hunscher, Helen A., Undergraduate Education in Public Health Nutrition, *J. Nutr. Educ.,* 4 Sum./72, Supp. 1, 134.
9. Kane, Robert L., ed. *The Challenges of Community Medicine,* Springer Publishing Co., New York, 1974, 124.
10. Lumsden, James E., Kathleen Zolber, Peter Strutz, Shirley T. Moore, Albert Sanchez, and David Abbey, Delegation of Functions by Dietitians to Dietetic Technicians, *J. Am. Diet Assoc.,* 69 8/76 143.

11. *Personnel in Public Health Nutrition,* The American Dietetic Association, Chicago, 1976.
12. Position Paper on the Dietetic Technician and the Dietetic Assistant, *J. Am. Diet. Assoc.,* 67 9/75 246.
13. Pye, Orrea F., The Master's Program in Public Health Nutrition, *J. Nutr. Educ.,* 4 Sum./72, Supp. 1, 137.
14. Skrovan, Clarence, Elizabeth T. Anderson, and Janet Gottschalk, Community Nurse Practitioner, *Am. J. Public Health,* 64 9/74 849.
15. Tapp, J. W., Jr., and K. W. Deuschle, The Community Medicine Clerkship—A Guide for Teachers and Students of Community Medicine, *Milbank Mem. Fund Q.,* 47 1969 411.
16. Tinkham, Catherine W., and Eleanor F. Voorhies, *Community Health Nursing,* Appleton-Century-Crofts, New York, 1972, 114.
17. U.S. Dept. of Health, Education, and Welfare, *Forward Plan for Health FY 1977–1981,* Aug. 1975, 15.
18. U.S. Dept. of Health, Education, and Welfare, *Guide Class Specifications for Nutritionist Positions in State and Local Public Health Programs,* Government Printing Office, Washington DC, February 1971.

5 HOW THREE COMMUNITY NUTRITION PROGRAMS DEVELOPED

While some specially funded community nutrition programs, particularly those established in response to political pressure, are developed in a short time, most broad community nutrition programs established on a permanent basis in health agencies develop slowly over a considerable period of time. The histories of three such permanent programs will be reported to show how community nutritionists work in different kinds of programs as they develop. These programs provide examples of how nutritionists apply their knowledge, perform the basic tasks, and utilize the concepts of community nutrition. One program is in Cooperative Extension, one in a voluntary association, and one in a health department.

PROGRAM IN COOPERATIVE EXTENSION

Cooperative Extension (formerly called Agricultural Extension) is an educational agency jointly sponsored by federal, state, and county governments.

This Extension home advisor, who has had graduate study in nutrition and public health, conducts a community nutrition program so she will be called a nutritionist in this report. This nutritionist joined the Extension staff six years ago with the mission of developing a food and nutrition public education program maximizing minimum resources, mainly working through the mass media, but also in other direct and indirect ways to reach the public. The first steps were (1) to become informed about the ongoing nutrition and related programs in the community and to let others know about this new service of Extension, (2) to get acquainted with the community and the audience, (3) to identify problems and resources, and (4) to plan a long-range program and set priorities.

As this is a large urban community, the nutritionist thought it might take six months to accomplish these objectives. Her first goal was to make contacts that would lead to opportunities for service. The first step was to meet key persons, so she introduced herself by telephone and visited each by appointment. These included the chief nutritionist in the county health department, the heads of home economics and health education in the county school office, the director of family services in the local welfare agency, the food editors of the local newspapers, and program directors of television and radio stations. Her open-ended question to them was: What activities or programs are there in your organization that are designed for health improvement through food and nutrition? She explained her own role as that of making the resources and expertise of Extension available and useful to them. The nutritionist obtained enough information to understand the current programs of the various agencies.

The public health department had an active nutrition program with a nutritionist responsible for each health district. The primary concerns were the promotion of health of mothers and children and the prevention of specific public health nutrition problems—especially coronary heart disease, hunger and malnutrition, and obesity. Each nutritionist in the various health districts conducted a community nutrition program, the activities differing according to the demands and needs of the specific community. Each program was focused primarily on the clientele known to the health center and community programs were planned to meet their needs.

The schools had an extensive nutrition component in the health education curriculum that was a part of regular classroom teaching, especially in the child care courses. Nutrition was integrated into classroom teaching rather than taught as a separate program.

The major nutrition program in a voluntary health agency was that conducted by the Heart Association, which had a nutritionist on its staff. The two nutritionists agreed to serve as consultants to each other in their special fields, considered the kinds of referrals each might make to the other, and discussed work on cooperative programs.

The public welfare agency had no nutrition component, but the director was pleased to have the Extension nutritionist available for help on food and nutrition problems.

There was a large active local dietetic association and an area public health association, with a small group of nutritionists and dietitians among the members.

Several local newspapers carried articles or columns on food and nutrition, but only two had regular food sections with staff members knowledgeable about food and nutrition. All were interested in receiving information on food and nutrition and in using the nutritionist as a resource.

Armed with this information about the community, the nutritionist planned her program, deciding to work through the community "thought-leaders," teachers, and mass media. The thought-leaders were those in positions to influence the thinking of groups, such as presidents of women's clubs, various spokesmen for parent-teacher groups, and the Director of Nursing and Health in the local American Red Cross.

The nutritionist received many calls from teachers and early recognized that she could provide some help to those who wanted to teach nutrition but hesitated to do so because they felt their information might be inaccurate. The nutritionist discussed the calls and the problems with the principal in one district and as a result was asked to participate in training for teachers in the child care program. She conducted a ten-lesson series to a number of groups of teachers and parents. This occupied much of her time in the latter part of her first year.

Meantime the nutritionist became active in the local dietetic association, home economics association, nutrition council, and public health association, and continued to get acquainted with community leaders in nutrition. As a member of the State Dietetic Association Continuing Education Committee, which was responsible for approval of continuing education programs for members, she was able to influence the quality of such programs. She participated in the activities of the local nutrition council, was a member of the organizing group for a nutrition section in the area public health association, and was later the first nutritionist elected to membership on the governing council of the association that has provided a way to give nutrition a greater influence in programs and committee activities.

One of the nutritionist's priorities has always been answering requests for information from professional persons, especially dietitians, home economists, public health nutritionists, and the media. The resources at her disposal include the State and Federal Extension offices, with specialists in nutrition, home management, and food technology. She has been especially careful to provide immediate answers to requests of newspapers, television, and radio for facts, opinions, or policy statements on food and nutrition questions in the news, such as nutritional value of ready-to-eat cereal, increasing the iron enrichment of breads, and the safety of food additives such as red dyes and nitrates.

The major emphasis in this long-range program is on community professional education through joint projects with other professionals and through consultation by telephone and mail. One channel is a monthly newsletter with about 2000 copies distributed to dietitians, nutritionists, home economists in public utilities, newspaper editors, university and secondary teachers, social workers and physicians. The second emphasis is on services as a resource to the Cooperative Extension staff and as a trainer for the personnel of the Expanded Food and Nutrition Education Project. The third emphasis is on cooperative programs with other agencies in public education, such as nutrition programs for the elderly and nutrition classes for the general public.

This nutritionist has developed a program with significant ways to reach the community and with a potential to improve nutritional status. She derives job satisfaction from working with both professionals and the public, and likes the agency policy, which permits her to develop the programs that are, in her own judgment, of benefit to the nutritional health of the community.

PROGRAM IN A LARGE HEALTH DEPARTMENT

The activities in this large health department over a sixty-year period are typical of the gradual development that takes place in any public agency over a period of time. A smaller agency has fewer problems and fewer resources, but utilizes the same program concepts and methods, and many of the specific activities could be adapted for use in community nutrition programs in smaller agencies.

The earliest activities in this agency were concerned with improving the nutrition of mothers and children, primarily by classes and individual counseling. Educational work in nutrition started about 1918 as one of the duties of the Child Hygiene Director, probably with patient counseling by physicians and nurses. The first nutritionist joined the staff in 1928 to work with parents of undernourished children for prevention of tuberculosis. A few years later, two more nutritionists were added to counsel pregnant women and mothers who brought their children to the well child conferences for preventive care, and an additional nutritionist was assigned to the tuberculosis control program. These nutritionists counseled individuals and groups in the health center or in the home and sometimes gave talks to parent-teacher or other groups.

In the early 1950's, although there was no change in the goal of improving the nutrition of mothers and children, a change took place in the concepts of how health education could best be conducted. The major responsibility for the health education of individuals and families who were recipients of departmental services was delegated to the public health nurse as the primary educator in all aspects of health. There were many more nurses than nutritionists, and because the nurses had regular contacts with the clients, this change provided the potential of reaching more persons.

The function of the nutritionist changed from patient education to staff education, particularly with the nutritionist's providing the public health nurses with information, techniques, skills and tools for instructing individuals or groups in health centers and homes. The nutritionist's responsibilities included identification of community needs and the development of programs to meet them.

Conforming to this trend, the department established, in 1953, a Nutrition Division with a head nutritionist and two staff nutritionists. This Division's mission was to improve the nutrition of the population, with first attention being paid to the nutrition of pregnant women, infants, preschoolers, and school children. The primary functions were staff education, preparation of leaflets and illustrative materials for teaching clients, development of resource materials for use of nurses, physicians and others, and participation with others in the community for a combined attack on identified problems. The latter was done through committees and task forces attacking nutrition problems in tuberculosis and dental caries, correcting misinformation among professional persons and the public, and in many other ways.

By 1960, nutrition activities were proceeding in three general categories:

1. Individual and group education by public health nurses for tuberculous patients, pregnant women, mothers of well children, and parents of children in church-sponsored schools. Nutrition information was integrated rather than taught as an entity; for example, in the prenatal classes the place of meat, milk, and eggs was related to the need for strong muscles during delivery, and the need for milk for fetal bone development was stressed.

2. Group education and consultation for physicians, nurses, dentists, dental hygienists, health educators, medical social workers and teachers.

3. Community activities that arose from the community's expression of needs, such as requests from teachers for advice on how to remove soft drink machines from school premises. The machines were sometimes sponsored by school-related groups as a source of

funds for athletic uniforms, motion picture projectors, and other unmet needs. Nutritionists tried to help teachers and parents find alternatives, such as selling fruit juices instead of soft drinks, or other ways to raise money.

About this time, there was an increase in proportion of senior citizens, so another goal was added: to improve the food consumption of older persons. The first activity was a specially funded research project on the effect of management practices on food acceptability and nutrient content of food consumed in nursing homes. The results indicated a need for better preparation of administrative and supervisory personnel before staff practices could be changed. It was some time before steps were taken in this direction. The second activity was improvement of the food practices of senior citizens living in their own homes by means of a community approach of state, county, and city nutritionists and the staff of the county agency responsible for senior citizens' affairs. Education was conducted in groups, by a community fair, a newsletter, and other methods.

By this time, the staff had increased to four nutritionists and functions were changing. The head nutritionist worked with the Department's executive personnel on joint planning for overall programs, such as new health facilities and comprehensive health care, and with voluntary agencies, such as the Heart Association to add nutrition programs to its activities. Staff nutritionists began to assume comprehensive responsibilities as specialists in child health, maternal health and tuberculosis control, and to develop resource materials on food money management, cultural food practices, and other overall topics. Through an interdepartmental agreement with the public welfare agency, extra staff was employed to price foods in 150 markets to obtain data for revision of the welfare food allowances.

There was a constant need for printed educational materials for use in classes and counseling and as a resource for professionals. Printed materials from other agencies and organizations were used when suitable ones were available, but there was a need for materials adapted to local practices, so staff began to make more of their own. A pamphlet on family food money management developed at that time for staff education is still in use after periodic price revisions, illustrating the long-range value of well-conceived and carefully prepared resource materials.

Several requests from staff nurses for information about food practices of local Mexican-Americans led to a study by one of the nutritionists and the preparation of a pamphlet in 1963. This was later followed by similar works on the food practices of blacks, and of certain national groups, such as Arabians, Samoans and Chinese; all these studies have become permanent educational materials in the Department. Recently leaflets for patient instruction were prepared for Japanese and Korean food patterns. Other printed materials and policy statements on diet counseling and other activities were developed in cooperation with nurses, physicians, and other staff.

As the poverty programs developed in the late sixties, the nutrition staff added a new goal, that of helping poor families find or create new resources. They encouraged more and better use of food stamps and cooperated in training personnel and providing consultation for Head Start and other poverty programs. The staff also participated in the development of nutrition training for homemakers and home health aides. A community worker was made available to the program, who, after appropriate training, assisted in taking food histories, preparing teaching materials and showing films.

A number of new programs, some specially funded, developed in the late 1960's, including comprehensive care for children, care for high-risk mothers and infants, and the counseling of young people living in the counterculture. Nutritionists participated in planning the nutrition component of lunch programs for senior citizens, a parent-child center, and a smoking-withdrawal clinic. They also participated in training of personnel for the Peace Corps and Vista, in preparing a project proposal for a family coronary prevention program, and in planning for a new comprehensive health care center.

Many of the young persons who attended the youth clinics followed unusual diets, most of which were nutritionally inadequate. Some were interested in a vegetarian diet, so staff prepared teaching and resource materials to show how various diets could supply adequate nutrients. The extensive use of drugs by many who came to the clinics resulted in concern about the nutrition of drug addicts, and as the emphasis on alcoholism and drug abuse increased, more attention was given to the relationship of nutrition to the prevention and treatment of these problems.

Weight control and weight reducing have always been popular topics. In recent years the prevention of obesity has been made a major goal, beginning with the infant. Nutritionists work toward this in many ways, organizing and conducting weight control clinics, developing some of the local TOPS (Take Off Pounds Sensibly) groups as a resource by presenting training courses for the leaders, developing an exercise component as a part of all weight control programs, and incorporating weight control into all nutrition teaching.

Another regular goal during this period of time was keeping staff and other nutritionists and dietitians up to date by inservice education in nutrition, techniques, and resources, so staff participated in planning conferences, lectures and other group events. Some of the topics covered were interviewing and counseling, program planning, coronary heart disease, high blood pressure, exercise, and revisions of the recommended dietary allowances.

During the last five years, a reorganization of the agency with decentralization of services and emphasis on treatment as well as prevention has resulted in an increase in direct services when the condition and prescribed diet need the particular skills of the nutritionist. This is limited to selected cases in which diet is a critical part of care, such as diabetes, high-risk pregnancy and failure-to-thrive infancy or programs in which the nutrition component is mandated by state or federal law. Nutritionists have mobilized students and volunteers to assist in getting dietary histories and to provide immediate counseling in some programs. Perhaps the most significant current activity is the initiation and development of a nutritional surveillance system to provide data on the local population that can be used for program planning and evaluation.

This 25-year history has been marked by a cycle in which emphasis in nutrition programs moved from direct patient service by dietitians through an era when nutritionists conducted community programs and provided subject matter and techniques enabling public health nurses to counsel patients, to the present, when nutritionists are conducting preventive activities as program managers and community organizers and participating directly in patient care.

PROGRAM IN A SMALL VISITING NURSE AGENCY

In early March 1963, an internist who was on the board of directors of this Visiting Nurse Agency (VNA), which covered a city of 50,000 and some adjoining territory, requested that the local health officer help the agency develop a resource for counseling patients who were referred to the VNA by local physicians. The VNA had a nurse-director and three public health nurses on its staff. The health officer arranged a conference of the VNA director, the president of its board, a community leader who was a retired nurse, the Health Department's Director of nursing, the health educator, the part-time public health nutritionist, and the internist to consider the problem and some possible solutions.

At the meeting the problem was presented by the internist, who expressed need for a qualified diet counselor to whom he could refer patients for instruction on therapeutic diets, mainly for diabetes, arthritis, heart disease, stroke, ulcer, and cancer, with an occasional diagnosis of gout or anemia. He said that other physicians in the area could also refer their patients to this service. The patients could not afford to pay a dietitian in private practice for this service, and even if they could, there were no dietitians in private practice in the city. He suggested that the service be provided through the VNA, although he knew there was no money in that year's budget for additional services.

The VNA nurses said they were aware of their patients' need for some help about diet and that they had observed that many patients did not follow the diets prescribed. The nurses thought that at least in some cases recovery was delayed because of this. They said that in other cases the patient and family would benefit from help to improve the regular family diet, especially on food budgeting, even though no therapeutic diet had been prescribed.

Various suggestions were made and discussed, such as having a part-time nutritionist on the VNA staff, having the staff nurses counsel the patients they visited, having the public health nutritionist provide this service, and referring the patients to the dietitian in the local hospital. It was agreed that having a part-time nutritionist was a good idea and should be considered in planning the budget for the next fiscal year. The nurses indicated that they were willing to counsel the patients and had already helped as much as they felt they could, but did not feel confident of their knowledge. Thus diet instruction was left to the physician and to the hospital dietitian, who were sometimes able to counsel patients or families at the time of discharge. But the nurses said that the patients needed detailed instruction after they returned home and followup as their recovery progressed.

The nurses said that if there could be good initial instruction and a detailed copy of the diet, they would undertake to monitor and followup the diet. The public health nutritionist offered to teach a series of classes on the various diets to help the nurses gain more confidence for this work, if a local dietitian could be found to assist on a volunteer basis.

The health educator asked for evidence that the other physicians would utilize the service; she had read an article about a community which had developed such a service, but the project failed because the physicians did not refer their patients. The health officer suggested that the internist, who was a leader in the local medical society, find out the extent of its members' interest and try to get the group to support the project. The VNA director pointed out that if the service was to be budgeted the following year, the agency would need community support to raise more money.

As the problems and solution appeared to be defined, it was decided to investigate the matters suggested and to meet again after the next meeting of the local medical society, since it was the concensus that the society's support was necessary for the success of the service. Other members of the group agreed to pursue some other channels for help and to report at the next meeting.

When the group met again three weeks later, the internist reported that the medical society was interested in the project and would give it publicity among the physicians in the area. The public health nutritionist had talked with three dietitians who were interested in part-time work, one of whom was willing to participate on a volunteer basis for an indefinite period, at first helping with the series of classes. She had been at home with her five children for 15 years, but had maintained her membership and interest in the local dietetic association, and felt that by participating in the sessions under the direction of the nutritionist she would be prepared to assume responsibility for the counseling service and to answer questions the nurses might have about individual patients. As soon as money could be found, she would be willing to work regularly on a 10-hour-a-week basis. The retired nurse had looked for a place to hold the classes, and found that the local electric company would allow use of their kitchen and meeting room and would donate part of the food. The dates had been set for the sessions and time was allowed in the nurses' schedules for them to attend. The director had decided to invite the staffs of the VNA's in three adjoining cities, so there were 12 nurses to attend the sessions.

The program developed as planned, the sessions were held, five physicians referred their patients, and the nurses counseled the patients with help from the volunteer dietitian. Before the end of the year, money was found to pay the dietitian and she worked 10 hours a week counseling patients on the more difficult diets and giving consultation to the nurses about the problems they encountered. She conferred with the dietitians in the three hospitals from which most of the patients had been discharged so that she knew ahead of time what some of the needs were. This interested the dietitians in improving the discharge instruction and they sent the VNA dietitian copies of the diets that were prescribed for the patients. As the need for the service grew the VNA increased the dietitian's time to 16 hours per week.

This service continued for about five years with a change of dietitians when the first one accepted a full time position in a local hospital. Again the public health nutritionist helped orient the new dietitian. After five years the VNA was no longer able to finance the project because of policy changes and changes in the health care delivery system in the area. However, the physicians felt that the service was very beneficial and arranged for a local hospital to enlarge its dietetic staff so that a dietitian would be available to handle the referrals and advise the nurses. Several times a year on request, the public health nutritionist and the dietitian conducted a refresher session for the nurses. The program still continues after 13 years.

COMMENT

The three community nutrition programs that have been described illustrate how programs can be developed. All three programs went through the same steps in development, that is, recognition or identification of needs and resources, plans for initiating the activities, development of the activities and, in the VNA, plans to phase out the program when this was indicated. The more limited and better defined VNA program developed in answer to an expressed, specific community need, and was implemented in a short period of time due to its limited nature and a cooperative community effort that required a minimum expenditure of money and time. The Extension program set up to provide a service that would meet a general need recognized by the agency, had a much slower development because the nutritionist had to lay the groundwork, identify specific needs, select priorities, and make the service known. The public health nutrition program developed in a public agency that had long accepted the need for a nutrition program in its structure along with many other programs with which it had to cooperate and compete for attention. The program developed slowly, and provided ongoing services that changed to meet changing needs.

The community nutritionist selecting a position needs to assess how the program in question will develop and whether the progress and eventual nature of the program are consistent with the nutritionist's own career objectives and most effective methods of working.

SUMMARY

The development of three community nutrition programs has been reported. One program was conducted by a nutritionist in a Cooperative Extension office, another by a nutrition director and staff in a large health agency, and a third was the program in a small visiting nurse agency. Each of the three programs developed in a different way, but all included assessment of needs, getting acquainted with the community, and program interactions with the community. These programs show some of the ways in which community nutritionists apply their knowledge to solve problems.

2 THE STRUCTURE

In the United States, health services are provided through a complex network of government health and welfare agencies and hospitals; private agencies, hospitals, and practitioners; voluntary agencies; schools; professional associations; philanthropic foundations; and other groups. In addition, health programs are affected by government regulation agencies.

Many of these organizations conduct community nutrition programs or have a nutrition component. Besides those named above, other organizations conduct activities related to nutrition. These include trade associations, food marketers, food processors, and other organizations of business and industry. There are also a number of consumer-oriented organizations of recent development that exert influence on food and nutrition, especially by publicizing food-related hazards and food laws.

The community nutritionist needs to understand the community structure and know how to use it for the improvement of nutrition. The nutritionist must also keep informed about new groups, evaluate their activities, support those that contribute to good nutrition and be a resource for advice to others on reacting to their activities.

6 GOVERNMENT AGENCIES

The Constitution of the United States does not specifically mention *health,* but it requires that the government promote the *general welfare* and empowers it to levy taxes for that purpose and to make laws necessary to carry out its power. *Welfare* has been interpreted to mean all matters that affect well-being, including health. This responsibility is carried on by *official agencies* established by the federal government and financed with public moneys. There are similar official agencies at state, county, and city levels, each of which has a specific structure and method of funding, usually through taxes.

Structure in the federal government has become very complex in the attempt to meet the needs of the citizens. Sometimes a new agency is created for a specific purpose even though the function could be appropriately performed by an existing agency. Legislation, that is, making the laws, is a very complicated process, starting with a bill, introduced in the Congress by a senator or representative, designed to accomplish a specific purpose, for example, to establish a child nutrition program.

In addition to the power of making laws about health and welfare, Congress has the power to investigate, regulate, and act on behalf of the individual. Congressional dissatisfaction with agency programs, with changes that are too slow, or pressure from constituents has frequently resulted in investigation followed by new legislation, amendments to existing laws, or strengthening enforcement; for example, in the 1960's public concern over hunger and malnutrition in the United States resulted in investigation by the Senate Select Committee on Nutrition and Human Needs that gave rise to important changes in the food stamp program, food distribution policies, and activities for the elderly.

Many federal and state laws that deal with the health of individuals are passed every year. A considerable number of them affect nutrition either directly or indirectly. In addition to bills that deal specifically with nutrition, there may be provisions for nutrition programs in larger bills, such as the Older Americans Act. The community nutritionist needs to be informed about existing laws of significance to nutrition, and should analyze bills for their impact on community nutrition and take appropriate action to support or defeat them.

Community nutrition programs exist in many governmental agencies and at many levels. The usual operating arrangement in health agencies has been bureaucratic, with many independent units hierarchically organized, each worker responsible to a higher level. In some agencies, there is under way a change replacing the bureaucratic structure with a systems approach, or arrangement of activities and values that contribute in various ways to a common objective. This has significant implications for future programs because it could change the placement of specialized programs such as nutrition by incorporating them into many other programs.

Another important change is the trend toward consolidation of agencies, resulting in the combination of city and county health departments, of health and welfare agencies, or of public health agencies, mental health agencies and hospitals. These consolidations are traumatic for staff and confusing to the public, but they may also provide better service at less cost to the taxpayer. Like all other changes, these must be accepted with the knowledge that it takes five to ten years to determine the benefits and that if there are none, further changes will take place. In the process of change, nutritionists, as individuals and taxpayers as well as professionals, should exert their influence to maintain the best possible nutrition services for the public. Consolidation of agencies may help streamline organizations, and simplified administration may make it easier for governors, mayors, and county executives to function, but the long-range effects on health service delivery and on preventive health are not yet available.

The purpose of this chapter is to help the reader develop a concept of the kinds of agencies in which nutrition programs may be found and an understanding of how various programs may operate. Likewise, the descriptions of agencies and programs are intended to inform the reader about some current operations as a background rather than to provide an extensive report. The nutritionist needs to be aware that structure, details of operation, and names of programs and agencies vary with place and time, necessitating a constant effort to keep informed.

FEDERAL AGENCIES

Most nutrition programs of the federal government are conducted or sponsored by either the Department of Agriculture or the Department of Health, Education, and Welfare. The structure and function of these Departments will be described with emphasis on the branches where most food and nutrition programs are found, along with a review of the activities and programs of some other governmental and quasi-governmental agencies that should be known to the community nutritionist. The major current nutrition programs themselves will be covered in the next chapter.

Though changes are always taking place, this review will give an idea of possibilities and point the way to understanding future programs. The community nutritionist needs to know about these programs because they are widespread; in some areas they are the only community programs, but in all areas they are important resources for handling problems and extending programs.

Department of Agriculture (USDA)

This agency acquires and diffuses general and comprehensive information about agriculture and conducts programs that include research, education, marketing, regulatory work, agricultural adjustment, surplus disposal and rural development. (25) It has a number of programs for improvement of nutrition and health that should be known to the community nutritionist. Two of the Department's five main divisions are of particular interest: Marketing and Consumer Services, and Conservation, Research and Education. (Figure 6.1)

Marketing and Consumer Services.   This unit conducts programs that protect producers, handlers, and consumers of agricultural products, especially farm fruits and vegetables. Some of the programs control marketing conditions for milk, fruits, vegetables and nuts by regulating market supplies, establishing minimum prices and other measures. *Section 32 Programs* use funds from certain customs receipts to encourage the consumption of foods that are in surplus or that have other marketing difficulties and to purchase surplus foods for school lunch and institutions. The *Food and Nutrition Service* (FNS) administers the food assistance programs in cooperation with state and local agencies. These include the Food Stamp Program and the five areas of the child nutrition programs.

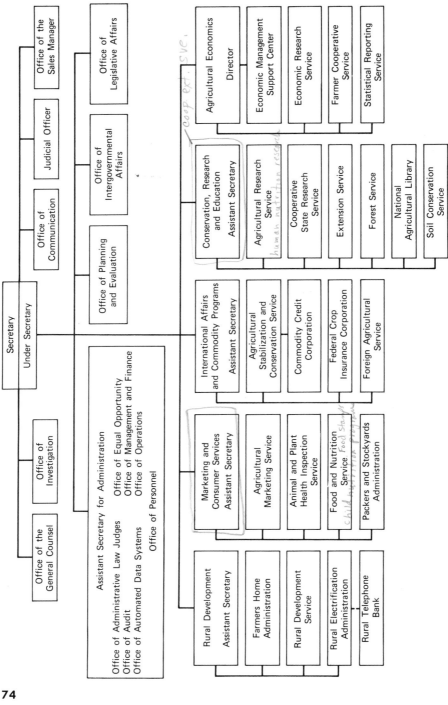

Figure 6.1 Organization Chart: United States Department of Agriculture. (From United States Government Manual 1975–76, p. 99)

Conservation, Research and Education. This Division conducts research and education to help agriculture meet the food and fiber needs of the country, to conserve soils, forests, water and other national resources, and to help the public benefit from technology by application to everyday problems and opportunities.

Extension Service, an educational agency, cooperates with state governments and county governments to comprise the Cooperative Extension Service.

Extension home economists, sometimes called home agents or home advisors, are members of the staff of the state land grant university. The three agencies, state, county, and university, work together in financing, planning and conducting education to show the public how to apply the latest technology to everyday living. Home economics and nutrition make up one of the major programs, designed to inform the public how to apply recent research to improve home and family living. Information is presented in person, by telephone, by mail, at meetings, and through newspapers, radio, and television.

Extension at the federal level has home economists and nutritionists who provide assistance to State Extension specialists, who in turn interpret research and prepare educational materials for counties. There are area staffs in almost all counties of the 50 states, with about 3000 offices.

Extension workers cooperate in many community programs helping to analyze needs and resources and to organize the community for solution of family and home problems. There are extensive 4-H programs for boys and girls and special programs in which aides trained by Extension staff work with low-income families in their own homes.

Agricultural Research Service (ARS) was established in 1953 to provide knowledge and technology to farmers so they can produce efficiently, conserve the environment, and provide food for the country. ARS conducts human nutrition research, including food consumption studies and the investigation of human needs for foods, nutrients, and meal content.

Department of Health, Education, and Welfare (USDHEW)

This Department was created by act of Congress in 1953. Its major functions are concerned with the availability of health services, the quality of education, and the administration of the Social Security system. (26) Most of the programs with which the community nutritionist may be involved are under the Public Health Service, the Office

of Human Development, or the Education Division. The Department
has 10 regions, each of which has a regional office and a director. One of
the director's functions is to represent the Department in contacts with
state and local officials (See Figure 6.2).

Public Health Service (PHS).   Though the PHS actually originated
in 1798, its responsibilities have been greatly broadened in the last 30
years. Its general responsibility is to promote and insure the highest
attainable level of health for all persons. Its major functions are "To
stimulate and assist States and communities with the development of
local health resources and to further development of education for the
health professions; to assist with improvement of the delivery of health
services to all Americans; to conduct and support research in the
medical and related sciences and to disseminate scientific information;
to protect the health of the Nation against impure and unsafe foods,
drugs and cosmetics, and other potential hazards; and to provide
national leadership for the prevention and control of communicable
disease and other public health functions." (28) These functions are
carried out by the seven subdivisions of the Public Health Service,
which are the following: Alcohol, Drug Abuse, and Mental Health
Administration; Center for Disease Control; Food and Drug Administration; Health Resources Administration; Health Services Administration; National Institutes of Health; and President's Council on Physical
Fitness and Sports.

The *Alcohol, Drug Abuse and Mental Health Administration*
(ADAMHA) provides leadership to the federal effort to ameliorate
health problems caused by abuse of alcohol and drugs and to improve
the mental health of Americans. It supports research and training and
provides technical assistance to state and regional agencies.

The *Center for Disease Control* (CDC) was established in 1946 as the
Communicable Disease Center of the U.S. Public Health Service. It was
renamed Center for Disease Control in 1970 because of its broadened
responsibility toward a wide range of preventable diseases. In 1973 it
became a full-fledged agency of the Public Health Service. Today it
administers programs concerned with communicable and vector-borne
diseases, lead poisoning, urban rat control, safe conditions for working
people, and the relationship of smoking to health.

An activity of the CDC that is of major significance to community
nutritionists is the development of a method for nutritional surveillance
now in use in ten states and one major urban area. States are advised
and assisted in developing their own systems for a continuous monitoring of the nutritional status of a specific population. (3)

The *Food and Drug Administration* (FDA) was established in 1930,

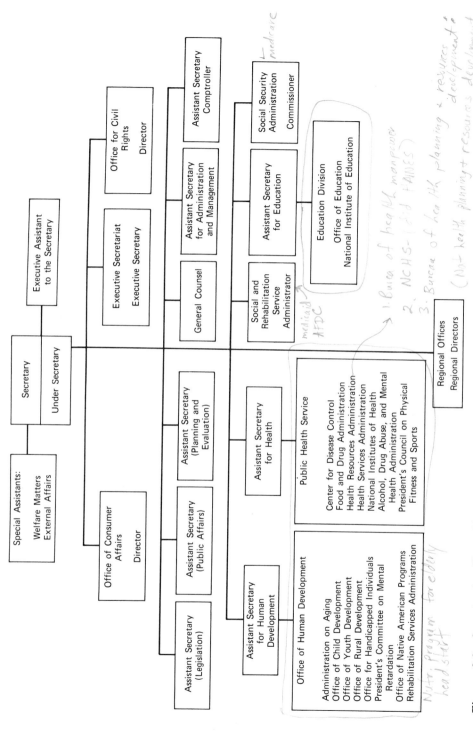

Figure 6.2 Organization Chart: United States Department of Health, Education, and Welfare. (From United States Government Manual 1975–76, p. 230.)

77

although its forerunners date to 1907. Its purpose is to protect the health of the nation against impure and unsafe foods and other hazardous substances. It carries out its field operations through the 10 DHEW Regional Offices and has laboratories and administrative offices in 19 major cities in the United States and Puerto Rico. In 1974 it had 6500 employees and a budget of about $160 million.

Its responsibilities cover most foods marketed in interstate commerce except meat, poultry, and processed eggs. These responsibilities include inspection of plants where foods are made or stored to assure safety of the products, approval of new food additives before they are used, setting standards for consumer products made under a standard of identity (specified ingredients) and developing regulations for nutrition labeling. (6)

The FDA works in two ways to prevent violations of the food laws (5), by educating and informing the food companies how to conform with the laws, and by seeking court action when the companies fail to adhere to the laws. When the FDA determines that a product in violation of the laws has crossed state lines, the product can be seized so that it will not get onto the market. The seized product may be relabeled, reconditioned, given to charity, or destroyed. Sometimes criminal charges are brought against the person or firm responsible for the violation, or a restraining order or injunction may be used to keep the unsafe product out of interstate shipment. The current concern about nutrient content and food additives makes the activities of this agency a frequent subject for controversy.

The Health Resources Administration is responsible for three units of importance to community nutrition. The Bureau of Health Manpower is responsible for programs on development and use of health personnel. The National Center for Health Statistics collects and analyzes statistics that reflect the health status, needs, and resources. The Bureau of Health Planning and Resources Development is responsible for development, administration, and financing of national, state, and area health planning and delivery systems under P.L. 93-641. (36)

PL 93-641, The National Health Planning and Resources Development Act of 1974 (18) was enacted into law on January 4, 1975. It establishes the structure for a nation-wide system of health planning. Title XV, the first part of the Act, establishes in the DHEW the National Council on Health Planning and Development to advise the Secretary of DHEW about national guidelines, implementation of the Act, and a new health delivery system. (Section 1503) It provides for the division of the country into *health service areas,* which are geographic areas with populations of 500,000 to 3 million, with exceptions for areas that are sparsely or heavily populated. (Section 1511)

Each health service area must have a special governing body called a *health systems agency* (HSA). (Section 1512) The HSA prepares the establishing plan and an annual implementation plan. The governing body must have at least 10 members, but not more than 30. A majority of the members are to be *consumers* of health care, broadly representing the various segments of the population. The rest of the members represent *providers* of health care (physicians, dentists, nurses, other health professionals, hospitals, health maintenance organizations, health insurers, health professional schools, and allied health professionals).

The HSA is required to have from 5 to 25 staff members providing expertise in administration, data collection and analysis, health planning, and development and use of health resources.

The functions of the HSA are to improve the health of residents, to increase accessibility, acceptability, and quality of health services, to control increases in costs, and to prevent duplication of services. (Section 1513) The HSA receives a yearly grant to meet the costs of carrying out its planning responsibilities, but is not permitted to use the money for health services or resources. (Section 1516)

The act also provides for a grant to each state for a State Health Planning and Development Agency to implement the state health planning and development function. (Section 1521) This function is to conduct state health planning activities, and to make a state health plan composed of the plans of all HSAs within the state. Another function is to determine need for proposed new health facilities and approve or disapprove the requests. There is also provision for a Statewide Health Coordinating Council of at least 16 representatives appointed by the governor and representatives from each HSA. (Section 1524)

Title XVI, the second part of the Act, provides for development of health resources by modernizing existing medical facilities, building new outpatient facilities, building new inpatient facilities, and remodeling existing facilities so they can provide new services (Section 1601).

The *Health Services Administration* provides professional leadership in delivery of health services. Through its Bureau of Community Health Services, it initiates and supports new ways to provide health services to specific groups, especially mothers and children and migrant workers and their families. It has a Health Maintenance Organization program that promotes development of prepaid health care systems. Starting July 1, 1974, the Bureau required each state to have programs for maternity and infant care, family planning, children's dental care, and comprehensive health services for preschool and school age children. (24)

Another function of the Health Services Administration, through its

Bureau of Quality Assurance, is to provide leadership for recognized standards of care in federal medical programs, including Medicare and Medicaid. The Indian Health Service provides comprehensive health services with a variety of nutrition programs for American Indians and Alaska natives.

The *National Institutes of Health* (NIH) works through 11 Institutes to improve the health of Americans, primarily by research, training and communication of biomedical information. Some Institutes that have special interest for the community nutritionist are Heart and Lung, Arthritis, Metabolism and Digestive Disease, Child Health and Human Development, and Aging.

The NIH has established the NIH-Nutrition Coordinating Committee for coordination of all NIH nutrition activities, including the development of a nutrition plan for NIH and the exchange of information among the Institutes of NIH and PHS agencies concerned with nutrition. (22)

The *President's Council on Physical Fitness and Sports* was established in 1970 by executive order to develop and coordinate a national program for physical fitness and sports. (32) It established the President's Fitness Program, a special program for men and women over 18, and urged that schools de-emphasize competitive athletics in favor of individual and noncompetitive forms of exercise that can be continued throughout life. It established Presidential Sports Awards in 38 sports activities in recognition of regular exercise that meets specific standards in various activities. The awards are for regular participation in and completion of specific programs for the various sports rather than for excellence of performance.

Office of Human Development.   This agency and its branches are concerned with groups of Americans identified as having special needs, namely, children, youth, the aged, handicapped persons, American Indians, Alaska natives and persons in rural areas. The purpose of the Office is to be sure that overall planning for the Department gives special attention to the needs of these disadvantaged groups. The Nutrition Program for the Elderly and Head Start are under this agency. (27)

Social and Rehabilitation Service. (SRS) This agency administers federal programs that provide financial and technical assistance to states to help them in turn to provide medical care for the needy. The *Medicaid* or Medical Assistance Program, administered by the state, provides funds for medical care for low income persons of all ages. Information about the Medicaid program in a specific state can be obtained from the state welfare department. Eligibility is determined by the state, so it differs in the various states. Expenditures for Medicaid for FY1975 were $13 billion (16).

Persons who receive federal assistance under programs for the aged, blind, disabled, or dependent children are eligible for Medicaid, along with some persons not eligible for those other programs because of unmet requirements as to age or residence. A state may also provide help for the "medically needy," that is, persons who can meet their other needs, but need help with medical expenses. One of the current problems about Medicaid is that under the present regulations it does not provide for ambulatory care in comprehensive health centers (CMC) or comprehensive mental health centers (CMHC). Thus, care in some of the most accessible locations is not covered.

SRS is also responsible for Aid to Families with Dependent Children (AFDC), the program that provides financial and other help for families with inadequate incomes. Most of these families are composed of mothers and children. In February, 1976, SRS paid benefits of almost $813 million to over 11 million persons in more than 3½ million families. (40)

Social Security Administration. (SSA) This agency administers the national Social Security program of social insurance through which covered employees contribute a portion of their earnings along with employer contributions, and monthly cash benefits are paid on retirement, disability, or death. *Medicare,* the federal government's health insurance system for persons over 65, is financed by part of the contributions and is administered as part of the Social Security program. (29)

Hospital insurance, the first part of Medicare, helps pay bills for hospital, nursing home, and home health care. The second part of Medicare is medical insurance, which helps pay for doctor's services, other services, and supplies. The individual pays a part of the costs of both programs.

The Medicare legislation covers only care that is "reasonable and necessary" and controls have been developed to prevent excess use of services. The decision as to what hospital care is reasonable and necessary is made in the hospital by a Utilization Review Committee. A Professional Standards Review Organization (PSRO) composed of physicians may review the care prescribed by other physicians.

Medicare payments are handled under government contracts by private insurance organizations known as *intermediaries* (for hospital care) and *carriers* (for medical insurance). The patient pays a certain fixed amount of the bills and Medicare pays other covered services for a 60-day period.

Expenditures of the Federal Government for Medicare for FY 1975 were $15 billion, mostly for hospital care and physician's services. Persons who cannot make the required payments are sometimes eligible for help from Medicaid. (16)

Federal Trade Commission

This independent administrative agency of the federal government operates under the public policy of support for the free enterprise system, preventing monopoly, trade restraints, and unfair and deceptive trade practices. (30) The main functions that are of immediate concern to the nutritionist are its control over advertisements and labeling of foods, drugs, and other household items, and its responsibility for matters pertaining to consumer credit such as credit cards and credit ratings, including the Truth in Lending Act. The Act applies to all credit, but has been especially important to low-income people, helping them avoid uninformed and excessive uses of credit. On loans, it requires expression of credit costs in terms of dollars and the annual percentage rate on the unpaid balance, providing a definitive way to compare costs from different sources.

Federal Information Center (FIC) Program

This branch of the General Services Administration operates 37 Centers in major metropolitan areas and has toll-free telephone connections to 37 other cities. The purpose of these Centers is to help a citizen find out what federal office can answer a question or solve a problem related to federal services or programs. These Centers can also answer some questions about state and local governments. Individuals may write, telephone, or visit the Centers, which also have helpful government publications available. (31)

Quasi-Governmental Agencies

Two *quasi-governmental agencies* (33) with which community nutritionists should be acquainted are *The American National Red Cross* and *The National Research Council.* These agencies have special charters from the federal government, perform officially delegated governmental functions, and receive funds and other support from federal agencies as well as funds from various private sources.

American National Red Cross (ARC).   While often classed as a voluntary organization, ARC operates under a special federal charter with responsibility for voluntary relief and communication between the American people and the armed forces, and for national and international disaster relief. Its activities are directed by a national Board of Governors with 50 members, 30 elected by the local chapters, 12 elected by the Board as members-at-large, and 8 appointed by the President of the United States, as is the Chairman of the Board. (35)

Red Cross encompasses four broad geographic areas, Eastern, Midwestern, Southeastern, and Western, each with a manager who directs the area activities. (1) For administrative and service purposes, there are divisions within the areas, each responsible for providing leadership and assistance to the chapters in a specific geographic area. In the early 1970's, there were 3300 chapters with about 1.7 million volunteers and 7 million students in school programs. Funds for agency activities are raised by an independent campaign with 35 to 40 million contributors.

Red Cross conducts relief operations in major disasters such as hurricanes, tornadoes and floods, and in many smaller local emergencies such as fires in homes and apartments. In addition, local chapters may carry on various programs that are broadly designed for the promotion of health and the prevention of disasters; these programs are developed according to community needs and chapter resources.

Two activities under the Supportive Volunteer Services are of particular significance to community nutritionists: preparation and service of food in quantity and under emergency conditions, and provision of public education and advisory assistance in food and nutrition. (1) One chapter organized a committee of nutritionists who train volunteer teachers (home economists and dietitians) to teach nutrition to interested groups of the public. There is also a course called "Fitness for the Future" designed to help individuals maintain health throughout life. There are many other activities that may include nutrition and diet, such as "Mother and Baby Care" and "Preparation for Parenthood." Other well-known services of the Red Cross are its blood bank and safety programs.

National Research Council (NRC). The NRC is one branch of the National Academy of Sciences. (34) The Academy was established by special charter from the U.S. Congress, signed by President Lincoln in 1863, its purpose being to serve upon request and without fee as an official adviser to the federal government on any question of science or technology, investigating, experimenting, and reporting. The Academy is responsible for all work done by the NRC. The expenses are paid from appropriations for specific purposes, usually through government contracts.

The NRC organizes broad attacks on various scientific problems of national importance by bringing eminent scientists together to exchange information and devise ways to deal with problems. NRC has no laboratories of its own but stimulates and supports work that deals with the problems with which it is concerned. It receives other funds from industry, foundations, scientific societies, and individuals. NRC has about 500 committees, boards and panels with members mainly from the academic world.

The branch of NRC best known to nutritionists is the Food and Nutrition Board, which was organized in 1940 at the request of the federal government for the purpose of advising about nutrition needs. (7) One of its first tasks was to prepare the initial plan for the Recommended Dietary Allowances (RDA) which was issued in mimeographed form in 1941. (11) Revision of the RDA is now carried on by the Food and Nutrition Board, whose scope has expanded greatly in recent years. The Board now has 15 members eminent in the nutrition field. Its function is to evaluate the evidence and findings of nutritional science and their application to food processing and public health. A major objective of the Board is to promote development of good food use practices by the U.S. population for attainment of the best health. There are many other committees under the Board that work on other food and nutrition matters such as safety of foods, dietary standards, dental health, and international nutrition programs.

In 1975, 80 percent of its funds came from federal agency grants and contracts and 20 percent from uncommitted funds provided by industry grants.

STATE HEALTH AGENCIES

The community nutritionist needs to know the state agencies that are responsible for programs and services related to nutrition. Some of these responsibilities will be under the state health agency, some under other regular or special agencies. A recent addition at the state level is the State Health Planning and Development Agency. (p. 79).

Local nutritionists need to know who in the state structure is responsible for nutrition programs and their coordination, food inspection, health programs for the elderly, consumer information, and other significant programs. Acquaintance with the appropriate personnel and the lines of communication will facilitate the nutritionist's work.

There is much variety in the structure and function of state health agencies because of differing needs and demands. Some states are mainly rural, some urban, some have large numbers of migrant workers, while others have sizable colonies of recent immigrants of various ethnic groups. Also, there is great variation in per capita income and in the prevalence of disease. In some states, the traditional "health department" that concentrated on preventive health has given way to a combination of health with welfare or with agencies mainly concerned with care of the sick.

The traditional programs of public health concerned with prevention were communicable disease, maternal and child health, laboratories, and environmental health. Alcohol and drug programs are some of the more recent additions. Some of the traditional programs of disease prevention and health promotion have given way to programs of treatment and rehabilitation with emphasis on community-wide planning for complete health care in the neighborhood health center backed up by hospital acute care services.

The state agency is generally concerned with policy, planning, legislation, standard-setting, consultation, financial support, organizational relationships, and research and evaluation.

It may arrange or provide resources for its local agencies, such as training or funds for training. It enforces the state laws and regulations, sometimes delegating this responsibility to a local agency. It may provide overall direction for programs and services conducted by local units in its jurisdiction and coordinate their programs.

The duties of the staff may include ongoing surveillance and evaluation, analyzing needs, preparing or locating teaching tools and resource materials, providing consultation to institutions, and enforcement of the regulations, as well as providing inservice education for professionals in schools and community, and cooperating in research and activity planning. The structure of the health agency varies greatly in different states and the nutrition unit may be in various administrative units of the agency.

Most states have public health nutrition directors, who have an organization called the Association of State and Territorial Public Health Nutrition Directors. (4)

The ASTPHND has a membership of 55 members, limited to such directors. It was founded in 1953 and is an affiliate of the Association of State and Territorial Health Officers (ASTHO). Its functions include making recommendations to the ASTHO on matters of legislation and public policy, facilitating communication among the members, and serving as an official body to work with related professional groups on mutual interests.

Nichaman and Collins have reviewed the activities of state public health nutrition programs. (14) They give a total of 173 nutritionists in identifiable state and local units (May, 1973) and discuss their programs and sources of funds. They name four major program areas as the foundation for programs within a state. These are (1) establishing a nutrition surveillance system, (2) setting nutritional standards, (3) providing nutritional consultation, and (4) conducting applied nutrition research. The surveillance program includes a continuous or periodic collection of data to assess the nutritional status of the population, which can be used to identify the needs of a specific area. Nichaman and Collins point out the advantages of first utilizing data that may already be collected by epidemiology, vital statistics, or maternal and child health programs, and they further note that these data may be the source of valuable facts about nutritional status that are not currently being used. These data may include height, weight, hemoglobin and other parameters. The authors emphasize the need for ongoing surveillance that can be used as a before-and-after evaluation survey as compared with a survey that describes only a one-time situation.

Nutritional standards or guidelines are needed for various programs, institutions, personnel, nutrition education, and evaluation, and the authors emphasize the need to develop standards for new programs. Nutrition consultation is an appropriate responsibility of the state nutritionists to other state agencies and to the state legislature about nutrition needs in the state, as well as to personnel in the local agencies. Applied nutrition research should be directed to the development of successful model programs that can be established at the local level. The authors also emphasize the need for a constant program review and reconsideration of priorities, and the discontinuation of outmoded approaches.

Community nutritionists in both public and private organizations need to be informed about the state health programs; they should support a strong state program that can provide leadership and information helpful in conducting meaningful local programs. Several nutrition developments in state agencies have been described in recent literature. In Massachusetts a State Board of Nutrition was established in 1974, largely due to a five-year effort of the Massachusetts Dietetic Association. (2)

In 1969, Louisiana designated severe undernutrition as a reportable disease that must be followed by an epidemiologic investigation. A number of states have also established statewide nutritional surveillance systems with assistance of the Center for Disease Control (9)

Recent reorganization and changes in programs in some agencies have resulted from the pressure on health agencies to adjust to the changing needs and demands of health consumers. This kind of adjustment is necessary to keep programs in step with the changing times.

LOCAL HEALTH AGENCIES

The community nutritionist should know the local agencies responsible for decisions about health-related programs that affect nutritional care.

These include county and city official health agencies and the newly developed health systems agency (HSA). (p. 79)

Official health agencies are established at the county and city level to assume responsibility for the health of the population within the jurisdiction served. The authority for establishing a county agency is delegated to the county by the state. In some states there is a county board of health responsible to county supervisors or commissioners; in others the director of the health agency is directly responsible to the county government.

The relationship between the state health agency and its counties also varies. In some states the county agencies are operated as subdivisions of the state agency; in others they operate as autonomous agencies, receiving funds from the state, conducting programs that meet state policies and standards, and seeking consultation and other services when needed.

Generally a city may establish its own health agency rather than be a part of the county unit so long as it conforms to the policies established by the state. It may then provide more or fewer services than other units and control its own tax rate for this purpose. The usual reason for a combination of county and city agencies is to avoid duplication of services; the usual reasons given for a city's withdrawal from the county agency are to save money and provide only the services needed. Often the actual reason is to relieve a smaller city of the burden of taxation to support the poverty areas of an adjacent large city.

The main activities of a local health department have a direct effect on the health of every individual and family residing within the jurisdiction. Though the services vary in each agency, there are certain ones that are usually provided. They include preventing and controlling preventable diseases; controlling tuberculosis, venereal disease, and other communicable diseases; preventing chronic disease and helping to rehabilitate its victims; safeguarding the health of mothers and children; maintaining the cleanliness and safety of water, milk, and food; controlling rats, insects and other vectors of disease; monitoring the health of employees in industry and the quality of care in hospitals and extended care facilities; keeping records of births, deaths and disease; and conducting other programs that affect the health and well-being of the citizens.

Since everybody eats, nutrition should be a component of all disease prevention and the care of every individual; when viewed as such, nutrition makes a direct contribution to the health and well-being of all. Community nutritionists in other agencies and also dietitians can be of great influence in establishing and supporting a strong nutrition program in the local health agency.

In recent years, many cities have opened neighborhood health centers (also called family health centers and ambulatory care clinics) in poverty areas to bring primary health care closer to the people. These centers are usually funded with federal moneys. This trend and the increase in overall health planning for all health needs in the community will produce further changes as implementation is accomplished.

Nutrition programs in local health agencies vary according to agency policies and the source of funding. Some local positions have been entirely funded from specific sources, especially maternal and child health or chronic disease funds. Usually in a specially funded program, the emphasis and type of activities that may be conducted are limited to a specific group such as the chronically ill or low income children of a certain age. The funding processes are in a period of change and the nutritionist needs to keep informed about sources for funding of specific programs. When a nutrition program is funded as a part of the local government, the content is sometimes determined by the impact nutrition has made on the members of the governmental body or administration. Often there are conflicting pressures from professional nutritionists, consumer groups, commercial interests, and other sources.

In some agencies, nutrition programs emphasize education for professionals in the agency and community, activities for the public and the community leaders, and community cooperative programs. In some agencies, the emphasis is on patient service, usually individual or small group counseling; in others little or no direct service is provided.

The community nutritionist needs to know about other programs in the same governmental structure that are related to nutrition; for example, a county or city government may have an office dealing with consumer affairs that takes action on food quackery, or a sanitation unit that issues advice about cooking and storage of food, and the public welfare agency may have homemaker or other programs with a food and nutrition component.

SUMMARY

The official health agencies of federal, state, and local governments constitute a complex network that is responsible for the health of United States citizens. Numerous laws that affect health and nutrition are enacted each year. The community nutritionist needs to know the laws that apply to the specific areas of the nutritionist's work.

Most nutrition programs of the federal government are under the Department of Agriculture or the Department of Health, Education, and Welfare. A brief description has been given of each agency that has nutrition programs or other programs about which the nutritionist should be informed.

National health planning, authorized under PL 93-641, is under way as a structure for a nation-wide health plan. The annual Forward Plan for Health contains the recommendations and guidelines of the Secretary of Health, Education, and Welfare as required by PL 93-641. Medicaid is the federal program of medical care for low income persons of all ages, and Medicare, a part of Social Security, is the health insurance program for persons over age 65.

Two quasi-governmental agencies, the American National Red Cross and the National Research Council carry out specific responsibilities assigned under their special federal charters.

REFERENCES CITED

1. American National Red Cross, Red Cross Service Programs, Rev. 1965, pamphlet, Washington DC, 13.
2. Board of Nutrition Established in Massachusetts, *J. Am. Diet. Assoc.* 66 3/75 241.
3. Center for Disease Control. U.S. Dept. of Health, Education and Welfare, Personal Communication from Gordon Robbins, Aug. 1976.
4. *Encyclopedia of Associations* 9th ed., Vol. I, *National Organizations of the U.S.,* Gale Research Co., Detroit. 1975, 740.
5. Food and Drug Administration, FDA Consumer Memo, leaflet, DHEW Pub. No. (FDA) 74-1018, 3/74, U.S. Dept. of Health, Education, and Welfare, Rockville MD.
6. Food and Drug Administration, We Want You to Know About Today's FDA, leaflet, DHEW Pub. No. (FDA) 74-1021, 1974, U.S. Dept. of Health, Education and Welfare, Rockville MD.
7. *Food and Nutrition Board,* pamphlet, 1/76. National Academy of Sciences, Washington DC.
8. Fuchs, Victor R., *Who Shall Live? Health, Economics and Social Choice.* Basic Books, Inc., New York, 1974, 141.
9. Langham, Rose Ann, A State Health Department Assesses Undernutrition, *J. Am. Diet. Assoc.,* 65 7/74 18.
10. Miller, C. Arden, Issues of Health Policy: Local Government and the Public's Health, *Am. J. Pub. Health,* 65 12/75 1330.
11. Mitchell, Helen, Recommended Dietary Allowances Up To Date, *J. Am. Diet. Assoc.,* 64 2/74 149.
12. National Research Council, Food and Nutrition Board, *Recommended Dietary Allowances,* 8th ed., National Academy of Sciences, Washington DC, 1974.
13. National Research Council, Food and Nutrition Board, *Activities Report,* 1975, National Academy of Sciences.

14. Nichaman, Milton Z. and Gretchen Collins, Nutrition Programs in State Agencies, *Nutr. Rev.,* 32 3/74 65.
15. Pickett, George, Toward a National Health Policy—Values in Conflict, *Am. J. Pub. Health,* 65 12/75 1335.
16. Social Security Bulletin, 39 2/76 6.
17. This Is Cooperative Extension, leaflet, U.S. Dept. of Agriculture, 1/73.
18. U.S. Congress, The National Health Planning and Resources Development Act of 1974, Pl 93-641, Jan. 4, 1975.
19. U.S. Dept. of Health, Education, and Welfare, *Forward Plan For Health, 1977–81,* Washington DC, Aug. 1975.
20. U.S. Dept. of Health, Education, and Welfare, *Forward Plan For Health, 1978–82,* Washington DC, Aug. 1976.
21. Ibid., 70.
22. Ibid., 108.
23. U.S. Dept. of Health, Education, and Welfare, Programs of the Maternal and Child Health Service, pamphlet, DHEW Pub. No. (HSM) 72-5005, 1/72, Government Printing Office, Washington DC, 1.
24. U.S. Dept. of Health, Education, and Welfare, *Promoting Community Health,* DHEW Publication No. (HSA)·75-5016, 1975, Government Printing Office, Washington, DC.
25. U.S. General Services Administration, Office of the Federal Register, *United States Government Manual 1975–76,* Government Printing Office, Washington DC, 1975, 96–127.
26. Ibid., 221–54.
27. Ibid., 231.
28. Ibid., 235.
29. Ibid., 244.
30. Ibid., 498.
31. Ibid., 512.
32. Ibid., 644.
33. Ibid., 648.
34. Ibid., 649.
35. Ibid., 651.
36. U.S. General Services Administration, Office of the Federal Register, *United States Government Manual, 1976–77,* Government Printing Office, Washington, DC, 1976, 296.
37. U.S. Office of Management and Budget, *1976 Catalog of Federal Domestic Assistance,* Government Printing Office, Washington DC, 38.
38. U.S. Office of Management and Budget, *1977 Catalog of Federal Domestic Assistance,* Government Printing Office, Washington DC, 178.
39. Ibid., 296.
40. *World Almanac, 1977,* Newspaper Enterprise Association, Inc., New York, 1976, 239.
41. *Your Medicare Handbook,* DHEW Pub. No. (SSA), 75-10050, U.S. Dept. of Health, Education and Welfare, Washington DC, March 1975.

CHAPTER 7

FEDERAL NUTRITION PROGRAMS

The National School Lunch Program was established in 1946, and some food distribution programs were started even earlier. Many of the present programs have arisen more recently, some developing from the poverty programs of the 1960's, which arose in a period of great social unrest.

A U.S. Senate Subcommittee on Employment, Manpower, and Poverty started an investigation on the problems of hunger in April 1967, making observations during visits to Mississippi and other areas. In April 1968, dramatic attention was focused on the problem by a television feature program "Hunger in America". (1) A month later, *Hunger, USA,* the report of a Citizen's Board of Inquiry into hunger and malnutrition in the United States, was published. (7) These presentations were based on observations, reports, and opinions rather than on objective studies since at that time there was little information on the extent of hunger and malnutrition in this country. They served the useful purpose of drawing attention to hunger and malnutrition as a national problem.

This was followed by the appointment of a Senate Select Committee on Nutrition and Human Needs in 1968 and the White House Conference on Food, Nutrition and Health in December 1969. The Select Committee hearings of 1968–69 attempted to evaluate the nation's programs in food, nutrition, education, health and welfare, especially as to delivery of services at state and local levels. Their purpose was to study the adequacies and shortcomings of these programs in order to find ways to meet the nutrition and other basic needs of Americans. Some of the topics addressed were (1) whether lack of nutrition education, health services, and adequate sanitation contribute to malnutrition and hunger, (2) the relationship between farm policy, food distribution programs, and nutrition needs, and (3) whether it is possible to supply a nutritionally adequate diet to people with limited funds through the private sector at a price yielding a fair return to the food producer and distributor. (15) The reports of these hearings constitute an extensive reference library on many nutrition topics and programs since they include much subject matter along with reports of local programs nutritionists can use in program planning and preparation. (15,16)

WHITE HOUSE CONFERENCE ON FOOD, NUTRITION, AND HEALTH

This Conference, held in December 1969, was called by the President to advise on the elimination of hunger and malnutrition due to poverty. Almost 3000 delegates participated in the Conference while 2000 other persons attended the plenary sessions. The delegates included many poor persons and consumer advocates along with nutritionists, government officials, executives of food companies, representatives of social organizations, and others. This was one of the first times that the poor participated in a national meeting of great import.

The various panels considered the social and political issues as well as the problems of food and nutrition, delineated the relationship between these two broad areas, and made about 450 recommendations on food assistance for the poor, nutrition and health programs, regulation of food production and supply, nutrition education, and other pertinent topics.

Some of the specific recommendations were:

1. Establishment of a nutrition surveillance system under the USDHEW for monitoring the effectiveness of nutrition programs.
2. Improvement of health services for all people, including the means for adequate food and nutrition education.
3. Provision of services as well as food for older persons.
4. Innovative uses of the media for nutrition education.
5. More adequate food programs including free food stamps and free school lunch or a system of cash supplementation to maintain all incomes at a specified level.

Measures taken by the federal government in response to the recommendations of the White House Conference included revision and extension of the food stamp program, replacement of most of the commodity programs by food stamps, expansion of the school lunch program with better provision for free and part-pay lunches, improvements in food labeling including a new labeling law, and enactment of measures for greater food safety. However, attempts to reach some long-term goals such as the production of more healthful foods, institution of effective nutrition education on a wide scale, and development of a national nutrition policy have made limited progress, as has the resolution of the problem of hunger due to poverty.

CURRENT NUTRITION PROGRAMS

The federal government conducts or sponsors many food and nutrition programs, delegating the responsibility to a state or other agency or providing funds to the state for use in carrying out programs that meet standards for eligibility, operation, matching funds, and so forth.

School Lunch and Child Nutrition

The *National School Lunch Program* was established by the National School Lunch Act of 1946, which has had several major amendments. (20,33) One in 1970 was designed to assure a free lunch to every child from a low income home, and one in 1976 established guidelines for determining eligibility for free and reduced price lunches. (2,10)

The Program, which is administered by the USDA Food and Nutrition Service, is designed to improve the nutrition of children, especially those from low income families, and to increase the use of foods that are in surplus production.

The Program provides cash grants and food donations to public and nonprofit private school lunch programs. The money is used to reimburse schools on the basis of the number of meals served, with additional funds provided for free and reduced-price meals for needy children. The reimbursement rate is revised periodically according to changes in cost. The amount of funds depends on several factors, and matching state funds are required for some of the federal money.

To qualify for participation, a school must serve a Type A lunch, which contains specific kinds and amounts of food providing about one-third of the Recommended Dietary Allowances for each child. The food requirements are (1) one-half pint of milk served as a beverage, (2) two ounces of cooked lean meat or the equivalent, (3) and (4) At least ¾ cup of fruits and vegetables, and (5) one slice of whole-grain or enriched bread or the equivalent in other breadstuff. In addition, two teaspoons of butter or fortified margarine must be available. These amounts are considered to be appropriate for a child age 10 to 12; smaller amounts may be served for younger children and larger amounts for children over 12.

The current trend is to modify the Type A lunch pattern to permit the use of new types and other forms of food and different methods of service. One of the most significant changes is permitting the use of lowfat or nonfat milk instead of whole milk. (10) This conforms to the wish of some parents and recommendations of some physicians for reduced use of saturated fats.

There is general agreement among nutrition educators that more nutrition education is needed in the School Lunch Program; however, there is divided opinion as to whether the entire meal should be served to each child or whether foods not desired by the child may be omitted on request. In 1976 the regulations were amended so that high school children need accept only three of the five foods that make up the Type A pattern.

More than 4 billion lunches were served in 1975 in 88,804 schools, with over 1.8 billion lunches free or at a reduced price. The total expenditures for 1975 exceeded $3.8 billion. (16)

The *Special Breakfast, Special Milk* and *Nonfood Assistance Programs,* authorized under the Child Nutrition Act of 1966, are also administered by the USDA Food and Nutrition Service, as are the *Summer Food Service* and *Child Care Food Programs,* which are, however, authorized under the School Lunch Act. (20,32)

The *School Breakfast Program* provides cash and donated foods to help public and private schools establish nonprofit nutritious breakfast programs. Preference is given to schools in low income areas, and to schools where many children have problems such as getting an appropriate breakfast, traveling long distances to schools, or having working mothers. All children may participate; those who can pay are expected to do so, while free or reduced-price meals are provided for those who lack enough money to pay. In fiscal year 1975, 294 million breakfasts were served in 14,293 schools. The estimate for 1976 is 354 million breakfasts. (31)

The *Special Milk Program* pays part of the cost of extra milk for needy children in schools and day care centers. All public and nonprofit private schools and other nonprofit child care institutions are eligible. In fiscal year 1975, 2.2 billion half-pints of milk were served under the Program. (31)

The *Nonfood Service Assistance for School Food Programs* provides cash grants to help schools in low income areas obtain equipment for preparation and serving of the lunch. (32)

The *Summer Food Service Programs for Children* provide meals similar to school lunches for children during the summer at public and nonprofit private institutions that operate organized recreational programs for children from low income areas. Meals must meet minimum nutritional standards and must be supplied free or at reduced cost to needy children. The estimate of participation for fiscal year 1976 is 3 million children. (31)

The *Child Care Food Program* supports public and nonprofit food service programs for children receiving child care in institutions such as day care centers, recreation centers, neighborhood houses, and day care services for handicapped children. Breakfast, snacks, lunch, and supper may be served with reimbursement based on the number of meals of each kind. The meals must meet certain criteria established by the Department of Agriculture. The estimated participation for fiscal year 1976 is 490,000. (31)

Special Supplemental Food Program for Women, Infants, and Children (WIC)

WIC was authorized by an amendment to the Child Nutrition Act of 1966, first for 1972–73, and extended by later amendments through 1978. (11, 40) The Program, administered by the USDA Food and Nutrition Service, provides federal grants-in-aid to state and local governments to provide nutritious foods for pregnant women and for six months postpartum, for women who are breast-feeding until the infant is 1 year old, and for infants and children until the fifth birthday.

The foods included are those that supply nutrients believed most likely to be low in the diets of the recipients, that is, protein, iron, and vitamin C. The foods for infants include iron-fortified formula or whole milk or other specified alternatives; iron-fortified infant cereal; and fruit juice fortified with vitamin C. The foods for older children and women are the following: whole milk, or specified alternates, including cheese; fruit juice fortified with vitamin C; and fresh or dried eggs.

The food may be provided by means of food vouchers and direct distribution or by other methods selected by the state. The cost of nutrition education to help recipients make good use of the foods may be met as a part of the administrative expenses. One of the objectives of the Program is to make a medical evaluation of the benefits of the food distribution.

Public or nonprofit health agencies may operate the program provided they give free or reduced-cost health services to residents of low income areas, have the personnel, expertise and equipment to perform the specified tests and measurements, and can maintain adequate records.

The state must designate areas that are most in need of extra food, determine eligibility of agencies, establish standards, and monitor programs. Applicants must live in low income areas, be eligible for free or reduced-cost medical care, and be at nutritional risk because of inadequate nutritional pattern, anemia, underweight, obesity, or other conditions specified in the Act.

Risk must be evaluated by an agency staff member by criteria that include a medical examination. Minimal data include height, weight, and head circumference (for infants), and hemoglobin or hematocrit, if equipment is available. Information about food intake from a history and 24-hour recall may be used, but should be accompanied by other data. A nutritionist, dietitian, physician, or nurse may evaluate nutritional risk and prescribe the food package. Certification must include evidence of medical, economic, and residential eligibility for the program.

Nutrition education services must be provided to all women in the program and to parents or guardians of children. The legislation specifies that minimum nutrition education must explain the nutrients needed and how to provide them with food as well as information on how to use the WIC foods.

It is required that the state agency that administers the program employ at least one trained nutritionist or dietitian. (40)

In the initial phases of the program, 52 state agencies were approved for operation of the program in 48 states, 2 Indian agencies, Puerto Rico, and the Virgin Islands. During fiscal year 1975, the peak caseload was 497,000. (34)

Food Distribution and Food Stamps

The *Food Distribution* (Food Donation) *Program* is administered by the USDA Food and Nutrition Service. (29) It distributes food directly to needy individuals, families, schools, summer camps, nutrition programs for the elderly, and charitable institutions that serve the needy. The programs are designed to improve the diets of the participants and to increase the market for foods included in surplus removal or price support programs. Eligibility for the Program is determined by designated state, federal, or other agencies. Distribution programs have operated since the 1930's, covering both families and group food service facilities, but the family program has been largely replaced by the Food Stamp Program. The only families who now receive donated foods live in a city, county, or Indian reservation that already has the Program. During fiscal year 1975, 763.8 million pounds of food were distributed. The food is provided free but some agencies pay part or all of the distribution costs.

The present *Food Stamp Program* was authorized under the Food Stamp Act of 1964 although there had been other stamp programs before that time. (17, 18) It is the major form of food assistance in the United States and has been established in all counties of all states. The objective of the Program is to increase the purchasing power of low income persons so that they can buy more food in a greater variety. Families and single persons who meet the nationwide eligibility standards can buy stamps that are worth more than the purchase price; the very poor receive their stamps free. The stamps are used at a participating market to buy food, or to buy seeds or plants for producing food. Alaskan natives may also use stamps to purchase hunting and fishing equipment.

Stamps cannot be used to buy nonfood items such as pet food, soap, cigarettes, alcoholic beverages, or paper goods.

Elderly persons can use the stamps to pay for meals served by authorized establishments, or if not able to prepare their own meals, can use the stamps to purchase home-delivered meals. Drug addicts and alcoholics in rehabilitation programs may use food stamps to buy meals prepared by authorized nonprofit organizations.

Eligibility of individuals and families is determined according to nationwide standards based on income, resources, and registration of family members for work. The amount paid for stamps is limited to 30 percent of the net income of the household. Most food markets participate in the Program.

State and local welfare agencies administer the Program, determining eligibility, figuring the amount of stamps according to family size and income, and issuing the stamp books. Plans for the Program include education in food planning, buying, and storage and preparation, conducted by Federal-State agencies with help from other groups and individuals. (17)

Volunteers and other community resources help explain the benefits of the Program to prospective participants and help with transportation, interpretation, and other problems.

The coupon allotment or amount of stamps for a family is based on the cost of the "Thrifty Food Plan" (Figure 7.1) published by the Department in November 1975. (21) The Act requires that the amount of stamps be adjusted twice a year to conform to changes in food prices.

Family Member	Milk, Cheese, Ice Cream²	Meat, Poultry, Fish¹	Eggs	Dry Beans and Peas, Nuts⁴	Dark-Green, Deep-Yellow Vegetables	Citrus Fruit, Tomatoes	Potatoes	Other Vegetables, Fruit	Cereal	Flour	Bread	Other Bakery Products	Fats, Oils	Sugar, Sweets	Accessories⁵
	Qt	Lb	No.	Lb	Lb	Lb	Lb	Lb	Lb	Lb	Lb	Lb	Lb	Lb	Lb
Child:															
7 months to 1 year	4.95	.39	1.2	.15	.41	.55	.09	2.49	1.02⁶	.02	.08	.04	.04	.19	.05
1–2 years	3.30	.83	3.3	.17	.22	.89	.65	2.26	1.02⁶	.31	.78	.24	.11	.30	.37
3–5 years	3.54	.95	2.5	.28	.20	.92	.88	2.28	1.03	.37	.94	.53	.38	.74	.59
6–8 years	4.22	1.27	2.4	.49	.22	1.10	1.23	2.50	1.12	.62	1.42	.79	.51	.94	.84
9–11 years	4.92	1.61	3.4	.53	.28	1.52	1.48	3.38	1.34	.81	1.82	1.10	.60	1.20	1.10
Male:															
12–14 years	5.18	1.79	3.6	.67	.33	1.45	1.59	3.30	1.22	.81	2.07	1.13	.77	1.21	1.45
15–19 years	5.08	2.35	4.0	.43	.32	1.70	2.10	3.43	.98	.99	2.36	1.46	1.00	1.05	1.73
20–54 years	2.57	3.03	4.0	.44	.39	1.80	2.02	3.69	.89	.92	2.29	1.33	.95	.86	1.24
55 years and over	2.37	2.45	4.0	.25	.51	1.85	1.75	3.77	1.09	.80	1.90	1.12	.79	.94	.73
Female:															
12–19 years	5.35	1.80	3.8	.28	.42	1.74	1.22	3.61	.72	.76	1.49	.84	.51	.74	1.36
20–54 years	2.81	2.41	4.0	.27	.52	1.86	1.51	3.39	.90	.67	1.41	.67	.57	.57	1.18
55 years and over	2.85	1.84	4.0	.19	.60	2.02	1.26	3.73	1.12	.68	1.30	.58	.37	.45	.66
Pregnant	5.25⁷	2.69	4.0	.42	.56	2.17	1.89	4.03	1.13	.58	1.41	.66	.59	.58	1.48
Nursing	5.25⁷	3.00	4.0	.38	.57	2.36	1.92	4.27	.98	.63	1.56	.82	.80	.75	1.54

Figure 7.1 USDA Thrifty Food Plan: Amounts of Food for a Week.[1]

[1] Amounts are for food as purchased or brought into the kitchen from garden or farm to prepare *all* meals and snacks for the week. Amounts allow for a discard of about 5 percent of the *edible* food as plate waste, spoilage, etc.

[2] Fluid milk and beverage made from dry or evaporated milk. Cheese and ice cream may replace some milk. Count as equivalent to a quart of fluid milk: Natural or processed Cheddar-type cheese, 6 oz.; cottage cheese, 2½ lbs.; ice cream or ice milk, 1½ quarts; unflavored yoghurt, 4 cups.

[3] Bacon and salt pork should not exceed ⅓ pound for each 5 pounds of this group.

[4] Weight in terms of dry beans and peas, shelled nuts, and peanut butter. Count 1 pound of canned dry beans—pork and beans, kidney beans, etc.— as .33 pound.

[5] Includes coffee, tea, cocoa, soft drinks, punches, ades, leavenings, and seasonings.

[6] Cereal fortified with iron is recommended.

[7] For pregnant and nursing teenagers, 7 quarts is recommended.

Source: USDA, The Thrifty Food Plan, CFE (Adm.) 326, Sept. 1975.

The extent of the Program is shown by participation of over 19 million people in March 1975. They paid $267 million, receiving $420 million worth of free stamps. There were 234,000 authorized retail food stores and 4875 sites approved for purchase of meals. (30)

Expanded Food and Nutrition Education Program (EFNEP or ENEP)

Like other programs of the USDA Cooperative Extension Service, EFNEP is funded by grants to land-grant universities that assist counties in program development for the improvement of home and family life. (12, 19, 28, 38)

Established in 1968, EFNEP has had a far-reaching effect through teaching by nutrition aides who are trained and supervised by professional home economists. The purpose is to help economically and socially disadvantaged families to improve their food practices as a way to a more adequate diet.

Most of the aides work in their own communities on a one-to-one basis in homes, or with small groups, teaching low income families how to improve their diets. This may include meal planning, food selection and purchasing, and food preparation, as well as housekeeping problems such as storage and sanitation that interfere with food and nutrition management. (3) Information is provided about community resources and eligible families are encouraged to apply for food stamps or donated foods.

In June 1974, 8000 aides were working in over 1200 locations, supervised by 800 home economists. At the end of fiscal year 1975, there were 320,186 families in the program. (28) Program evaluation has shown an increase in the number of homemakers who serve one or more servings from each of the four food groups and also of those who provide the recommended servings from each group. That this program reaches the low income group it was designed to serve is shown by a 1969–71 study of family incomes, when 60 percent of the families had less than $3000 income and 90 percent less than $5000. It was also found that 65 percent were families from minority and ethnic groups with homemakers who had less than an eighth grade education. However, after participation in the program, even though there was improvement in the diet, many homemakers and some other family members still did not eat an adequate diet.

A related program of nutrition education for young people in city poverty areas employed 300 professionals and had the help of 44,000 volunteers. (14) This program is similar to 4-H programs for farm youth, conducted mainly through volunteer leaders working with groups of young people.

Early and Periodic Screening, Diagnosis and Treatment (EPSDT)

The EPSDT program was part of the Social Security Amendments of 1967 with the final regulations effective in 1972. It is administered by the USDHEW. The program requires each state to provide preventive medical care for all Medicaid beneficiaries under 21 years. The preventive care includes health screening during preschool period for early identification and correction of problems that may lead to later physical or mental disability, and periodic screening until age 21, for the purpose of reducing the number of handicapped persons. (25, 37)

The program pays the cost of the screening, which is conducted by existing health care resources such as child health clinics, Head Start, nursery schools, day care centers, or private physicians or clinics. The examination includes specific parameters; those of main significance to nutrition are height, weight, and hemoglobin or hematocrit. Though assessment of nutritional status is included at every age, the law specifies only evaluation for underweight, low stature, and overweight. No provision was made to evaluate the diet.

Some health agencies have arranged to take a food record and counsel the mother, but in others there is not enough personnel to do this. Nutritionists should work for a more adequate nutrition component so that nutrition screening and services are available in all areas. Though it is intended that the problems identified should be treated, there is no provision for followup to see that this is done, and, in some communities, resources for followup are limited or not available.

It has been estimated that at least 1.9 million children were screened from 1971 through 1974. The potential national cost saving in five years was estimated at $5.3 billion, and in 20 years at $34.5 billion, most of it from the potential lifetime earnings of the children saved by the program. Some states have specified objectives for the nutritional screening, for example, to identify children who exhibit or are in danger of developing growth retardation, dental caries, obesity, anemia, or other manifestations of malnutrition. (37)

Early reports from selected programs showed that 47 percent of the children were referred for further diagnosis and treatment, 24 percent for dental care, 10 percent for vision problems, and 3 percent for hearing problems. (9, 37)

Head Start

This program was established in 1965, created by the Congress under the Economic Opportunity Act of 1964. (6, 22) Continuation was authorized by the Community Services Act of 1974 and authority for appropriation of funds was extended through 1977. The program is administered by the USDHEW Office of Human Development. It provides nutritional, medical, dental, mental health, educational and social services, mainly for children from age 3 to school age but including some younger children.

The objective of Head Start is to help children from low income families achieve social competence by overcoming the handicap imposed by poverty. It is concerned with all aspects of child development and the approach requires the participation of parents and community. Ten percent of the enrollment opportunities must be offered to handicapped children. Programs may be part-time or full-time, and each program must be operated by a local governmental or nonprofit agency in a poverty area. It is the responsibility of the local program to find and use community services so it can provide the required services. Some community nutritionists have been able to participate in staff training and consultation, or in other ways.

Nutrition in Head Start has three major mandates: to provide food that meets nutritional needs in a safe, sanitary manner, to provide a physical and emotional environment conducive to development of good food habits, and to help staff and parents understand the contribution of nutrition to the child's total development.

Head Start programs are eligible for federal food programs, either the Child Care Food Service Program or the National School Lunch Program, providing they meet the requirements.

Head Start has one nutritionist at the national level and a few in the regional offices. Many local programs have staff nutritionists. New performance standards effected in 1975 require direction by a qualified full-time staff nutritionist or regular supervision by a qualified person. Qualifications may be (1) meeting membership requirements for the American Dietetic Association plus a year of experience in community nutrition, including services to preschool children, or (2) baccalaureate degree with a foods and nutrition major plus two years of experience as in (1). When the required supervision is on a part-time basis a minimum of eight hours of services per month per center is suggested. (22)

During fiscal year 1975, Head Start served 350,000 children. Since its beginning in 1965, it has served over 6 million children from the 50 states, Puerto Rico, the Virgin Islands, and the Pacific Trust Territories. It has improved the health, nutrition and quality of life and has provided other help to the children and their families. (35)

Maternal and Child Health Programs

Passage of the Social Security Act in 1935 included a commitment from the Federal government to help states improve health services for mothers and children. (5, 24) Since that time, the government has made grants to states for this purpose. These were formula grants made on the basis of population, income and other factors, with the requirement that the state provide some matching funds. (26)

In 1965, further amendments to the Social Security Act provided for grants for special projects for comprehensive health services for children and youth in low income areas.

Further changes in the law in 1967 put all child health activities under one authorization with formula grants to states for maternal and child health and crippled childrens services. In addition, grants were made for special projects for maternity and infant care, family planning, intensive infant care services, health services for children and youth, and dental services for children.

Important expansion of programs developed after enactment of PL 88-156, Maternal and Child Health and Mental Retardation Planning Amendments of 1963. This provided more grants to provide care for high risk mothers in low income areas. Before 1972, the projects were approved, funded, and monitored by the Federal government.

Starting in 1974, the Federal government delegated the responsibility for administration of programs of projects to the states. The programs are administered by the state maternal and child health program unit. The guidelines stress completeness and continuity of care and need for evaluation and monitoring. (24)

Since the inception of the program, the best-known projects have been those for maternity and infant care and children and youth. The major significance in these programs is the provision of comprehensive care, that is, attention to all factors that contribute to the provision of high quality care.

The *Maternity and Infant Care Projects* (M & I, MIC) are programs designed to help reduce the number of mentally retarded and physically handicapped children resulting from complications of pregnancy, and to reduce maternal and infant mortality by providing special care for high risk maternity patients and their infants from birth to one year. (4, 24, 26) The program is open to prospective mothers when there is high risk to their health or to that of their infants, accompanied by indications that there would be inadequate prenatal care because of low income or other reason beyond their control. High risk factors for the pregnant woman include anemia, malnutrition, hypertension, diabetes, age under 16 or over 36 years, history of premature birth, and other conditions. High risk factors for the infant include low birth weight, failure to thrive, metabolic abnormalities and other problems. (24)

M & I recommends that prenatal care should be provided by a multidisciplinary team of clinician, community worker, dentist, health educator, nurse, nutritionist, and social worker. Though the projects are sponsored by a variety of agencies—medical centers, health departments, university hospitals, and others—much of the care was given in neighborhood clinics, most of them in low income urban areas, all of them in areas that had a higher than average rate of infant mortality.

The nutrition services include evaluation of the diet of the pregnant woman, counseling, and other services as necessary to help the woman achieve a satisfactory nutritional status. This might include a diet history, individual or group nutrition education, referral for an emergency food order, interpretation of the value of food stamps, and advice about housekeeping, management, child care, or other problems that interfered with an adequate diet for mother and family. These services are provided by nutritionists, home economists and nutrition aides along with community workers, social workers, nurses, and other project personnel.

Services under these projects increased from 1964, the first year of the program, when the number of maternity admissions was about 57,000, to 1972 when there were 56 Projects, with about 141,000 maternal admissions and 48,000 high risk infants receiving services. In fiscal year 1974, it was estimated that 142,000 mothers and 48,000 infants benefitted from the programs. (34) One of the program objectives was to get the women under care during the first trimester, and that number increased from 14.5 percent in 1967 to almost 26 percent in 1973. (25)

Other evidence of the value of the Projects in the areas served by M & I was provided by a decrease in the infant mortality rate, indicating as association with these programs and perhaps a causal relationship. (8)

The *Children and Youth Projects* (C & Y) provide comprehensive health care for preschool and school children in low income areas. (4, 26) In 1972 there were 59 C & Y programs providing service to about 456,000 children, most of them in low income urban areas, whose medical care was limited because of low income or other reasons beyond family control. It was estimated that 550,000 children would receive services in 1974.

The comprehensive medical, dental, and mental health services include screening, diagnosis, treatment, correction of defects and after-care. It is required that care provided under the C & Y must be coordinated, with care provided by cooperative arrangements with other agencies serving the same area, such as M & I, schools, and social service agencies; for example, if adequate vision screening is provided at school, the C & Y might only assume responsibility for necessary care of occasional eye infections and followup. The C & Y program stresses prevention; the value was evident after several years, when it was found that the hospital admission rate had dropped among the Project children who had received preventive care.

Nutrition services are provided by the multidisciplinary Project staff, similar to the provision for the M & I Projects. The exact services vary with the project, but usually comprehensive nutrition care includes nutritional status assessment by physician and other staff, a dietary history with nutritional care plan and nutrition education based on the findings, referrals for help in obtaining foods, food stamps, supplements, and equipment. Personnel and specific programs are planned according to the needs of the people, with individual or group instruction as indicated by analysis of needs and resources. To minimize transportation problems, much of the care is provided in neighborhood health centers, with clinics arranged so that waiting time is minimal.

One of the related objectives is to find the best ways for paraprofessional workers to contribute to total health care, and the kind of training and supervision needed. (34) In the nutrition program, they are used to prepare visual materials, conduct food demonstrations and teach homemaking skills. Some of the Projects have developed innovative ways to provide services, for example, developing emergency food supplies to keep families from going hungry and organizing a teenage weight control group in conjunction with a summer camp.

Nutrition Program for the Elderly

This Program was established in 1972 by Public Law 92-258, an amendment to the Older Americans Act of 1965. It is administered under the Office of Human Development of the U.S. Department of Health, Education and Welfare. (23, 36) It makes grants to the states to provide nutritionally adequate, low cost meals with social and rehabilitative services for persons over 60. The purpose of the Nutrition

Program is to assist low income persons to improve factors that cause malnutrition and contribute to their social problems. These include poor cooking skills, limited mobility, apathy, and lack of incentive.

Federal grants are made to the states to pay up to 90 percent of the cost of individual programs which may be operated by public or private nonprofit agencies, organizations or institutions, political subdivisions, or Indian tribal organizations. Each program must have a council that includes elected representatives from the group, and professional representatives of various disciplines such as nutrition and social work, who help plan and conduct the operation. Each program must serve at least 100 meals per day for five days a week except in sparsely populated areas, where a smaller number may be served. It must also provide nutrition education, socialization, and recreation, as well as transportation for persons who would otherwise be unable to participate. Home-delivered meals can be provided for a few homebound persons. Food stamps may be used to pay for the home-delivered meals but not for the meals served in the congregate setting. There must be an opportunity for participants to make a contribution for the cost of the meal, but if they do not do so the meal is provided free. No means test is permitted. Each program must contract for the services of a dietitian or a nutritionist to approve the menus and the content of nutrition education and to advise about other nutrition matters.

Each hot meal must provide: (1) 3 ounces of meat or a specified alternate; (2) Two ½-cup servings of different vegetables and fruits, one vitamin C-rich daily, and one vitamin A-rich several times a week; (3) 1 serving of bread or alternate; (4) 8 ounces of milk or the calcium equivalent in cheese; and (5) 1 serving from a dessert group, which includes fruit and simple desserts such as cake, pie and cookies. Menus must be planned ahead with consideration of the special needs of the elderly and the religious, ethnic, cultural, and regional needs of the group.

At the end of fiscal year 1975, the Program was providing 240,000 meals daily at 4200 sites. The estimate for 1976 was as many as 300,000 meals daily at about 5000 sites. (36)

SUMMARY

The federal government provides funding for a number of nutrition programs for mothers and children. These include the Child Nutrition Program, School Lunch Program, WIC, EPSDT, Head Start, Maternity and Infant Care Project, and Children and Youth Project.

The Food Stamp Program is a form of income maintenance that increases the purchasing power of low income families so that they can buy more food of greater variety. EFNEP, a part of the Cooperative Extension Program, provides nutrition teaching in home and neighborhood by nutrition aides. The Nutrition Program for the Elderly is a program of low cost meals for social and rehabilitative services to persons over 60.

Most of these programs are funded by a combination of federal and state or local moneys and are locally administered according to standards established by the federal government.

REFERENCES CITED

1. CBS, Hunger in America, 1969.
2. Child Nutrition Programs: Income Poverty Guidelines for Determining Eligibility for Free and Reduced-Price Meals and Free Milk, *Federal Register,* June 14, 1976, (41 F.R. 23988).
3. Cook, Frances, Nutrition Education Via People-to-People, *J. Nutr. Educ.,* 1 Fall/69 9-11.
4. Egan, Mary C. and Betty J. Hallstrom, Building Nutrition Services in Comprehensive Health Care, *J. Am. Diet. Assoc.* 61 11/72 491.
5. Hallstrom, Betty J. and Doris E. Lauber, Multidisciplinary Manpower in the Nutrition Component of Comprehensive Health Care Delivery, *J. Am. Diet. Assoc.,* 63 7/73 23.
6. Head Start Programs Performance Standards, *Federal Register* 40 No. 126, June 30, 1975, Part II.
7. *Hunger, U.S.A., A Report by the Citizen's Board of Inquiry into Hunger and Malnutrition in The United States,* New Community Press, Washington DC, 1968.
8. Komaroff, Anthony L. and Paul J. Duffell, An Evaluation of Selected Federal Categorical Health Programs for the Poor, *Amer. J. Pub. Health,* 66 3/76 255-261.
9. Mayer, Jean, ed. *U.S. Nutrition Policies in the Seventies,* W. H. Freeman and Co., San Francisco, 1973, 5.
10. National School Lunch Program: Child Nutrition Programs, *Federal Register,* 5/4/76 (41 F.R. 18426-18428).
11. Special Supplemental Food Programs for Women, Infants, and Children, *Federal Register,* 1/12, 1976 (FR Doc. 76-861).
12. Spindler, Evelyn B., Mary E. Jacobson and Carolyn B. Russell, Action Programs To Improve Nutrition, *J. Home Econ.,* 61 10/69 635.
13. This Is Cooperative Extension, leaflet, U.S. Dept. of Agriculture, 1/73.
14. U.S. Congress, Senate, Select Committee on Nutrition and Human Needs, Hearings, *National Nutrition Policy Study, Part 7—Nutrition and Government,* 93rd Congress, 2d session, 1974, 3354.
15. U.S. Congress, Senate, Select Committee on Nutrition and Human Needs, Hearings, *Nutrition and Human Needs, Part I—Problems and Prospects,* 90th Congress, 2d session, Dec. 17, 18, 19, 1968, 5.

16. U.S. Dept. of Agriculture, Food and Nutrition Service, Child Feeding Program Fact Sheet, rev. 6/22/76.

17. Department of Agriculture, *1961–75 Food Stamp Program,* Food and Nutrition Service, FNS-118, rev. 1/76. Washington DC, leaflet.

18. U.S. Department of Agriculture, *Food Stamp Program,* Food and Nutrition Service, PA-1123, August, 1975, Washington DC, pamphlet.

19. U.S. Dept. of Agriculture, *Impact of the Expanded Food and Nutrition Education Program on Low-Income Families,* Agricultural Economics Report No. 220, 1972, Government Printing Office, Washington DC.

20. U.S. Dept. of Agriculture, *National School Lunch Program: Background and Development,* FNS-63, Government Printing Office, Washington DC, 1971, 14.

21. U.S. Dept. of Agriculture, *The Thrifty Food Plan,* Consumer and Food Economics Institute, CFE (ADM.) 326, Sept. 1975, Hyattsville MD.

22. U.S. Dept. of Health, Education and Welfare, *Handbook for Local Head Start Nutrition Specialists,* USDHEW, June 1975.

23. U.S. Dept. of Health, Education and Welfare, *Manual of Policies and Procedures for the National Nutrition Program for the Elderly,* 45 CFR 909, Office of Human Development, Washington DC.

24. U.S. Dept. of Health, Education, and Welfare, *Maternal and Child Health Services, Programs of Projects, Guidelines,* Public Health Service, Rockville MD, Sept. 1976.

25. U.S. Dept. of Health, Education and Welfare, *Promoting Community Health,* DHEW Pub. No. (HSA) 75-5016, 1975, 10, 33.

26. U.S. Dept. of Health, Education, and Welfare, Maternal and Child Health Service Programs: Administering Agencies and Legislative Base, Public Health Service, Maternal and Child Health Service, Rockville MD, 1972, 57.

27. U.S. General Services Administration, Office of the Federal Register, *United States Government Manual 1975/76,* Government Printing Office, Washington DC, 1975, 107.

28. U.S. Office of Management and Budget, *1976 Catalog of Federal Domestic Assistance,* Government Printing Office, Washington DC, 38.

29. Ibid., 39.

30. Ibid., 40.

31. Ibid., 41.

32. Ibid., 42.

33. Ibid., 43.

34. Ibid., 145.

35. Ibid., 290.

36. Ibid., 303.

37. Wallace, Helen M., Hyman Goldstein, Allan C. Oglesby, The Health and Medical Care of Children Under Title 19 (Medicaid) *Am. J. Pub. Health,* 64 5/74 501.

38. Wang, Virginia L., and Paul H. Ephross, ENEP Evaluated, *J. Nutr. Educ.,* 2 Spring 1971 148.

39. *White House Conference on Food, Nutrition and Health,* Final Report, Government Printing Office, Washington DC, 1970.

40. WIC Program Regulations, *Federal Register,* Doc. 76-861 Title 7-Agriculture, Ch. II, Part 246.

ADDITIONAL REFERENCES

Bowering, Jean, Mary A. Morrison, Ruth L. Lowenberg and Nilda Tirado, Role of EFNEP Aides in Improving Diets of Pregnant Women, *J. Nutr. Educ.,* 8 7–9/76 111.

Kirk, Thomas R., Gerald Rice, and Paul M. Allen, EPSDT—One Quarter Million Screenings in Michigan, *Am. J. Public Health,* 66 5/76 482.

Lucaczer, Moses, The National School Lunch Program in 1973: Some Accomplishments and Failures, *Nutr. Rev.,* 31 12/73 385–88.

Rada, Edward L., Medicating the Food Stamp Program, *Amer. J. Pub. Health,* 64 5/74 477–480.

CHAPTER 8

NONGOVERNMENT ORGANIZATIONS THAT MAY HAVE NUTRITION PROGRAMS

There are a number of nongovernment organizations that have community nutrition programs or other nutrition component. They include voluntary health agencies, professional organizations, organizations connected with business and industry, and foundations. Some have a nationwide network of services, others cover a limited territory, or have offices only in major population centers.

The community nutritionist needs to know the health and welfare agencies that serve the area and cooperate with them in sharing resources, developing activities, and coordinating programs. Some organizations set standards or perform special services for the profession or the field. Some are sources of teaching materials or funding for community projects. Community nutritionists and nutrition or other personnel from various organizations may join forces on professional or community committees, or advisory bodies, developing a useful symbiotic relationship.

VOLUNTARY HEALTH AGENCIES

A *voluntary health agency* is a private, nonprofit organization, chartered and licensed by an appropriate government agency, conducting activities designed to mitigate a specific health problem, and funded by contributions from individual citizens or private organizations. Most voluntary agencies have national organizations with state affiliates and local branches. Funds are raised locally, either as part of a united drive, or by the individual agency. (5, 6, 14, 16)

Perhaps the most important characteristic of the voluntary agency is that to a large extent its work is carried on by volunteers. Frequently the service of an executive is loaned to a voluntary agency by a business or industry for a period of time for fund-raising or another specific activity, or an individual is granted time from a regular job to serve as chairman of the board or in some other capacity which demands much ability and time. Many of the larger units of voluntary agencies have staffs of paid professionals who carry on the day-to-day work. Most voluntary agencies are governed by boards of directors or trustees responsible for policy-making, program planning, fund-raising, and overall direction. Usually the board of directors or trustees includes prominent individuals from the professions, business, industry, the social community, politics, and so forth.

The public's increased awareness and sophistication about health programs has resulted in changes in voluntary agencies due to reconsideration by the agencies of their proper roles in the health community and of the need to represent all segments of the community. This has resulted, in several agencies, in a change from an entirely medical-and-physician-oriented program to one that includes other health disciplines, among them nutrition. It has also brought representation of various minorities—black, Latin-American, Asian, and others as appropriate in a specific community—and of women in policy-making positions.

The voluntary agency fills some unique needs in our society, being organized to provide services not offered by official agencies, and to improve the quality of care by demonstration programs, professional education, personnel training, and the improvement of facilities. Frequently voluntary agencies assist official agencies by providing expert consultation, assessing community needs, helping start new programs, supporting research, and stimulating legislation, and by directing attention to emerging needs so that these can later be met by the public agencies. In addition, voluntary agencies provide a way for individuals and groups to use their own resources in meaningful ways by contributing time, money, and prestige to a cause in which they have a particular interest.

Most voluntary health agencies fulfill a useful role in the total health agency structure by providing needed services, by cooperating with government agencies on specific projects or by conducting programs, that, for political reasons or lack of funds, a government agency cannot pursue. However, some voluntary agencies have narrow objectives, spend too much of their funds on administration and too little for actual programs, or have overlapping objectives, programs, and fund-raising activities.

Standards and ethical guidelines have been established by the National Health Council for national voluntary agencies. To meet these standards, the agency must be directed by a board of volunteers from a wide geographical area with a rotating membership, and must have guidance for activities in the public interest from committees that include specialists in pertinent subject matter fields.

In theory, a voluntary agency should go out of existence when the need to which it administers no longer exists. In practice, very few are dissolved, but some have successfully changed their functions. For example, the former National Tuberculosis and Health Association is now the National Lung Association, and the National Foundation for Infantile Paralysis is now the National Foundation-March of Dimes, each attacking a new set of problems.

In many states, the major program activity is at the state level. However, programs in the large metropolitan areas may be even more extensive. One of the reasons for the present interest in support of voluntary organizations is an increased awareness by individuals of the tax-deductible nature of contributions to these nonprofit organizations. Politicians and government officials are aware that money given as tax-free contributions is channeled away from the public treasury, but they also recognize the value of the agency work.

Though only a few voluntary health agencies have notable nutrition programs, they provide an important resource; the community nutritionist should find out about those in the specific area and cooperate with them for mutual benefit. The nutritionist should also be aware of the need for participation in coordinating their efforts with those of official health and welfare agencies. Present broad health planning includes the coordination of programs and use of funds by all health agencies, both governmental and private, and the advancement of health through efficient use of both tax moneys and private funds.

Wilner (16) lists three kinds of focus for the voluntary health agency: a specific disease (cancer, lung); a part of the body (heart, kidney); and a specific group (children with birth defects, pregnant women). Usually the goals are to improve the quality of care by training personnel and improving facilities, to inform individuals about recognition, prevention and treatment, and to sponsor or conduct research. Three agencies that have nutrition programs and are likely to be found in many areas will be described.

American Diabetes Association (ADA)

This Association was founded in 1940 to improve the care and treatment of all persons with diabetes and to conduct research on ways to prevent and cure the disease. (1, 2) Until 1975, the professional membership was limited to doctors of medicine, but a bylaws change at that time opened it to nutritionists, dietitians, podiatrists, nurses, diabetic educators, and all others who participate in the care and treatment of people with diabetes. In 1975 the Association had 53 affiliates with over 200 branches and a membership of 3000 professionals, 25,000 affiliates, and about 80,000 subscribers.

The present activities of the ADA are under four major programs: (1) public education and detection, to alert the public to the early signs of the disease and to find unrecognized cases; (2) patient education, to teach the patient about the disease and its control; (3) professional education, to provide information to physicians and other professional health workers on treatment; and (4) research, to find methods of prevention and cure.

The ADA publishes *Diabetes Forecast,* a bimonthly for diabetic patients and their families, and a professional journal, *Diabetes.*

American Heart Association (AHA)

Heart was founded in 1924, at first as an organization for physicians and physician education, but in 1948 it became a voluntary health agency. Membership is now 105,000 (40,000 physicians and 65,000 others) with 55 affiliates and 1190 local subdivisions. (3) The directors include physicians, scientists, nurses, nutritionists, dentists, and representatives of other professions and of business, unions, and many other groups. The objective is to support research, education, and community service programs to reduce death and disability from heart disease. Fund-raising is by an independent campaign. *Heart* has a program of education for the public and for various professionals; it finances research and carries on many kinds of community services, publishes pamphlets and professional journals, and provides films and speakers. The national Association has a nutrition and weight control program with a small nutrition staff at headquarters. Some local chapters also have staff nutritionists and conduct public service programs in both prevention and treatment. (4)

National Foundation-March of Dimes (MOD)

The MOD is the successor to the National Foundation for Infantile Paralysis, founded in 1938. After the conquest of that disease, the agency changed its name and focus. (9, 10, 11) It now has approximately 2000 chapters in the United States with most of the work conducted by volunteers.

It sponsors research, health service, and education programs to prevent birth defects and otherwise improve the outcome of pregnancy. A birth defect is defined as an abnormality of structure, function, or metabolism existing at birth and resulting from a genetic or an environmental cause. (12) MOD considers malnutrition during the prenatal period as a major factor in low birthweight and mental retardation, and emphasizes the importance of diet.

MOD conducts its work through grants to medical services, professional education, and public and school health education programs. Among the programs supported are genetic counseling and care of high risk pregnant women and the critically ill newborn. In 1975 MOD and the American Home Economics Association cosponsored an Institute on Maternal and Newborn Health for home economics leaders.

Coordinating Bodies

These constitute another kind of voluntary agency, which includes health councils, community councils, nutrition councils, and similar groups at national, state, and local levels. They are concerned with broad scale planning or liaison for a community to integrate programs and avoid duplication of services. Generally a coordinating council membership is composed of representatives from the various agencies in a community. Among those of special significance to nutritionists are nutrition councils, which exist in most states and many local areas; however, the functions may differ from those described here. Community nutritionists need to understand the role of coordinating bodies and play an active role in leading such groups into meaningful activities. (5, 14)

Interagency Committee on Nutrition Education (ICNE). This important Washington, D.C., group is supported by USDA. (8, 15) Its membership includes representatives of local official and quasiofficial agencies that have a nutrition component in their programs. The purpose of the ICNE is to exchange information among the agencies and to coordinate activities. Among its major accomplishments was the formulation in 1964 of a set of basic nutrition concepts that have been widely used and are known to most nutritionists. Another was publication of *Nutrition Program News,* which provided information about the activities and programs of the represented agencies. A third was sponsoring the National Nutrition Education Conferences that were held at five-year intervals. The last one, held in 1971, dealt primarily with teenagers and their nutrition. (15)

Nutrition Committees and Councils. These groups exist in many states and at some local levels as groups of professionals, usually with representation from community leadership groups. (7, 13) The Committees conduct various coordinating and educational functions. Some of the publics through which a nutrition council can function are communications media, food makers and marketers, school curriculum makers, and professional groups. Some activities in 1974 that won Nutrition Action Awards from the National Nutrition Exchange were compiling a guidebook to services and programs, conducting an innovative nutrition education program, and preparing a study guide for PTA groups.

PROFESSIONAL ORGANIZATIONS

Every discipline that is a health-related profession has at least one professional association to which the members owe allegiance and on which they depend for professional support. Recently unions for professionals have developed, which may have an increasingly important influence in the future. A union may be for one profession as teachers or physicians, or for all professions in a particular agency or institution. As yet the unions have a relatively small significance for community nutritionists in most places, but where they are established, they play an important part in negotiations for salaries and fringe benefits.

The larger professional associations for health personnel have national organizations with state and local affiliates. They establish standards for membership, credentials and certification, serve as a source of information to the members through professional journals, newsletters and other publications, and hold annual meetings for exchange of current information, discussion of issues, reports of research, and solving of problems. Many of them now conduct or assist with programs for continuing education for members or for other professions.

Financing for these organizations comes mainly from membership dues, exhibits at annual meetings, and journal advertising. Many of them now have affiliated tax-free foundations, established because of recent changes in income tax laws.

Professional associations are usually a good influence on their members, advancing their particular field of health care and encouraging research and innovation, but sometimes they devote too much attention to self-interest and aggrandizement of the profession. Yohalem and Brecher (31) comment that the training and utilization of allied health manpower has been complicated by the organization of health workers into professional associations and unions because the professional groups press for certification and raise entry standards while the unions try to upgrade positions and increase wages.

Either professional groups or unions may increase job requirements, making it hard to qualify and hard for the educational institutions to provide the training. (31) For the most part however, both types of organizations are genuinely concerned with maintaining a high standard of patient care. The increasing complexity and scope of knowledge required for the practitioner emphasize the need for ever higher standards and more preparation. In most organizations the leadership has shown a willingness to respond to the expressed wishes of the membership.

Organizations for Community Nutritionists

Most disciplines have a number of professional organizations relating to their particular fields. Though there are several of interest to the community nutritionist, there is at present no organization that *limits* membership to persons actually engaged in community nutrition programs, which is necessary to make it possible to focus on community nutritionists' specific needs, the first being to establish an identity.

There have been several attempts to establish a separate association for public health nutritionists but no such attempts for community nutritionists. One of the problems in such an organization is the small number of persons in this highly specialized group, making it difficult to form a viable, productive organization. A professional organization for community nutritionists would need to focus on the field of community nutrition, with a membership of persons in programs primarily concerned with interaction with the community.

Many community nutritionists belong to one or more of the organizations that will be discussed.

American Dietetic Association (ADA). The ADA is the professional organization of over 26,000 dietitians and nutritionists from hospitals, military, government agencies, colleges and universities. (17, 18) It has affiliated associations in all 50 states. The goals of the ADA are (1) to improve the nutrition of human beings, (2) to advance the science of dietetics and nutrition, and (3) to promote education in these and allied areas. The qualifications for membership are a baccalaureate degree in a program specified by the Association and the completion of an approved internship or an equivalent clinical experience coordinated with academic work or a traineeship. A master's or doctoral degree may also meet the requirements. The Association has recently established a Dietetic Technician membership class for a person who has completed a two-year college level course (associate degree program) according to the standards established by the ADA. The position was discussed on p. 54.

The Annual Meeting includes scientific sessions with lectures and other educational activities, and commercial and educational exhibits. In 1967 ADA established a registration system for members, with an examination required after that time to attain registered status. In 1976 registration was made independent of ADA membership. ADA is the accrediting body for coordinated dietetic internship programs. The Association is active in legislation, maintaining a Washington representative. It publishes position papers on matters of concern to dietitians and establishes the academic and experience requirements. The monthly *Journal of the American Dietetic Association* publishes scientific and research papers and reports of activities in the field. An Association pamphlet of special value to the community nutritionist is *Food Facts Talk Back.*

The ADA was formerly oriented to the work and needs of the hospital dietitian with emphasis on administration and diet therapy, but it has broadened its interests to the entire community, working to develop programs related to nutrition in the broad issues of health and welfare. Community nutritionists are now attempting to form an interest group within the framework of the ADA. Both national and affiliated state and local groups have many activities of interest to the community nutritionist, who should be a participant and leader in them.

American Home Economics Association (AHEA). This is the organization for professional home economists, that is, the college graduate with a degree in home economics or two years of experience in the field. (19, 20) Founded in 1909, it had in 1975 52,000 members in 52 state groups. Its major objective is to improve the quality of individual and family life. It covers all areas including foods, nutrition, and consumer education. Few nutritionists are members, but more might well consider the advantages of a continuing contact with home economists in teaching, business, and other fields.

The Association has several divisions of particular interest to the community nutritionist: Food and Nutrition, Human Services, Extension, Family Economics-Home Management, Consumer Interest, and Aging. AHEA has established the Center for the Family, which has as its first project the publishing of a fact book on the family to include quantitative data on nutrition. It is also working on problems of the aging and is cooperating with the National Foundation-March of Dimes on projects in maternal and child health. It publishes the monthly *Journal of Home Economics* and the quarterly *Home Economics Research Journal.*

American Public Health Association (APHA). Membership in APHA is open to persons in all community health specialties and to interested consumers. The 26,000 members also represent 53 regional groups. The Association promulgates standards, establishes uniform practices and procedures, creates testing methods for selection of professional public health workers, establishes minimum education qualifications, and explores other matters of significance to public health. (26) Some standards important to nutritionists are those for training public health nutritionists and those for nutritional assessment. (23)

The APHA Food and Nutrition Section includes nutritionists, food technologists, and others interested in the field. The scope of interest is indicated by the resolutions passed at the 1974 APHA Annual Meeting that related to National Nutrition Policy, Multiple Risk Factors in Coronary Heart Disease, and Nutritional Assessment in Health Surveillance. (22) A recent poll of members of this Section indicated concern for the coordination of its purposes with those of other nutrition organizations. (21)

Society for Nutrition Education (SNE). The goal of SNE is to make nutrition education more effective. It conducts activities in education, communication, and research. Persons with nutrition training who are concerned about nutrition education may apply for membership. (28)

The Society was organized in 1968 and in 1976 had almost 4000 members from all over the world, with the majority from the United States. Regular publications include the quarterly *Journal of Nutrition Education* and a newsletter, *SNE Communicator.* It publishes extensive reviews of materials in the field and operates the National Nutrition Education Clearing House, which is a collection of more than 5000 items including books, journals, pamphlets, and audiovisual aids available for reference and loan. (24)

Other Nutrition Organizations

There are a number of other organizations for persons with different primary interests in nutrition. A brief discussion of some of them follows:

American Board of Nutrition. The Board has 240 members who are certified physicians qualified to treat nutritional and metabolic disorders and scientists who conduct scientific work on human nutrition and nutrient requirements. (25)

American Institute of Nutrition. This group is made up of 1500 experimental nutrition scientists from universities, government, and industry. One of its divisions is the American Society for Clinical Nutrition, which has 350 physician members. The Institute publishes the *American Journal of Clinical Nutrition* and the *Journal of Nutrition*. (25)

National Nutrition Consortium. The Consortium was founded by the American Dietetic Association, American Institute of Nutrition, American Society for Clinical Nutrition, and Institute of Food Technologists, but has since been joined by the American Academy of Pediatrics, the Food and Nutrition Board of the American Academy of Sciences, and the Society for Nutrition Education. It now represents the combined membership of seven organizations, over 50,000 persons. It consults on nutrition matters, with government and industry leaders, recommending action and supplying technical information and advice. (17, 26)

Nutrition Today Society. This is "a cooperative organization devoted solely to acquainting the world with the new science of nutrition." (27) It is open to health professionals and others who are interested in its goal. Members represent the professional fields of agriculture, biochemistry, dentistry, dietetics, food technology, home economics, medicine, nursing, nutrition, paramedical, and school food service. One of its 17 Founding Officers was a dietitian. The journal *Nutrition Today* is the principal benefit of membership, but the Society also produces teaching materials for use in professional and public education. Among the best are their slides and printed materials on diagnosis of nutritional disorders.

Other Professional Organizations

The associations of many other professionals, for example, American Medical Association, American Dental Association, and American Association for Physical Health and Recreation, have an interest in nutrition just as nutritionists incorporate the subject matter of medicine and other fields into their own work. Cooperation will help to assure that the subject matter is authentic.

The American Medical Association (AMA) has a Department of Foods and Nutrition with a staff of nutritionists and dietitians. It has assumed some of the functions of the Council on Foods and Nutrition, which was established in 1936 and terminated in 1975. The Council disseminated nutrition information to the medical profession and the public, sponsored educational symposia, published scientific reports, and issued policy statements. One of the best known was the joint statement with the NRC Food and Nutrition Board on Improving the nutritional quality of foods. In recent years the Council had carried on programs concerned with improvement of nutrition teaching in medical schools, clinical nutrition, nutritional management of patients, and the physician's role in the community. (29)

The American Academy of Pediatrics has a Committee on Nutrition to advise the Academy on nutrition. The Committee's recommendations are prepared with assistance from a technical advisory group, one or more consultants, and liaison representatives from other organizations including the American Dietetic Association, Food and Nutrition Board, and the Food and Drug Administration.

ORGANIZATIONS SPONSORED BY BUSINESS AND INDUSTRY

The community nutritionist will find that considerable support and many useful services are provided by business and industry. The nutrition program may be a resource to them providing guidance about the development of materials, explaining the needs and possible uses of materials in nutrition programs, or suggesting sources for more detailed information.

The kinds of services provided by business and industry change with economic and social conditions such as, the availability of products and money, and the need to promote products. Some services and goods that have been provided by business in the past are nutrition education materials such as leaflets, pamphlets, posters and films; pamphlets, books, and films for use as professional resources; sponsorship and funding of workshops, lectures and symposia; and financing prizes or awards for contests or scholarships. The cost of these professional helps is usually part of the advertising or public relations budget of an organization. The organizations which provide most of the services useful to the community nutritionist may be divided into four groups.

Trade Associations

These are generally nonprofit, voluntary associations of business competitors in the same trade or industrial operation, formed to provide services to members, especially on stabilization of production and prices, and expanding production and sales. (32, 33) Services to members may include (1) advertising and marketing, such as developing and promoting a seal or emblem, furnishing copy, photos, or mats for advertising or publicity, sponsoring advertisements, and conducting market surveys; (2) staff education, such as sponsoring workshops and short courses, and preparing manuals and texts, and (3) liaison with government to keep members informed of changes in laws and to keep government informed about the problems of the industry and its position on matters of public policy, and to provide government with models for industry-related legislation.

Food Cooperatives or Marketing Groups

These groups have a promotional thrust with less emphasis on an educational component. Many are concerned with only one product, for example, apples, citrus fruit, potatoes, turkey, or lamb. Some cover only a local or regional area. These groups sometimes offer support for nutrition programs as a means of public relations and community visibility.

Food Vendors

These include both companies that make or distribute food products, and other companies, such as pharmaceutical houses, that produce infant formulas and other products used as food. Many of these companies supply recipes that contain their products. Some companies have also supplied resource materials for professionals, and professional samples of their products, and have supported various activities of professional associations and other local groups.

Retail Market Chains

Some chains prepare or distribute leaflets and other informational materials on food buying, meal planning, and nutrition; some employ home economists as consumer representatives to establish good will, to help consumers, or to promote particular kinds of foods; and some participate in developing new programs such as food labeling, or in local programs for consumer education. The home economist with a food chain may provide customer services in consumer education, food product information and food purchasing. The home economist also provides services to the employer such as staff education, product testing, store design, and community services (e.g., education by printed materials and television programs). (35)

Other Companies

These include insurance companies, public utilities, and equipment manufacturers, which disseminate information of food preparation and related subjects or on nutrition and health. Their community services provide an indirect way of publicizing their products or services. Some of these companies have provided other help such as advice on speakers or facilities for meetings.

Resources for Community Nutrition

Some of the trade associations that can provide services of use in nutrition programs will be discussed briefly.

American Institute of Baking (AIB). This is a research and educational organization, founded in 1919, now with 450 members who are representatives of baking and allied trade companies. It has a staff of 60 conducting basic education in nutrition, baking science, and technology; maintaining an extensive library in the field; and preparing materials suitable for use in community nutrition programs. The AIB can supply nutritional data and other information about breads and other bakery products. (34)

Cereal Institute. Founded in 1943, it now has seven members and a staff of seven. It conducts research and education on nutrition and the role of cereals in the diet. It can supply filmstrips, leaflets, pamphlets, posters, and other teaching materials to schools, health organizations, and similar agencies as well as nutritional data on cereal products. (34)

Evaporated Milk Association. There are 11 members (manufacturers of the product) and a staff of three. It prepares printed materials and filmstrips for nutritionists, teachers, and others, covering uses of evaporated milk, labeling, and infant feeding. (34)

Manufacturing Chemists Association. Founded in 1872, this Association now has about 200 members in the United States and Canada, representing manufacturers of basic chemicals who sell a substantial portion of their production to others. It conducts technical symposiums and workshops for the trade and publishes manuals, guides, and technical bulletins. Its materials on additives have been of special value to community nutritionists. (34)

National Canners Association.   Founded in 1907, the Association has a staff of 140 and about 500 members who are commercial packers of food products processed by heat in hermetically sealed containers. It has a consumer services department that prepares educational materials for home economists, food editors, and teachers. They give information about the nutritional value of canned foods and their use in the diet. The Association publishes pamphlets, charts, manuals, and books about canning and canned foods and holds training sessions for the industry. It is a source for information about canned foods. (34)

National Dairy Council (NDC).   Founded in 1915, this is the trade association for milk producers and dealers and manufacturers in the industry. There are affiliated Dairy Council units with offices in 105 cities in 43 states. Most of the state and local groups have staff nutritionists who conduct community nutrition programs in their areas. Programs are developed to fit local needs, such as sponsoring or helping plan educational events for nutritionists, dietitians, teachers, and other professionals, providing speakers, preparing printed materials, and participating in community planning.

The NDC conducts research and educational programs on eating habits using the four-food group approach with emphasis on dairy products. It has recently developed prepared programs in nutrition and dental health, food labeling, and the economics of dairy foods for local use.

NDC has two publications of particular interest to professionals, *Nutrition News* and *Dairy Council Digest,* and it publishes other materials for schools and the industry. (34)

National Livestock and Meat Board.   It was founded in 1922 and now has a staff of 59. As the service organization for the meat industry, it promotes, educates, and provides information about meats. Over a period of 55 years, it has supported nutrition research studies at medical schools, universities, and hospitals with a total of 425 grants. It does recipe testing, supplies materials to the media, and publishes teaching materials for classroom use. It has a Home Economics Department and a Nutrition Research Department, and is establishing a Department of Education. Five times a year it publishes a newsletter, *Food and Nutrition News,* which is available to professional nutritionists. (34)

United Fresh Fruit and Vegetable Association. The Association was founded in 1937 by the merger of two produce organizations that dated back to 1904. Its 24 staff members serve a membership of 2600 growers, shippers, brokers, carriers, wholesalers, retailers, and others who handle fresh fruits and vegetables. Association activities include (1) working with government agencies on existing and proposed regulations and watching legislative developments and keeping members informed; (2) conducting training sessions for member firms on retail merchandising, telephone selling by wholesalers, and so forth; (3) maintaining a promotion program that provides material and releases for newspaper food editors, TV and radio stations, and syndicated columnists; (4) setting up meetings for various segments of the trade so they can work out their problems; and (5) publishing a variety of materials for the trade and others.

Of general interest to professional nutritionists is *Nutrition Notes,* an eight-page newsletter, issued quarterly, that reviews information on nutrients, especially those significant in fruits and vegetables. Menu planners for institutions and other large organizations may find useful the eight-page *Monthly Supply Letter,* which gives expected supplies of produce for the coming month. Although the Association does not maintain an information service as such for nutritionists, some questions can be answered. (34)

Using the Resources

Many other businesses and industries supply educational materials or services useful in community nutrition programs. The nutritionist can keep informed about them through news notes and advertisements in professional journals, through promotional materials and publications received in the mail, and through visits by representatives of companies who offer services. An opportunity to meet personnel and to see materials and products is provided at the annual meetings of the American Dietetic Association, American Home Economics Association, and other organizations.

The services of these companies offer an important resource for the nutritionist, some providing information not readily available elsewhere, especially about the selection, storage, use, and nutritional value of their products; however, merit must be judged by an objective evaluation for each item. Some educational materials emphasize the nutritional values of the product, suggest ways it can be used, provide authentic nutrition information, and promote the product within useful limits, but others overemphasize the brand, product, and company at the expense of the nutrition message. Some promote the nutrient content of basic foods, but others may concentrate on selling a product that supplies mainly calories while having little nutritional benefit. A list of organizations with addresses is given on page 129.

FOUNDATIONS

Foundation is defined in *The Foundation Directory* as "a nongovernmental, nonprofit organization, with funds and program managed by its own trustees or directors, and established to maintain or aid social, educational, charitable, religious, or other activities, serving the common welfare, primarily through the making of grants." (39) Parrish has defined it more succinctly as "a nongovernmental institution which makes grants." (44) The foundation has also been characterized as a channel through which private wealth can be contributed to public purpose. In 1965 foundations were characterized as the "only important agencies in America free from the political controls of legislative appropriations and pressure groups and free from the necessity of tempering programs to the judgments and prejudices of current contributions." (42) The role of the foundation has been innovation since it has fewer constraints than other agencies to do research, demonstration, train personnel, or try new programs. (46) Parrish (44) gives two basic characteristics that distinguish the foundation from other charitable organizations: (1) the funds are received from a single person or a small group, and (2) the major function is making grants rather than conducting programs.

The *Foundation Directory* does not list organizations called foundations which have other primary purposes. Some appeal to the public for funds, some are trade organizations for industrial or other groups, and some function as endowments set up for special purposes within organizations governed by groups from the organizations. The last are classified as *community foundations*.

Because foundations had become a permanent repository for vast amounts of wealth, estimated in 1965 at 14.5 billion dollars, with grants of about 800 million dollars annually, the Congress passed the Tax Reform Act of 1971. Before the enactment of the Tax Reform Law, there was limited reporting and it was difficult to obtain information about the types or amounts of grants made, or even to obtain a list of grants. There was less consideration of social responsibility than desirable, and meager information was available on new foundations or on those which went out of existence. It will be some time before more complete records will be available. (38)

The change in the tax law will probably inhibit development of new foundations and cause many small ones to dissolve because it requires a greater flow of funds. Market conditions and general state of the economy affect the amount of available funds by increasing, or recently, reducing the value and return of investments. The records for 1971–1973 showed that about 50 percent of all grants were under $1,000, 30 percent were from $1,000 to $5,000, and 20 percent were $5,000 or more, with some over $1 million. The large foundations distributed 80 percent of the total dollar value.

Most of the money goes to education; the second largest amount goes to health, the third largest to welfare, and the fourth largest to science. *The Foundation Directory* contains some suggestions for preparing grant proposals and shows where in each state there is a collection of information on foundations. The Foundation Center estimates that there are 26,000 foundations, 82 percent of them having less than $200,000 in assets. Some have large endowments; some receive funds and distribute all of them in the same year.

Community foundations are characterized by multiple sources of funding rather than by a single endowment fund; for this reason they are classified under the law as *public charities.* Since they are considered as publicly supported, they are subject to fewer governmental controls, pay no excise tax, and have fewer limitations on gifts of new funds. As a professional grantmaking organization, a community foundation can offer an advantageous way to administer many different kinds of charitable funds. Their programs are essentially the same as those of other foundations. Some have been organized as offshoots of governmental agencies or professional organizations to accept funds or conduct activities that would not otherwise be possible because of tax status, conflict of interest, and so forth.

Nutritionists should be aware of foundations as a possible source of funding for innovative programs. Many are interested in food and in health, some specifically in nutrition. Many have specific, defined objectives that should be investigated before a grant is requested. Some that have made grants to nutrition related programs or have nutrition related objectives will be mentioned briefly.

The Kellogg Foundation gives aid mainly for application of knowledge, with health as one of its program interests. (40)

The Rockefeller Foundation has as one of its primary purposes "the conquest of hunger and its attendant ills." (41)

The Foundation Directory mentions nutrition among the interests of several lesser known foundations, such as Esmark Foundation (Chicago), Research Corporation (New York), and United Brands (New York).

Some foundations that should be known especially to nutritionists are:

The American Dietetic Association Foundation, which administers funds for awards, scholarships, grants, donations, bequests and gifts, and directs research and educational activities. Its goal is to advance education and science in nutrition and dietetics. (36)

The American Home Economics Association Foundation, which administers funds for fellowships and international scholarships and finances workshops, conferences, research, and production of educational materials. (37)

The Nutrition Foundation, which was previously supported by contributions from the food industry, established new goals in 1972. These were stated as "to take an active role in the stimulation of public education programs, in focusing objective scientific attention on current issues in food safety and nutrition and in hammering out research priorities." (43) It expects to support research in nutrition of young infants and pregnant women and on food safety questions. The Foundation will now have public representatives as a majority of its controlling body and will be able to obtain grants from other foundations and from the government. It has been suggested that large food companies allocate 1 percent of their advertising budgets to the Foundation for nutrition education (45) The Foundation has 59 members and publishes a monthly journal, *Nutrition Reviews.*

SUMMARY

Associations for health professionals are usually national in scope with state and local affiliations. They establish standards, publish technical journals and educational materials, hold meetings for exchange of information, and conduct continuing education for members and other professionals. There is no one association that meets all the needs of community nutritionists.

Business and industrial organizations may conduct nutrition programs or provide services for community nutrition programs. They offer a valuable resource for the community nutritionist.

Foundations are nongovernmental and nonprofit private organizations that usually operate by conducting or funding innovative programs.

The community nutritionist needs to know local organizations that are active in nutrition and to cooperate with them to enhance progress toward the objective of good nutrition.

REFERENCES CITED

Voluntary Health Agencies

1. American Diabetes Association, *Annual Report: 1974—The Year of Momentum,* American Diabetes Association, New York, 1974.
2. American Diabetes Association, Personal communication from Ernest M. Frost, 9/4/75.
3. American Heart Association, *Heart Facts 1976,* American Heart Association, Dallas, 1975.
4. American Heart Association, Personal communication from Mary Winston, 8/22/75.
5. Anderson, C. L., *Community Health,* C. V. Mosby, St. Louis, 1973, 339.
6. Brager, George, and Harry Specht, *Community Organizing,* Columbia University Press, New York, 1973, 33.
7. Hill, Mary M., Nutrition Committees and Their Role in Community Action Programs, *Nutrition Program News,* Jan.–Feb., 1964, U.S. Dept. of Agriculture, Washington DC.
8. Hill, Mary M., Personal communication, 1975.
9. National Foundation-March of Dimes, All About the March of Dimes, leaflet, White Plains, NY, n.d.
10. National Foundation-March of Dimes, Leaders Alert, 29, leaflet, White Plains NY, n.d.
11. National Foundation-March of Dimes, Personal communication from Gabriel Stickle, 7/16/76.
12. National Foundation-March of Dimes, Los Angeles County Chapter, Genetic Counseling, leaflet, Los Angeles, n.d.
13. Nutrition Council as a Tool for Change, *J. Nutr. Educ.,* 6 10-12/74, insert i-iv.
14. Osborn, Barbara, *Introduction to Community Health,* Allyn and Bacon, Boston, 1964, 327.
15. Robinson, Meredith, Interagency Committee on Nutrition Education (ICNE) *Nutrition Program News,* 11-12/73, 1.
16. Wilner, Daniel M., Rosabelle P. Walkley, Lenar S. Goerke, *Introduction to Public Health,* Macmillan, New York, 1973, 54.

Professional Organizations

17. ADA News, *J. Am. Diet. Assoc.,* 69 9/76 311.
18. American Dietetic Association, All About the American Dietetic Association, pamphlet, The American Dietetic Association, Chicago, n.d.
19. American Home Economics Association, AHEA Fact Sheet, leaflet, Washington DC., June 1974.
20. American Home Economics Association, What Does AHEA Offer the Professional Home Economist?, leaflet, American Home Economics Association, Washington DC, n.d.
21. *APHA Newsletter,* Food and Nutrition Section, April 1975, American Public Health Association, Washington DC.

22. Association News, Resolutions and Position Papers, *Am. J. Pub. Health,* 65, 2/75, 188.
23. Christakis, George, ed., Nutritional Assessment in Health Programs, *Am. J. Pub. Health,* 63, Nov. 1973, Supplement, 82 p.
24. *Encyclopedia of Associations,* 9th ed., Vol. I, *National Organizations of the U.S.,* Gale Research Co., Detroit, 1975, 472.
25. Ibid., 739.
26. Ibid., 762.
27. Nutrition Today Society, announcement, in *Nutr. Today,* 9 3–4/75, 17.
28. Society for Nutrition Education, *J. Nutr. Educ.,* 7 4–6/75 46.
29. White, Philip L., A Brief History of the AMA's Council on Foods and Nutrition, *Nutrition Today,* 10 1–2/75 10.
30. Wilner, Daniel M., Rosabelle P. Walkley, and Lenar S. Goerke, *Introduction to Public Health,* Macmillan Co., New York, 1973, 60.
31. Yohalem, Alice M., and Charles M. Brecher, The University Medical Center and the Metropolis: A Working Paper, in Ginzberg, Eli M., and Alice M. Yohalem ed., *The University Medical Center and the Metropolis,* Josiah Macy, Jr. Foundation, New York, 1974, 8.

Business and Industry

32. *Ballentine's Law Dictionary,* 3d ed., Wm. S. Anderson, ed., The Lawyers Co-Operative Publishing Co., Rochester NY 1969, 1288.
33. Bradley, Joseph F., *The Role of Trade Associations and Professional Business Societies in America,* Pennsylvania State University Press, University Park PA, 1965, 4.
34. Correspondence with the organization, 1976.
35. Olmstead, Agnes R., Superwoman for the Supermarket, *J. Home Econ. Assoc.,* 64 10/72 9.

Foundations

36. All About the A.D.A., pamphlet, American Dietetic Association, undated, 8.
37. *Encyclopedia of Associations,* 9th ed., Vol. 1, *National Organizations of the U.S.,* Gale Research Co., Detroit, 1975, 544.
38. Foundation Center, *The Foundation Directory,* 5th ed., Columbia University Press, New York, 1975, ix.
39. Ibid., xi.
40. Ibid., 157.
41. Ibid., 272.
42. *Foundations: 20 Viewpoints,* Russell Sage Foundation, New York, 1965, 108.
43. Nutrition Foundation Announces New Goals and New Leadership, *Nutr. Rev.,* 30, 1/1972, 1.
44. Parrish, Thomas, The Foundation, A Special American Institution in *The Future of Foundations,* Prentice-Hall, Englewood Cliffs, NJ, 1973, 10.

45. Ullrich, Helen D., and George M. Briggs, The General Public, in Mayer, Jean ed., *U.S. Nutrition Policy in the Seventies*, W. H. Freeman and Co., San Francisco, 1973, 184.
46. Wilner, Daniel M., Rosabelle Price Walkley, and Lenar S. Goerke, *Introduction to Public Health*, Macmillan, New York, 1973, 60.

Some Organizations Sponsored by Business and Industry

American Institute of Baking (AIB)   (312) 944-6577
400 E. Ontario Street, Chicago IL 60611

Cereal Institute   (312) 782-7140
135 S. LaSalle Street, Chicago IL 60603

Evaporated Milk Association (EMA)   (202) 223-6820
910 17th Street N.W., Washington DC 20006

Manufacturing Chemists Association   (202) 483-6126
1825 Connecticut Ave., N.W., Washington DC 20009

National Canners Association   (202) 331-7070
1133 20th Street, N.W., Washington DC 20036

National Dairy Council   (312) 696-1020
6300 North River Road, Rosemont IL 60018

National Livestock and Meat Board   (312) 346-6465
36 So. Wabash Avenue, Chicago IL 60603

United Fresh Fruit and Vegetable Association   (202) 293-9210
1019 19th Street, N.W., Washington DC 20036

3 THE TOOLS AND SKILLS

The community nutritionist uses many tools and skills in conducting programs. Both are used in various ways in the broad techniques of community organization, management and planning, and professional and public education.

Many kinds of tools are available from a variety of sources, but they must be evaluated before use. The nutritionist will need to prepare others to have appropriate ones for all occasions.

The work of the nutritionist will be facilitated by an early mastery of the basic skills so that those that are used often can be applied effectively in different situations. The important thing about tools and skills is finding the ones that will work in a particular situation. The nutritionist is constantly confronted by different situations and must decide quickly which skills and tools will be the most effective.

CHAPTER 9

TOOLS

A *tool* is anything necessary to the carrying out of an occupation. The nutritionist uses many tools such as tables of nutrients and food quantities, food patterns and guides, food records and diet histories, recipes, measuring equipment, and food itself. The background and uses of some of these tools will be discussed.

RECOMMENDED DIETARY ALLOWANCES (RDA)

The Eighth Revised Edition of the book *Recommended Dietary Allowances* was prepared by the Committee on Dietary Allowances of the Food and Nutrition Board of the National Research Council in 1974. "The Recommended Dietary Allowances are the levels of intake of essential nutrients considered, in the judgment of the Food and Nutrition Board on the basis of available scientific knowledge, to be adequate to meet the known nutritional needs of practically all healthy persons." (19)

All nutritionists and dietitians need to be thoroughly familiar with the scientific basis for the RDA and should use the book as a resource for scientific information and a conservative operating guide and standard. Teaching and materials should be updated to conform with the changes as each edition is published. It is especially important to note the changes and additions and the basis for them. As the Allowances represent the concensus of a group of our most able nutrition researchers working in a quasiofficial capacity (p. 84) they provide a depth of knowledge, a considered judgment, and a compromise which the community nutritionist should use for the stated purposes. The Board has access to much information not readily available to others and is best able to weigh the evidence and make a decision on its meanings.

The major uses the community nutritionist will make of the RDA are (1) as a guide for planning meals and buying food, (2) as a tool for evaluating the nutrient intake of the food consumed by an individual or group, and (3) as background for developing diet instruction. Other uses are to establish standards for public assistance, to evaluate the adequacy of the total national food supply, and to establish guidelines for nutritional labeling of foods.

The amounts of nutrients in the RDA tables are estimates of amounts recommended for daily consumption by each individual. It is important to note that the Allowances are for well individuals and that they are believed to cover the needs of 95 percent of all well people in the United States. There are a number of practical points that have specific implications in application of the RDA by the nutritionist.

1. Intakes of individual nutrients fluctuate from day to day; for most nutrients, intake should be evaluated over a week's time to see that the average consumption provides the RDA. Each day's food should provide some of each nutrient and a day of low consumption should be followed by one with a substantial amount. The major exception is vitamin C, which should be provided every day. Judicious use of high nutrient foods such as pork (for thiamin), citrus fruit or dark green leafy vegetables (for vitamin C), and liver (for iron, riboflavin, niacin, and vitamin A) can be used to compensate for a day of low intake.

2. Food intake of higher amounts of specific nutrients than the RDA should not be regarded as a waste or as luxury consumption. In fact, frequent oversupply of some nutrients will occur as adequate amounts of others, especially the trace elements, are planned. It is unlikely that ordinary foods used in customary ways will provide harmful amounts of any nutrients. However, control is needed especially to avoid over-fortification with vitamins A and D since excessive consumption of these vitamins may be harmful. There has been a recent tendency to add nutrients to many foods, especially snack foods that are often consumed in excessive amounts, so fortification of these foods should be carefully monitored.

3. Small surpluses of nutrients are not harmful, but small deficits over a long time will lead to deficiency and depletion. Continued monitoring and evaluation are necessary.

4. The Allowances can be applied to the food intakes of individuals. In the past, some nutritionists have believed that the Allowances should be applied only to group averages. Harper has stated (12) "... the Recommended Dietary Allowances are estimates of amounts of nutrients that, if *consumed* daily by each individual in a specified population group, should insure that the needs of nearly all individuals in the group who are well will be met." Thus the Allowances apply to the individual whether living alone, in a family situation, or in an institution. Nutritionists need to make frequent calculations of nutrients from actual consumption figures, and food plans and menus should be judged in the same way to be sure the recommended amounts of nutrients are supplied each day.

5. Use of a variety of foods is an important safeguard because of the natural variability in foods, and there is increasing evidence that nutrients in addition to those included in the RDA tables are necessary for humans and that there are possible as yet unknown interrelationships between nutrients.

6. Some of the safety of the RDA lies in diets that include a wide variety of foods. Sometimes the diet over a long period is made up of a restricted number of foods, as may be the case with infant diets and weight control diets. Careful monitoring is needed to be sure such diets are nutritionally adequate, especially in the trace elements.

7. The Board states that there is no specific need for fat except to supply fat-soluble vitamins and essential fatty acids and that this can be met by a diet containing 15 to 25 grams of food fats. (20) This amount is far below the present average consumption of fats as 40 to 45 percent of total calories, or 70 grams for the 1500 calorie diet and 90 to 100 grams for the 2000 to 2500 calorie diet. Limiting the fat calories to 35 percent means reducing fat to 70 to 80 grams, which necessitates a considerable change in foods. If lower fat diets are planned, the *kind* of fat might also be changed to meet the joint recommendation made by the Food and Nutrition Board, the American Heart Association, and the American Medical Association. Based on a 30 percent of total calories recommendation, they suggested less than 10 percent from saturated fat sources, less than 10 percent from polyunsaturated fat sources, and the rest from monounsaturated fat sources. Considerable adjustment in food fats would be necessary in many diets to achieve those proportions. (3) Reducing the total fat and the amount of saturated fats are necessary measures for weight control and are part of the best approach now known to the prevention of heart disease.

Leverton points out (15) that providing food and nutrients is neither an exact science nor an easy process, although wise food selection can be taught in broad terms so that persons with minimum nutrition knowledge can help others learn how to plan meals that provide the Allowances. The nutritionist must also remember that failure to consume the RDA does not mean that an individual or a group is malnourished, but indicates a need to consider the possibility of malnutrition when an individual consumes less over a period of time; for example, if the regular iron intake is far below the RDA, it would be wise to test for iron deficiency. As the Allowances are believed to provide generously for the needs of most individuals, it is possible that a particular individual may have lower requirements, hence a lower intake may meet the need.

Leverton discussed three pitfalls in using the Allowances: (1) using them to set risk levels so that dietaries can be judged good or poor, which is frequently done, but the Board did not make provision for such use; (2) failing to provide enough nutrients on a restricted calorie diet, which requires a greater nutritional density (i.e., more nutrients per 100 calories) than is needed in a higher calorie diet; (3) assuming that if the RDA are provided all other needed nutrients will also be provided, an especially fallacious idea when a diet contains many fabricated or synthetic foods.

OTHER DIETARY ALLOWANCES

Community nutritionists working in the United States will have little occasion to use tables, discussed below, prepared for use in other countries, but should know of their existence and how they differ from the Food and Nutrition Board's Recommended Dietary Allowances, which should be used in the United States.

Canadian Dietary Standard

This was formulated in 1968 and was designed for use as a guide in planning diets and food supplies. The amounts were generally lower than the 1968 U.S. Recommended Dietary Allowances. Possible changes in the recommendations have been under study. (6)

FAO-WHO Recommended Intakes of Nutrients

This table, intended for use in developing countries, gives values for energy, protein, seven vitamins, and two minerals. (11) The stated purpose is for use with food composition tables to prepare recommendations for present and future intakes of food for population groups as the necessary data for planning adequate food supplies to meet the needs of such groups. The amounts for various nutrients tend to be lower than the Food and Nutrition Board's Recommended Dietary Allowances.

U.S. RECOMMENDED DAILY ALLOWANCES (U.S. RDA)

These were developed by the Food and Drug Administration in 1973 to replace the Minimum Daily Requirements (MDR). They are not intended to replace or to be used instead of the Food and Nutrition Board RDA. The MDR were established in 1951 by the Food and Drug Administration as a basis for the mandatory labeling of dietary foods and vitamin preparations in accordance with the Federal Food, Drug, and Cosmetic Act.

The U.S. RDA are defined as ". . . the amounts of protein, vitamins and minerals people need each day to stay healthy . . .". (25) They were developed as reference standards for use in nutrition labeling and in labeling vitamin-mineral supplements. There are different sets of values for four population groups. One named "Adults and Children Over Four Years" is used on most food labels. The ones for infants and children are used only for labeling baby and junior foods, while the fourth is only for special use in relation to needs of pregnant and lactating women. The U.S. RDA are based on the 1968 RDA and will be changed only when there are substantial changes in the RDA. No changes were made for the 1974 revision.

The U.S. RDA are based on the highest value of the RDA for each nutrient for any sex-age group, but are higher for protein, ascorbic acid, vitamin E and vitamin B_{12}. Thus many of the U.S. RDA values are 30 to 40 percent or more above the amounts of nutrients for other sex-age groups. For example, niacin is set at 20 milligrams, the RDA for males age 15–22, which is 66 percent above the 12 mg allowance for the female age 57. Values for copper, biotin, and pantothenic acid, nutrients that are not in the RDA table, were formulated for use in labeling vitamin-mineral supplements.

FOOD LABELS AND NUTRITION LABELING

The community nutritionist must teach both professionals and the public what kind of information appears on the label, where it appears, and how the consumer can use it. A collection of food cans, boxes, and packages is easily assembled and provides a good teaching device. It is also a frequent source of information for the nutritionist. Another effective method is education carried out during a visit to a market where labels can be examined.

All food labels must contain the name of the product, weight or measure of the contents, and name and place of business of the manufacturer, packer, or distributor. Usually there is other information on the label, perhaps a description of the food, as "stewed" tomatoes. Often there is a list of ingredients, including additives such as sodium nitrate, BHA, or alginate. Lists of ingredients are not required for some 300 foods such as mayonnaise, which conform to a *standard of identity,* a standardized basic recipe. Some fruit and vegetable products may bear USDA grades that refer mainly to appearance. (26)

Nutrition labeling has been in effect since July 1, 1975, and is required for any food to which a nutrient has been added or that makes any claim about nutritional value. Other foods may also have nutrition labels at the option of the producer.

The law standardizes the layout of the label. (25) The upper part of the label shows serving size and number of servings in the container. It also shows calories in the designated serving and grams of protein, carbohydrate, and fat. The lower part of the label states the percentages of the U.S. RDA for protein, vitamin A, vitamin C, thiamine, riboflavin, niacin, calcium, and iron. This information is required.

The label may also give the percentage of the U.S. RDA for any of 12 additional vitamins and minerals, the percentage of calories from fat, and the amount of polyunsaturated fat, saturated fat, cholesterol, or sodium per serving. (18) There may be similar information for a serving of the food after it is cooked or prepared as directed on the label. It is important to note the serving size since this is designated by the producer. For example, the serving size of tuna may be the entire can of $6\frac{1}{2}$ ounces, an amount larger than is usually served.

There are many other important details in the regulations. When no nutritional claims are made about a specific nutrient, a note may indicate that the product contains less than 2 percent of the U.S. RDA. The values for protein are based on protein quality. If the quality is higher than that of casein, the U.S. RDA of 45 is used for the value, if lower than casein, the U.S. RDA of 65 must be used. (25)

The Food and Drug Administration has also instituted Nutritional Quality Guidelines to prescribe a basic level of nutrient composition for a class of food, such as a frozen dinner. When the product meets the specifications of the Guidelines, it may carry the statement, "This product provides nutrients in amounts appropriate for this class of food as determined by the U.S. Government." (8)

Consumers can use the nutrition labels to compare different brands or kinds of foods, to determine calorie intake, to avoid restricted items (such as sodium or cholesterol), and to learn about the nutritive values of new foods.

FOOD COMPOSITION TABLES

Calculation of the nutrient content, that is, the amounts of energy, carbohydrate, fat, protein, minerals, vitamins, and other constituents of a food, a meal, or a dietary requires tables that give such information about individual foods. There is no one table that can supply all the information needed by most community nutritionists, so they need to be acquainted with a number of publications for this purpose.

The basic source is the USDA publication *Nutritive Value of American Foods In Common Units.* (1) It contains about 1500 foods, almost 2500 items, giving values for household measures and market units. It is a technical publication designed for use of professional and technical personnel. It gives values for water, energy, protein, fat, carbohydrate, calcium, phosphorus, iron, sodium, potassium, vitamin A, thiamin, riboflavin, niacin, and ascorbic acid. A separate table gives information on fatty acids.

Nutritive Value of Foods is another USDA publication giving nutritive values for household measures and metric weights of commonly used foods, including ready-to-eat foods and basic products used in food preparation. It includes 615 items grouped under 10 classes, with values for proximate composition, fatty acids, calcium, iron, and five vitamins and much other useful information. It is a good reference for home economists, serious homemakers, and high school classes as well as nutritionists and dietitians. (24)

Food Values of Portions Commonly Used is a frequent reference for nutritionists. (7) The data are from many sources, mainly from publications and communications of the USDA, with data on commercial food products from the manufacturers. Data are given on energy, protein, vitamins, and minerals, a total of 26 constituents. The lists include basic foods, mixed dishes, and commercial food products with special tables showing nutrition labeling of some foods, nonnutritive ingredients, vitamin-rich products, cholesterol, foods used at various times in history, and so forth. There are also tables for height and weight and for metric conversions.

Community nutritionists will need other publications to obtain nutrient values for many foods now found in U.S. markets patronized by various ethnic groups from Latin America, South America, Mexico,

Samoa, East Asia, Africa and other parts of the world. Many publications are listed in a recent FAO publication. (10) Three that may be needed by the nutritionist will be described.

Food Composition Table for Use in Africa

This gives values for energy, proximate composition, three minerals, and five vitamins for 100-gram portions. (28) It contains 1624 items with the foods divided into 14 food groups, which are cereals and grain products; starchy roots, tubers and fruits; legumes and legume products; nuts and seeds; vegetables and vegetable products; fruits; sugars and syrups; meats, poultry and insects; eggs; fish and shellfish; milk and milk products; oils and fats; beverages; and miscellaneous. English names are used where available, otherwise scientific or local names are used. The data were obtained from published and unpublished materials, from local sources, and other references.

Food Composition Table for Use in East Asia

The table contains 1629 items in 100 gram portions, listed under the same 14 food groups as the Africa publication except that the meat group is meat, poultry and game. (30) The information was obtained from available local data with some analyses for this particular publication. It includes a table of amino acids in addition to the other values in the African table.

INCAP-ICNND Food Composition Table for Use in Latin America

It provides values for 729 items in 14 food groups—cereals and grain products, vegetables, fruits, dry legumes and their products, nuts, dried seeds, sugars and syrups, meat and poultry, eggs, fish and shellfish, milk and milk products, oils and fats, beverages, and miscellaneous. (29) Names are in both English and Spanish. Scientific names are also given. Values are given for proximate composition, energy, three minerals, and five vitamins. The data were compiled from available analyses from the areas where the foods are used and others added from other sources.

Other Sources for Food Values

Some composition data on new foods, brand-name foods, and special dietary foods can now be obtained from labels since labeling is required on any food which has an added nutrient or which makes a nutritional claim. However, specific amounts are required only for calories, protein, carbohydrate, fat, and sodium. Values for vitamins and minerals are given as percentages of the U.S. RDA, so food composition tables must be used for these items, or the amount can be calculated from the label as when the label shows that a food has 10 percent of U.S. RDA of iron. The U.S. RDA is 18 milligrams, so the content is 1.8 milligrams.

Most food manufacturers and distributors can supply useful information about the nutrient content of their products. The trade associations for various industries are another source for this kind of information. The present labeling laws will stimulate industry to provide more values that should add data on many items.

Watt and coauthors report (27) current activities that should lead to extensive, useful, and readily available data. The most important is a computerized Nutrient Data Bank (NDB), which has been established in the U.S. Department of Agriculture "to serve as an international repository for data submitted by industry and experiment stations, from government contracts and grants, and, as before, from literature searches." (27) This will provide a place where data for all nutrients from many sources will be assembled and computerized for storing and retrieval.

Some publications have been prepared to meet specific needs. One USDA publication that is useful for the nutritionist in preparing menus, meal patterns, market orders, and other materials is *Food Yields Summarized by Different Stages of Preparation.* (16) It gives the yield after preparation and the loss or gain in preparation. Losses reflect inedible parts (e.g., bone in meat) and parings and trimmings (e.g., potatoes). Gains include absorption of water, as in cooking rice or oatmeal, and fat, as in frying doughnuts. New data include changes in pork cooked to 77°C instead of 85°C, the previous recommendation, and data on losses in meats in microwave cooking.

FOOD EXCHANGE LISTS

The Food Exchange Lists were developed in 1950 by a joint committee of the American Diabetes Association, American Dietetic Association, and the U.S. Public Health Service to provide a practical way to estimate food values of diabetic diets. They were revised in 1976. (9) They are widely used by nutritionists and dietitians in work with diabetic, low calorie, fat-controlled, and other diets.

The principle of the Exchange Lists is that all exchanges in each group have approximately the same amount of calories, carbohydrate, protein, and fat. Each exchange contains similar minerals and vitamins.

It must be noted that considerable variations exist within the various groups and additional selections are necessary, for example, to select rich sources of ascorbic acid and carotene from the fruit and vegetable exchange lists.

The advantages of the Exchange Lists are the ease with which both professionals and patients can understand and put them to use, and their wide use, so that a patient who changes residence or medical provider can continue to use the same lists. Calculation of food values is still done when necessary.

The revised lists provide for modifications in fats, cholesterol, and calories, and give more information about trace elements and vitamins. They also provide more options within the food groups and a better framework for individualizing diets. Though the booklet is addressed to the patient, it is not intended to stand alone but to be used as a tool in counseling. One experienced nutritionist teaches the use of the Exchange Lists by first demonstrating the selection of a meal using food models, then having each patient select a diet with several possible exchanges.

USDA FAMILY FOOD PLANS, 1974

The three plans at different cost levels—low, moderate and liberal—are based on amounts of foods in each of 15 food groups that will provide a nutritious diet for 12 sex-age groups and for pregnant and lactating women. (21) The Low Cost and Moderate Cost Food Plans will be used frequently. (Figure 9.1, 9.2) A lower cost "Thrifty Food Plan" was discussed on page 98.

The major differences in the low-cost plan as compared with the moderate-cost plan are smaller amounts from the milk group, the meat group, the fruit and vegetable group, and bakery items, and larger amounts of potatoes, cereals, flour, and bread. For the low-cost plan, selections within food groups must be mainly among the least expensive foods and the meals have less variety; however, many families are able to serve palatable and attractive meals using foods consistent with the low-cost plan.

The liberal-cost plan (Figure 9.3) includes a greater variety of foods, more foods from animal sources, and more fruits and vegetables. It includes also more expensive foods and allows for more waste.

The community nutritionist should be familiar with the Family Food Plans because they are the basis for many dietaries and cost estimates, and for most calculations of welfare food budgets. All three plans may be used in estimating food amounts and costs for families and small groups, and for evaluating amounts and costs of foods used.

Family Member	Milk, Cheese, Ice Cream [2]	Meat, Poultry, Fish [3]	Eggs	Dry Beans and Peas, Nuts [4]	Dark-Green, Deep-Yellow Vegetables	Citrus Fruit, Tomatoes	Potatoes	Other Vegetables, Fruit	Cereal	Flour	Bread	Other Bakery Products	Fats, Oils	Sugar, Sweets	Accessories [5]
	Qt	Lb	No.	Lb	Lb	Lb	Lb	Lb	Lb	Lb	Lb	Lb	Lb	Lb	Lb
Child:															
7 months to 1 year	5.70	0.56	2.1	0.15	0.35	0.42	0.06	3.43	0.71[6]	0.02	0.06	0.05	0.05	0.18	0.06
1–2 years	3.57	1.26	3.6	.16	.23	1.01	.60	2.88	.99[6]	.27	.76	.33	.12	.36	.68
3–5 years	3.91	1.52	2.7	.25	.25	1.20	.85	2.95	.90	.30	.91	.57	.38	.71	1.02
6–8 years	4.74	2.03	2.9	.39	.31	1.58	1.10	3.67	1.11	.45	1.27	.84	.52	.90	1.43
9–11 years	5.46	2.57	3.9	.44	.38	2.13	1.41	4.81	1.24	.62	1.65	1.20	.61	1.15	1.89
Male:															
12–14 years	5.74	2.98	4.0	.56	.40	1.99	1.50	3.90	1.15	.67	1.88	1.25	.77	1.15	2.61
15–19 years	5.49	3.74	4.0	.34	.39	2.20	1.87	4.50	.90	.75	2.10	1.55	1.05	1.04	3.09
20–54 years	2.74	4.56	4.0	.33	.48	2.32	1.87	4.81	.93	.71	2.10	1.47	.91	.81	2.11
55 years and over	2.61	3.63	4.0	.21	.61	2.38	1.72	4.92	1.02	.62	1.73	1.23	.77	.90	1.16
Female:															
12–19 years	5.63	2.55	4.0	.24	.46	2.17	1.17	4.57	.75	.63	1.44	1.05	.53	.88	2.44
20–54 years	3.02	3.21	4.0	.19	.55	2.34	1.40	4.17	.71	.55	1.31	.94	.59	.72	2.13
55 years and over	3.01	2.45	4.0	.15	.62	2.54	1.22	4.57	.97	.58	1.24	.86	.38	.64	1.11
Pregnant	5.25	3.68	4.0	.29	.67	2.80	1.65	4.99	.95	.66	1.52	1.06	.55	.78	2.56
Nursing	5.25	4.16	4.0	.26	.66	2.99	1.67	5.33	.78	.61	1.55	1.16	.76	.91	2.70

Figure 9.1 USDA Low-Cost Food plan Showing Amounts of Food for One Week.[1]

[1] Amounts are for food as purchased or brought into the kitchen from garden or farm. Amounts allow for a discard of about one-tenth of the *edible* food as plate waste, spoilage, etc. Amounts of foods are shown to two decimal places to allow for greater accuracy, especially in estimating rations for large groups of people and for long periods of time. For general use, amounts of food groups for a family may be rounded to the nearest tenth or quarter of a pound.

[2] Fluid milk and beverage made from dry or evaporated milk. Cheese and ice cream may replace some milk. Count as equivalent to a quart of fluid milk: Natural or processed Cheddar-type cheese, 6 oz.; cottage cheese, 2½ lbs.; ice cream, 1½ quarts.

[3] Bacon and salt pork should not exceed ⅓ pound for each 5 pounds of this group.

[4] Weight in terms of dry beans and peas, shelled nuts, and peanut butter. Count 1 pound of canned dry beans—pork and beans, kidney beans, etc.— as .33 pound.

[5] Includes coffee, tea, cocoa, punches, ades, soft drinks, leavenings, and seasonings. The use of iodized salt is recommended.

[6] Cereal fortified with iron is recommended.

Source: U.S. Department of Agriculture, Agricultural Research Service, *USDA Family Food Plans, 1974.* Talk by Betty Peterkin, 12/12/74, p. 23.

Family Member	Milk, Cheese, Ice Cream [2]	Meat, Poultry, Fish [1]	Eggs	Dry Beans and Peas, Nuts [1]	Dark-Green, Deep-Yellow Vegetables	Citrus Fruit, Tomatoes	Potatoes	Other Vegetables, Fruit	Cereal	Flour	Bread	Other Bakery Products	Fats, Oils	Sugar, Sweets	Accessories [5]
	Qt	Lb	No.	Lb	Lb	Lb	Lb	Lb	Lb	Lb	Lb	Lb	Lb	Lb	Lb
Child:															
7 months to 1 year	6.46	0.80	2.2	0.13	0.41	0.49	0.06	3.98	[6] 0.64	0.02	0.06	0.05	0.05	0.19	0.08
1–2 years	4.04	1.69	4.0	.15	.29	1.24	.59	3.44	1.03	.26	.81	.33	.12	.26	.79
3–5 years	4.74	1.88	3.0	.22	.30	1.46	.85	3.51	.74	.27	.82	.73	.41	.81	1.42
6–8 years	5.79	2.60	3.3	.34	.37	1.94	1.17	4.39	.84	.39	1.14	1.11	.56	1.03	1.97
9–11 years	6.68	3.31	4.0	.38	.45	2.61	1.40	5.76	1.03	.51	1.47	1.51	.66	1.31	2.63
Male:															
12–14 years	7.02	3.77	4.0	.48	.48	2.44	1.52	4.66	.94	.56	1.69	1.54	.85	1.34	3.65
15–19 years	6.65	4.65	4.0	.29	.47	2.73	2.00	5.45	.80	.67	1.98	1.82	1.05	1.15	4.41
20–54 years	3.38	5.73	4.0	.29	.59	2.92	1.94	5.93	.76	.65	1.97	1.65	.95	.96	2.95
55 years and over	2.97	4.64	4.0	.19	.70	2.91	1.69	5.88	.89	.53	1.58	1.45	.87	1.05	1.50
Female:															
12–19 years	6.22	3.32	4.0	.24	.53	2.62	1.21	5.38	.68	.56	1.34	1.22	.56	.97	3.36
20–54 years	3.35	4.12	4.0	.19	.62	2.84	1.35	4.94	.54	.49	1.28	1.08	.65	.81	2.89
55 years and over	3.35	3.21	4.0	.14	.72	3.09	1.17	5.50	.81	.52	1.20	.98	.45	.73	1.39
Pregnant	5.44	4.57	4.0	.25	.91	3.52	1.60	6.13	.73	.83	1.77	1.28	.46	.85	3.50
Nursing	5.31	5.01	4.0	.26	.91	3.76	1.73	6.52	.74	.81	1.84	1.42	.69	1.00	3.79

[1] Amounts are for food as purchased or brought into the kitchen from garden or farm. Amounts allow for a discard of about one-sixth of the *edible* food as plate waste, spoilage, etc. Amounts of foods are shown to two decimal places to allow for greater accuracy, especially in estimating rations for large groups of people and for long periods of time. For general use, amounts of food groups for a family may be rounded to the nearest tenth or quarter of a pound.

[2] Fluid milk and beverage made from dry or evaporated milk. Cheese and ice cream may replace some milk. Count as equivalent to a quart of fluid milk: Natural or processed Cheddar-type cheese, 6 oz.; cottage cheese, 2½ lbs.; ice cream, 1½ quarts.

[3] Bacon and salt pork should not exceed ⅓ pound for each 5 pounds of this group.

[4] Weight in terms of dry beans and peas, shelled nuts, and peanut butter. Count 1 pound of canned dry beans—pork and beans, kidney beans, etc.— as .33 pound.

[5] Includes coffee, tea, cocoa, punches, ades, soft drinks, leavenings, and seasonings. The use of iodized salt is recommended.

[6] Cereal fortified with iron is recommended.

Source: U.S. Department of Agriculture, Agricultural Research Service, *USDA Family Food Plans, 1974.* Talk by Betty Peterkin, 12/12/74, p. 24.

Figure 9.2 USDA Moderate Cost Food Plan Showing Amounts of Food for One Week [1]

Family Member	Milk, Cheese, Ice Cream [2]	Meat, Poultry, Fish [3]	Eggs	Dry Beans and Peas, Nuts [4]	Dark-Green, Deep-Yellow Vegetables	Citrus Fruit, Tomatoes	Potatoes	Other Vegetables, Fruit	Cereal	Flour	Bread	Other Bakery Products	Fats, Oils	Sugar, Sweets	Accessories [5]
	Qt	Lb	No.	Lb	Lb	Lb	Lb	Lb	Lb	Lb	Lb	Lb	Lb	Lb	Lb
Child:															
7 months to 1 year	6.94	0.97	2.3	0.14	0.43	0.60	0.06	4.71	[6] 0.64	0.02	0.05	0.06	0.05	0.20	0.09
1–2 years	4.26	2.07	4.0	.17	.31	1.50	.59	4.10	[6] 1.07	.28	.82	.35	.13	.27	.95
3–5 years	5.08	2.35	3.1	.23	.32	1.77	.85	4.18	.76	.27	.79	.78	.45	.85	1.74
6–8 years	6.25	3.18	3.4	.36	.40	2.35	1.18	5.21	.85	.39	1.08	1.23	.60	1.08	2.41
9–11 years	7.21	4.04	4.0	.39	.48	3.15	1.41	6.83	1.04	.51	1.39	1.67	.71	1.38	3.21
Male:															
12–14 years	7.57	4.57	4.0	.50	.51	2.94	1.52	5.52	.95	.56	1.60	1.71	.92	1.40	4.47
15–19 years	7.18	5.59	4.0	.31	.50	3.29	2.01	6.45	.84	.69	1.92	2.05	1.07	1.20	5.36
20–54 years	3.64	6.83	4.0	.32	.62	3.51	1.95	6.99	.79	.66	1.91	1.86	.95	1.00	3.54
55 years and over	3.24	5.54	4.0	.19	.76	3.52	1.68	6.97	.89	.54	1.49	1.57	.94	1.09	1.82
Female:															
12–19 years	6.72	3.97	4.0	.25	.56	3.15	1.21	6.34	.71	.59	1.31	1.35	.54	.98	4.09
20–54 years	3.62	4.86	4.0	.20	.66	3.41	1.35	5.81	.56	.51	1.24	1.22	.66	.84	3.47
55 years and over	3.65	3.79	4.0	.15	.76	3.71	1.14	6.42	.74	.54	1.17	1.12	.48	.77	1.66
Pregnant	5.91	5.43	4.0	.26	.96	4.22	1.57	7.17	.70	.87	1.70	1.45	.46	.87	4.20
Nursing	5.76	5.97	4.0	.28	.97	4.51	1.72	7.66	.75	.84	1.76	1.58	.68	1.02	4.52

[1] Amounts are for food as purchased or brought into the kitchen from garden or farm. Amounts allow for a discard of about one-fourth of the *edible* food as plate waste, spoilage, etc. Amounts of foods are shown to two decimal places to allow for greater accuracy, especially in estimating rations for large groups of people and for long periods of time. For general use, amounts of food groups for a family may be rounded to the nearest tenth or quarter of a pound.

[2] Fluid milk and beverage made from dry or evaporated milk. Cheese and ice cream may replace some milk. Count as equivalent to a quart of fluid milk: Natural or processed Cheddar-type cheese, 6 oz.; cottage cheese, $2\frac{1}{2}$ lbs.; ice cream, $1\frac{1}{2}$ quarts.

[3] Bacon and salt pork should not exceed $\frac{1}{3}$ pound for each 5 pounds of this group.

[4] Weight in terms of dry beans and peas, shelled nuts, and peanut butter. Count 1 pound of canned dry beans—pork and beans, kidney beans, etc.—as .33 pound.

[5] Includes coffee, tea, cocoa, punches, ades, soft drinks, leavenings, and seasonings. The use of iodized salt is recommended.

[6] Cereal fortified with iron is recommended.

Source: U.S. Department of Agriculture, Agricultural Research Service, *USDA Family Food Plans, 1974.* Talk by Betty Peterkin, 12/12/74, p. 25.

Figure 9.3 USDA Liberal-Cost Food Plan Showing Amounts of Food for One Week.[1]

145

The Family Food Plans provide diets consistent with typical U.S. food patterns according to data obtained in the 1965–66 Household Food Consumption Survey (p. 21). However, modifications in the food groups are necessary to adapt them to some cultural food patterns, for example, when large quantities of rice are consumed instead of the bread and potatoes of most American diets. Foods and quantities in the 1974 food plans were modified to conform with changes in information about food values, new foods, relative costs of foods, and types of foods used, and to adjust for computer use. The Food Plans were based on the 1974 Recommended Dietary Allowances, with modifications in amounts of foods to provide the nutrients.

The completed food plans meet the RDA for energy, protein, calcium, iron, vitamin A value, thiamin, riboflavin, niacin, and ascorbic acid. Fat provides 40 percent or less of total calories. Iron amounts were based on the higher enrichment levels proposed by the Food and Drug Administration in 1973, but these were not adopted. Probably only 80 percent of the RDA levels for vitamins B_6 and magnesium are provided by the plans, but this was assumed to be acceptable in view of the limited food composition data for these two nutrients.

The Plans are used as the basis for updating costs in selected cities across the U.S. The list includes 100 foods that are priced routinely by the Bureau of Labor Statistics (BLS).

The Plans are used for regular estimation of costs for several cities following a specific procedure that involves collecting prices, weighing foods in each food group, and setting a price per weighed pound, quart, and so forth. It is anticipated that there can be a better estimate of the nutritional quality of the Food Plans when more complete food composition data are available from the Nutrient Data Bank now under development. (21, 27)

FOOD GUIDES AND FOOD GROUPS

Though much nutrition information is available in the media, in books, and in advertisements, planning meals that supply the proper nutrients begins with food. The usual method is to divide foods into groups according to the kind of nutrients they contain and their use in meals. All food guides and patterns should incorporate provisions for calorie and weight control.

A review by Hertzler and Anderson gives the history and development of food guides used in the U.S. starting with the one used by Atwater in 1894. (13) Ahlstrom and Rasanen have reviewed the food group systems used in 47 countries. (2)

History and Use of Food Guides

Many food groupings have been developed with three to eleven groups. Each guide has been planned to emphasize foods of particular importance to the country, ethnic group, or food industry for which it was developed.

Food guides have proved useful because they can be prepared to include all cultural foods and adjusted to all meal patterns, including the snacking and nibbling patterns common today.

Some early teaching guides in the U.S. were based on the eleven food groups then used by the USDA in its food consumption studies. A five-group guide used in Puerto Rico was described by Roberts. (23) One of the premises in its use was to emphasize foods that were being used in inadequate amounts while not emphasizing foods that were already being consumed in adequate amounts by most Puerto Ricans.

In the 1940's, after publication of the first Recommended Dietary Allowances, the Federal government developed the "Basic Seven" food grouping. This gave special emphasis to green leafy and yellow vegetables, citrus fruits and tomatoes; put eggs, dried beans and nuts into the meat group; and had a separate group for butter and fortified margarine. There was a group for whole grain and enriched breads and cereals while baked foods made with unenriched flour, such as crackers, sweet rolls, special breads, and many cereals were not included in the basic food groups. The Basic Seven groups have been largely replaced by the Four Food Group Plan.

The Four Food Groups

Hertzler and Anderson explain the use of the Four Food Groups as developed in the publication, *Essentials of an Adequate Diet.* (13) The meat, milk, and fruit-vegetable groups were intended to be major sources of one or two nutrients and to supply a significant amount (one-fourth or more) of another two or more nutrients. The bread-cereal group was expected to supply at low cost and on a regular basis important amounts of most nutrients. Since that time, a problem has arisen in use of food groups due to the increase in synthetic and fabricated foods because they do not supply the same basic amounts of nutrients as are supplied by the foods they replace. An example is use of spun soy products to replace meat.

Though the Four Food Groups are used as a teaching tool in elementary school and high school, with nurses and homemakers, and appear in advertisement in all forms of media, there are still some misconceptions about their use. Perhaps the most common are the following:

1. That using the recommended number of servings from each group assures that all needed nutrients will be supplied. Actually, careful selection of foods from the four food groups is necessary to make a food list that provides the daily RDA for individuals. Choosing oat or wheat cereals rather than corn cereals, pork rather than beef, cantaloupe rather than casaba melon, orange rather than tomato, make important differences in food value. Another important point about selection within groups is that this is the best way to get a variety of foods that helps to assure getting all trace elements.

2. That all nutrients will not be supplied unless the specified foods from each group are consumed. It is possible to get all the nutrients without having the specified number of foods from each group. Perhaps the best example is found when one of the "prize package" foods such as liver is used, since its high amount of iron, vitamin A, riboflavin, and niacin can compensate for lack of other sources of these nutrients.

3. That there is no reason to eat more foods than specified from each of the four groups. Actually, it is nutritionally advantageous to eat more basic foods as this will tend to compensate for selections of lower value from the groups, and to minimize consumption of sweets and other foods that provide only calories.

4. That the recommended amounts of foods from the four groups will lead to obesity. Actually, they provide about 1200–1400 calories so will not in themselves lead to obesity. Careful control of fat and sugar used in cooking and serving is necessary to avoid these high sources of calories. Limiting fat and sugar also reduces the amount of other foods consumed; for example, limiting butter reduces bread consumption, limiting meat fat reduces potato consumption, and limiting both fat and sugar reduces the use of high calorie desserts, such as pie, cake, cookies, and ice cream.

Food groups, including the four food groups much used in the United States, provide a convenient, adaptable tool for teaching most population groups. Nutritionists still need to make frequent calculations from the specific foods as a check on the practical use of food groups, the distribution of fatty acids, and to see that they supply fiber, trace elements, and vitamins of recently developed concern.

FOOD INTAKE RECORD FORM

This form is used to record the food intake of an individual or family. It may be used for either a *food recall* or a *food record*. The *recall* is made from the client's memory of food eaten in the preceding 24 hours, and written on the form by the client or by the interviewer. The *record* is kept by the client at home for a specified period, usually one day or sometimes three days.

In preparing the forms, care should be taken not to force the client into recording a three-meal-a-day pattern. The nutritionist may find a need for several kinds of food records and will need to develop special ones for particular situations, for example, one for the nibbling food pattern with no meal designations, or one for taking records on young children who are not in a three-meal-a-day pattern.

The first sample form (Figure 9.4), designed for the client to complete, has instructions and names of meals. The second (Figure 9.5) was designed for use in a prenatal clinic where the nurse regularly counsels the patients. The form may also be used by a nutritionist or physician. It has space for the nurse's notes and is filed in the patient's chart. The third (Figure 9.6) is for clients not on a three-meal-a-day plan.

The food record can provide information on food preferences, nutrient intake, amount spent on food, sources of calories, sources of sodium, amount and types of fat, use of cultural foods, and other information. Reviewing a number of records is a way to identify problems common to many clients. The information may be used in public education, for inservice education of nurses, and in teaching leaflets and resource materials.

A food record form for computer use was developed by Johnson and coworkers (14) with a computer program to process the data. They believe that the method can be used as a screening device to determine the adequacy of nutrients consumed by a low income population. The form comes with printed instructions and helps for interpretation and is completed by the client shading a half or whole box. The authors believe that the dietary information obtained can be used to guide education or intervention programs.

FOODS AND FOOD MODELS

Food and food models provide ideal teaching tools in community nutrition. When the objective is to encourage use of a new food or a new method of preparation, nothing surpasses real food to show selection and cooking and serving possibilities. Tasting the product is a most effective way to encourage use; for example, many persons have decided to eat liver regularly after trying it chopped and seasoned or made into a beef and liver loaf.

In teaching professionals or paramedical personnel about ethnic food practices, showing the difference between specific foods such as plain

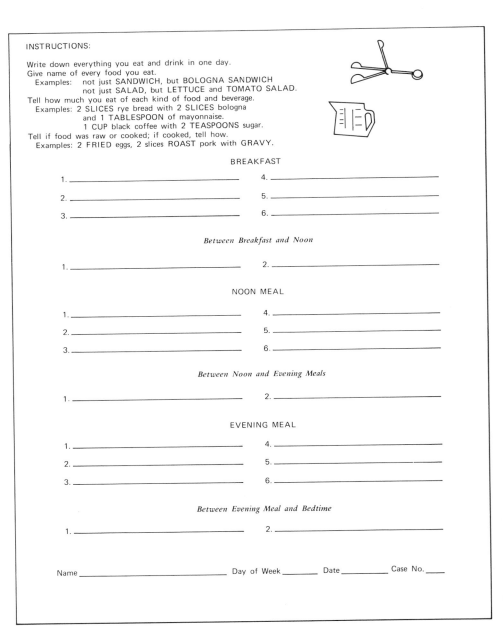

INSTRUCTIONS:

Write down everything you eat and drink in one day.
Give name of every food you eat.
   Examples: not just SANDWICH, but BOLOGNA SANDWICH
                  not just SALAD, but LETTUCE and TOMATO SALAD.
Tell how much you eat of each kind of food and beverage.
   Examples: 2 SLICES rye bread with 2 SLICES bologna
             and 1 TABLESPOON of mayonnaise.
             1 CUP black coffee with 2 TEASPOONS sugar.
Tell if food was raw or cooked; if cooked, tell how.
   Examples: 2 FRIED eggs, 2 slices ROAST pork with GRAVY.

BREAKFAST

1. _____   4. _____

2. _____   5. _____

3. _____   6. _____

Between Breakfast and Noon

1. _____   2. _____

NOON MEAL

1. _____   4. _____

2. _____   5. _____

3. _____   6. _____

Between Noon and Evening Meals

1. _____   2. _____

EVENING MEAL

1. _____   4. _____

2. _____   5. _____

3. _____   6. _____

Between Evening Meal and Bedtime

1. _____   2. _____

Name _____ Day of Week _____ Date _____ Case No. ____

Figure 9.4   Record of Foods Eaten in One Day.

INSTRUCTIONS:
- ☐ Write down everything you ate and drank in one day, OR
- ☐ Write down everything you served your family and yourself in one day.
  Give the specific names and amounts of foods, for example, write:
  - ½ cup orange juice, NOT JUST fruit juice;
  - 2 slices roast pork with gravy, NOT JUST meat;
  - 2 slices rye bread with 2 slices bologna and
  - 1 tablespoon of mayonnaise, NOT JUST sandwich.

NURSE'S RECORD	
Food Groups	Amounts Eaten
Milk	_____
Meat	_____
Vegetable-Fruit	_____
Vitamin A . .	_____
Vitamin C . .	_____
Other	_____
Cereal-Bread .	_____

BREAKFAST   Time of Day _____

amount   name of food   amount   name of food

BETWEEN MEALS   Time of Day _____

amount   name of food   amount   name of food

NOON MEAL   Time of Day _____

amount   name of food   amount   name of food

BETWEEN MEALS   Time of Day _____

amount   name of food   amount   name of food

EVENING MEAL   Time of Day _____

amount   name of food   amount   name of food

BETWEEN MEALS   Time of Day _____

amount   name of food   amount   name of food

Is this the way you usually eat?   ☐ YES   ☐ NO

Day: _____ Date: _____

OTHER INFORMATION

FOOD MONEY

$ _____ per week for _____ persons.

MODIFIED DIET

OTHER

CHANGES NEEDED

INSTRUCTIONS GIVEN

LEAFLETS GIVEN

NURSE'S SIGNATURE

DATE

CLINICIAN'S SIGNATURE

_____ M.D.

FOOD RECORD
Public Health Nutrition Division
County of Los Angeles Health Dept.
H-101 (Rev. 10-68)
76R208D—Cdb 11-71

PATIENT'S NAME

RECORD NUMBER

Figure 9.5   Food Record.

FOOD RECORD FOR _____

Name   Date

Please write down everything you ate and drank on the day named.

time   amount   name of food   time   amount   name of food

Figure 9.6   Food Record for Unstructured Eating Pattern.

and converted rice will make it clear there are real differences that account for the preferences of some cultural groups for the plain kind. A display of the bread types used by various cultural groups, for example, whole wheat bread, cornbread, flour tortillas, and pita bread, and showing how they are used provides an opportunity to discuss similarities in nutrient content.

Food models are available in a number of versions, three-dimensional in plastic and flat in cardboard. They can be used to show sizes of portions and appearance of the prepared product and for practice in food selection in groups. Plastic models of many foods are available while others can be custom made. Sources of food models are given at the end of this chapter. The nutritionist can also make a flat set or add to the commercial sets by mounting food pictures from magazines on cardboard to get foods that are not included in the sets. Related items can sometimes be used to get attention, for example, a paper fish, a toy plastic pig, or a giant inflated orange.

RECIPES AND PREPARATION METHODS

When using recipes in preparing teaching materials, it is important that they be tested, accurate ones, with the required equipment and ingredients likely to be available in the homes of the persons involved, and that they have simple, clear directions easily followed. The resulting product must be one that will be acceptable to the cultural group concerned. Sometimes a recipe can be developed with the group and group members encouraged to try it before the next meeting.

Nutritionists should know standard proportions and food preparation methods so they can suggest changes to fit a favorite family recipe into a special diet pattern and fit a modified diet for one member into the family meal pattern with a minimum of extra work and cost. The need for such a modification may arise when a family member is diagnosed as a diabetic, or one member needs a restricted sodium diet. The nutritionist can suggest plain fruit for dessert when the family has pie, or lemon and herbs as seasoning instead of the salt used in the regular family food.

Changes in preparation methods may also be needed when new information becomes available on nutrients, foods or meals, or when less expensive ingredients are to be substituted for commonly used ones, as nonfat dry milk for fresh whole milk. Sometimes it may be feasible to apply the modification for one person to the food for the whole family, as substituting a polyunsaturated oil for saturated fat in cooking in products where the substitution makes little difference in the physical characteristics of the finished product. A good basic cookbook and information about seasoning are an important part of the nutritionist's tools. A good source for general information about cooking is the AHEA *Handbook of Food Preparation,* which gives proportions, standard methods, substitutions, and similar information. (4)

RESOURCE MATERIALS FOR PROFESSIONALS

These consist of printed materials, films, programmed learning devices and other items designed to provide food and nutrition subject matter, related information for content, and information about program methods. Often when a teaching tool is prepared for use in instructing an individual, a group or a community, a companion piece is needed to help nutritionists, nurses, aides, or other persons use the tool effectively. This should concentrate on background information pertinent to the specific teaching tool, so it is frequently necessary for the nutritionist to prepare a special piece to meet the need. Something originally prepared for other use, or by persons not informed about the specific situation, will often contain extraneous material or lack pertinent information, or will not fit in with other materials in use, causing confusion for the person with limited nutrition background.

Another purpose of preparing resource material for a specific use is to synthesize ideas from a variety of sources. In one agency, staff nutritionists needed to know what they could appropriately say and do about exercise as a part of weight control. Two of them reviewed the literature, obtained other information, and, utilizing these sources, prepared a handbook on the subject for staff use.

TEACHING MATERIALS FOR NUTRITION EDUCATION

These include all devices for nutrition education, for instruction and counseling, general distribution, or other uses. Examples are leaflets on normal diet, prenatal diet, food money management, and ways to increase milk consumption.

Some of the newer types of equipment have been reviewed in "Audiovisual Methods for Nutrition Educators." (5) In some agencies and usually in schools, health educators and other specialists are available to help the teacher make effective use of audiovisual materials. Programmed learning and computer-assisted learning may be available in some agencies and schools. The small projectors designed for self-instruction or the cassette player-recorder may be very useful to provide repetition after teaching. They enable the individual learner to study and test until there is certainty that the subject has been mastered.

Audiovisual and printed materials should be used as tools by the educator, not as substitutes for teacher action. This applies as well to visiting speakers who come to a group to explain their programs; they should be considered as helping the teacher present a unified picture, rather than as substitute teachers themselves.

SUMMARY

Nutritionists need many tools to conduct their work. The NRC Recommended Dietary Allowances provide the foundation for selecting food for the diet. Everyone who reads labels is becoming acquainted with the U.S. Recommended Daily Allowances, which are the reference standards for labeling of foods and food supplements. The nutritionist makes constant use of the common food composition tables and frequently needs values for some exotic foods to answer questions of professionals and the public.

The Food Exchange Lists are a useful tool in normal nutrition as well as modified diets. The Low Cost Food Plan is used in teaching and calculating costs for low income families. When more money is available, the Moderate and Liberal Cost Plans are used in estimating food amounts and costs for families and small groups.

Many food groupings have been used in the past. Currently the Four Food Group Plan is the most widely used. Food records of various formats may be prepared to record food intakes. For example, they can be based on a three meal pattern or on an unstructured listing of foods.

The nutritionist needs skill in using recipes and should be acquainted with standard proportions and food preparation methods to help families adjust their food practices to meet requirements imposed by income, diet modifications, or limited facilities.

REFERENCES CITED

1. Adams, Catherine F., *Nutritive Value of American Foods in Common Units,* Agriculture Handbook No. 456, United States Dept. of Agriculture, Washington DC, 1975.
2. Ahlstrom, Antti, and Leena Rasanen, Review of Food Grouping Systems in Nutrition Education, *J. Nutr. Educ.,* 5 1–3/73 13–17.
3. Alfin-Slater, Roslyn, Fats, Essential Fatty Acids, and Ascorbic Acid., *J. Am. Diet. Assoc.,* 64 2/74 169.
4. American Home Economics Association, *Handbook of Food Preparation,* 7th ed., American Home Economics Association, Washington DC, 1975.
5. Audiovisual Methods for Nutrition Educators, *J. Am. Diet. Assoc.,* 63 11/73 550.
6. Campbell, J. A., Approaches in Revising Dietary Standards, *J. Am. Diet. Assoc.,* 64 2/74 175.
7. Church, Charles F., and Helen N. Church, *Food Values of Portions Commonly Used: Bowes and Church,* 12th ed., J. B. Lippincott, Philadelphia, 1975.
8. Dunning, H. Neal, and Ogden C. Johnson, Nutrient Labeling and Guidelines, in *Shoppers Guide, the 1974 Yearbook of Agriculture,* U.S. Department of Agriculture, Washington DC, p. 62.
9. *Exchange Lists for Meal Planning,* American Diabetes Association and American Dietetic Association, Chicago, 1976.
10. Food and Agriculture Organization of the United Nations, *Food Composition Tables: Updated Annotated Bibliography,* Rome, 1975.

11. Food and Agriculture Organization of the United Nations, *Handbook on Human Nutritional Requirements*, FAO Nutritional Studies No. 28, WHO Monograph Series No. 61, Rome, 1974.

12. Harper, Alfred E., Recommended Dietary Allowances: Are They What We Think They Are?, *J. Am. Diet. Assoc.*, 64 2/74 151.

13. Hertzler, Ann A., and Helen L. Anderson, Food Guides in the United States, *J. Am. Diet. Assoc.*, 64 1/74 18.

14. Johnson, Nancy E., Susan Nitzke, and Dina VandeBerg, A Reporting System for Nutrient Adequacy, *Home Econ. Res. J.*, 2 6/74 210.

15. Leverton, Ruth L., The RDA's Are Not for Amateurs, *J. Am. Diet Assoc.*, 66 1/75 9.

16. Matthews, Ruth H., and Garrison J. Young, *Food Yields Summarized by Different Stages of Preparation*, U.S. Dept. of Agriculture, Agriculture Handbook No. 102, Washington DC, Rev. 1975.

17. National Nutrition Consortium, Inc., with Ronald M. Deutsch, *Nutrition Labeling: How It Can Work for You*, National Nutrition Consortium, Bethesda MD, 1975, 68.

18. Ibid., 96.

19. National Research Council, Food and Nutrition Board, *Recommended Dietary Allowances*, 8th ed., National Academy of Sciences, Washington DC, 1974, 2.

20. Ibid., 35.

21. Peterkin, Betty, USDA Family Food Plans, 1974, *Family Economics Review*, 1975, ARS-NE-36, United States Department of Agriculture, 3.

22. Peterkin, Betty, USDA Family Food Plans, 1974, Talk at National Agricultural Outlook Conference, Washington, D.C., 12/12/74, United States Department of Agriculture, 15.

23. Roberts, Lydia, J., A Basic Food Plan for Puerto Rico, *J. Am. Diet. Assoc.*, 30 11/54 1097–1100.

24. United States Department of Agriculture, *Nutritive Value of Foods*, Home and Garden Bulletin No. 72, Government Printing Office, Washington DC, Rev. Jan. 1971.

25. United States Department of Health, Education, and Welfare, Food and Drug Administration, *Read the Label, Set a Better Table*, leaflet, Rockville MD, DHEW Pub. No. (FDA) 75-40001.

26. United States Department of Health, Education, and Welfare, Food and Drug Administration, We Want You To Know About Labels on Foods, leaflet, DHEW Pub. No. (FDA) 75-2008, Washington DC, 1973.

27. Watt, Bernice K., Susan W. Gebhardt, Elizabeth W. Murphy, and Ritva R. Butrum, Food Composition Tables for the 70's, *J. Am. Diet. Assoc.*, 64 3/74 257.

28. Wu Leung, W. T., F. Busson, and C. Jardin, *Food Composition Table for Use in Africa*, U.S. Dept. of Health, Education, and Welfare, Bethesda MD, and Food and Agriculture Organization of the United Nations, Rome, 1968.

29. Wu Leung, W. T., and Marina Flores, *INCAP-ICNND Food Composition Table for Use in Latin America*, Interdepartmental Committee on Nutri-

tion for National Defense, National Institutes of Health, Bethesda MD, 1961.

30. Wu Leung, W. T., Ritva Rauanheimo, and Flora Chang, *Food Composition Table for Use in East Asia,* United States Department of Health, Education, and Welfare, National Institutes of Health, Bethesda MD, 1972.

SOURCES OF FOOD MODELS

Address   Telephone

Nasco
901 Janesville Avenue   (414) 563-2446
Fort Atkinson, WI 53538

or
1524 Princeton Avenue   (209) 529-6957
Modesto, CA 95352

Vinyl plastic replicas of 200 foods in individual servings and market units. Can custom-make other items.

National Dairy Council
6300 North River Road   (312) 696-1020
Rosemont, IL 60018

Cardboard food models of individual servings, in color. Contact above office or local Dairy Council.

CHAPTER 10

BASIC SKILLS

Though the field of community nutrition is very complex, the work is accomplished by the application of a number of basic skills. By definition, *skill* is the ability to do something well as a result of knowledge, training, and practice. In a community nutrition program, there is a need for a nutritionist and other personnel who have many skills. The community nutritionist needs the ability both to perform the necessary skills and to teach them to others, sometimes requiring only a few skills and sometimes many, depending on the particular position. The skills are applied in the broad techniques used in community nutrition programs.

The nutritionist will learn some skills in college courses, but others must be learned in field work or in inservice education, or acquired on the job. Some nutritionists, especially those who enter the field in their middle years, will have the advantage of experience in child rearing, family management, food planning, and other home tasks.

EDUCATION IN COMMUNITY NUTRITION

Much of the work of the community nutritionist is education of individuals and groups. The work is with people of all ages, both the public and professionals. A course in educational methods should be part of the nutritionist's preparation. The emphasis here will be on certain principles and processes which are involved in the various skills and techniques of community nutrition. Much of the present material on changing practices is based on diet in disease treatment in the hospital setting. In community nutrition, similar methods must be applied to the maintenance of good nutrition and prevention of disease among well people, as well as to disease treatment.

The skills and techniques of community nutrition reflect both the educational process and the change process since the improvement of nutrition practices requires change. The community nutritionist must understand how to use these processes effectively. The skills of establishing rapport, teaching, instructing, interviewing, and counseling are also applied in many other skills; they will be discussed as general methods.

The Educational Process

The educational process is the development of the knowledge and skills of others for the purpose of producing changes in behavior. The community nutritionist is constantly engaged in teaching that is, helping others to learn something. Much of this teaching is in informal contacts or by indirect methods. Some teaching is by the instruction process in which knowledge is provided in a systematic, preplanned manner. Craig characterizes the educational process as "a process of creating and arranging situations that stimulate and guide learning activity toward desirable goals." (6)

Though most educators have observed that many people tend to resist change, it seems to be agreed that the educator can make it more acceptable in several ways. The teacher must make sure that the change is understood, having the individual participate in the process, and helping with the decision to change. The concept should be established first and the change developed from it. Learning should proceed from one small change that is comparatively easy to a bigger, more difficult one. The change should proceed as part of a plan rather than as an isolated action, with the teacher helping the learner see that important benefits will result.

Craig points out the need for four phases of teaching: (1) preparation, by both teacher and learner; (2) presentation, by teacher; (3) application and active involvement of the learner; (4) evaluation and checking to see if the learner has learned.

The good teacher is well informed about subject matter, enthusiastic about the benefits the learner will derive from the change, and able to get the individual or group to accept the teacher as both friend and helper.

Using the Change Process. The process of change, or learning, occurs in a number of phases that are not necessarily clear-cut or in this order. (6, 10, 28)

1. The individual recognizes that there is need for change and that it is possible as there are other foods to eat and other activity patterns, and that better food practices will benefit the family's health.

2. The individual is led to a belief that the change is worthwhile. Motivation may be achieved through giving information about nutrition or suggestions about food or by developing a desire for improvement in family health. The teacher must see the change through the eyes of the client and help identify the barriers to change. Selecting the right change is very important; it must be one that has a good chance for success. At this point, the teacher must interest the student in making a change by helping the student realize the benefits it would bring.

3. The individual looks at different ways change may be accomplished, considers how it can be done, and what the result will be. The teacher must help the individual answer these questions and decide what change to make.

4. At this point, the change should be tested by some action method such as performing it through simulation, by playing roles, or in another way.

5. The individual must decide to give the new idea further trial at home or at work. If the trial is successful, the change may be adopted.

6. When possible, the new practice is reinforced later by repetition, by application in a related situation or by means of a new method.

The change process can be applied in many situations in the education of the public and professionals and in producing change in self, peers, or professional colleagues. The nutritionist should note that the method may be applied in reverse as protection against changes others wish to make. Identifying the process when used by others, as in advertising or selling, can help the individual avoid an unwanted change by termination of the contact at an early stage.

Vargas has suggested ways to change habits and to motivate change, emphasizing the importance of using small steps. (28) She describes the teaching process as one in which emphasis is placed on what the students are doing rather than on what the teacher is doing. She suggests that the objectives should be stated in terms of what the student can do as a result of the teaching, for example, when studying a restricted sodium diet, the students can name compounds high in sodium (such as baking soda and salt), plan low sodium meals for a day and order a restaurant meal for the low sodium diet. Vargas also suggests that individual participation can be achieved even in a large group; for example, after showing a film on food preparation, each learner can complete a written exercise that covers the content and can suggest changes that could be made in the home to accomplish the same objectives. The nutritionist will need to find other methods for persons who do not read or write.

Frankle reports that in a youth program where activity or life style was a problem the counseling nutritionist needed to use three steps to produce change. These were (1) getting the individual to recognize that current behavior was a problem and that there was an alternative, (2) refuting erroneous information, and (3) initiating new learning. Before the third step, the existing practices were designated as beneficial, neutral, or harmful. Efforts to change were concentrated on the last. (8)

Leypoldt mentions (18) some points of special importance in changing adults. The learning process must be two-way between teacher and learner, and both must share the responsibility for success or failure of the learning process. The adult's ideas, attitudes, and knowledge are the result of a lifetime of experiences. The teacher needs to help the adult learner recognize this and challenge beliefs when necessary.

Many adults have food beliefs based on misinformation that must be changed before correct information can be taught. The nutritionist needs to develop ways to do this, watching for the right time to challenge incorrect ideas and the best way to exchange them for correct ones.

Adults learn best what they want to know, what is useful to them at the time, and what they can apply immediately. They must be personally involved, for example, keeping their own food records, calculating sugar and fat in their own meals, or making a food list for themselves.

In any group or community, either professional or public, there are leaders who are the first to change. Their reports on a positive experience cause others to change. The nutritionist should identify these people early and keep them informed so that they will lead the way in changes in food practices as well as support new programs.

Gifft and coauthors point out (11) the need for continued reinforcement of learning that results in making the necessary adjustments and in transfer of the learning to other experiences. Repetition, which is one way, may be accomplished by use of some of the newer tools such as programmed learning, or by role playing, exhibits, charts, or posters, or work with food or food models.

Repetition may also be provided in a series of counseling sessions or in a class with the counselor, or in further counseling by another person, usually the nurse or nutrition aide. Reed reports a situation in which reenforcement of dietary counseling was provided by a cassette recording of the counseling session that the patient took home to hear as many times as desired. Many patients brought their own cassettes for the recording. The hospital cassettes were loaned to others. When the patient did not have the necessary equipment, the library arranged to loan both cassette and cassette player. (25)

Establishing Rapport

The development of rapport, which is a sympathetic and friendly working relationship, precedes many activities or is one of the steps. (9, 13, 16) It must be done frequently under many circumstances and with a variety of people. It is an integral part of all educational processes—teaching, interviewing, counseling, consultation, and other activities in which change is desired, being applied in an appropriate way in each situation. Sometimes it entails little more than introductions, but in many situations all steps of the process are necessary. The general steps are:

1. Greet the client or group, being polite, friendly and personal, using names if possible.
2. Express interest and desire to help with the problem (e.g., evaluation of diet, need for weight loss, teaching misinformation).
3. Encourage the client to express fears and concerns about the problem or the pending changes, listen thoughtfully, be nonjudgmental and accepting. (Is client afraid of problem? Afraid of the medicine? Worried about cost? Does the nurse think there is not enough time to teach nutrition?)
4. Let the client know that the nutritionist understands the situation, has helped others with similar problems, and will help the client do what must be done.
5. Express confidence that the client can handle problems and progress toward a solution. Point out the expected benefits.

If the teacher is to help the learner, they must accept each other. The teacher must assume most of the responsibility for developing a friendly relationship. Many times the learner would rather not be seeing the teacher. A learner may come voluntarily into a teaching situation because of feeling a need to learn. Other learners come only because they think it is necessary, as is often true among persons who receive public assistance. Often the learner is very skeptical about the meeting, and has a set of preconceived ideas about food and a number of prejudices. Sometimes the learner comes with the intention of promoting some personal ideas about food and nutrition.

Methods for Individuals and Small Groups

There are two main steps in the process: first, interviewing, that is, getting the information that identifies the problem, and second, counseling, in which the actual teaching takes place.

Interviewing. Interviewing as used here means a conversation conducted by a member of the nutrition staff to gather information or data that can be used to help clients. The person being interviewed may be the client, a community leader, or a representative of some agency or governmental unit that can provide help for solving the problems of clients. The conversation is designed to achieve a specific purpose about some matter of mutual concern to the interviewer and the person interviewed. (9)

The purpose is usually to obtain information about the food eaten by an individual or family, often with additional information about accompanying practices (e.g., purchasing and preparation) or to obtain information about programs or activities of other agencies (e.g., asking a staff member of a local voluntary agency about its educational programs). Interviewing precedes counseling and will also be used by the nutritionist for many other purposes, such as to obtain information from a job applicant, to ascertain another person's views, to learn what a superior advises about a problem, or to learn about a staff member's activities. Because this method will be used so often, it is important that the nutritionist master the art and skill that facilitate its use.

The purpose of the interview determines the content, which is usually concerned with one subject and proceeds in a definite direction. The interviewer takes responsibility for seeing that the interview progresses in such a way as to achieve its purpose. Generally the interviewer asks questions and the interviewee answers them. Since an interview usually has a time limitation, the interviewer should plan the questions carefully.

In interviews between professional or paraprofessional and client, as in getting information about food practices, the interview is designed to lead ultimately to action that will be beneficial to the client, and the interviewer is the leader, asking questions that the client answers, providing pertinent information. The interviewer confines the conversation to subjects that will help resolve the client's problems. An interview should encourage the individual to discuss any negative feelings that are related to the purpose of the interview as well as to provide information.

The skills of interviewing can also be used in reverse, that is, when the nutritionist is being interviewed, by another nutritionist who wants information, or by a prospective employer, or by a student seeking general information about the nutrition field to help the interviewer achieve the desired purpose.

Steps in The Interview. The following steps are usually included but may proceed in a different order. (9, 16)

1. Introduce self and establish rapport.
2. Explain purpose of interview.
3. Ask questions pertinent to the particular interview. When taking a diet record, ask about the foods eaten, place where eaten, who prepared food, extent of activity, amount of sleep, client's perception of own condition and eating practices. When getting information on another program, ask about specific activities: who conducts them, their purpose, their value, and possible cooperation. Also explain own role and program, help or service provided, and help or service needed.
4. Check for understanding (e.g. restating and clarifying responses of interviewee).
5. Summarize the information gathered.

Counseling. Counseling is "the process of providing individualized professional guidance to assist a person in adjusting his daily food consumption to meet his health needs." (13) Like interviewing it is a conversation, directed by the counselor for a purpose, in this case to change the food practices of the client. The purpose of diet counseling may be to teach preventive care for the well individual or to teach a therapeutic diet for the patient with a health crisis. When a patient has been referred by physician or nurse, the nutritionist should read the patient's medical record before interviewing and counseling. (14)

The purpose of diet counseling is to change food practices so that all necessary constituents are provided (e.g., increasing the amount of foods high in vitamin A), or to modify the food intake for special needs (e.g., adding whole grains to increase fiber). The client or patient and the person who prepares the family meals should both be included when possible. The process of counseling is based on an interchange of opinions between counselor and client, which increases the client's knowledge about food and nutrition, modifies attitudes, and results in the client's making the recommended changes.

Counseling on nutrition usually starts with the record of food eaten, which is obtained as part of an interview that precedes counseling. In community nutrition the interview may be very brief, confined to getting minimal information about a food record kept by the individual or taken by someone else. Sometimes the counseling is planned ahead of time; sometimes it takes place spontaneously with little opportunity for planning. In either case, the counselor must get information about the purpose and background of the client before starting the change process.

Steps in counseling.   The steps may proceed in a different order or some may be combined.

1. Evaluate the food record available from the interview or supplied by the client. This may be done with the client by discussing food intake and encouraging the client to compare the kinds and amounts of foods eaten with those recommended on a daily food guide.

2. Help the client to see how the whole family can use the same basic foods. Identify the good practices and encourage their continued use.

3. Help the client to identify the poor practices, that is, the food groups for which intake is especially low.

4. Help the client to suggest ways to improve the diet by adding foods that fit the client's cultural pattern and family preferences, and can be obtained with available money.

5. Help the client decide on one or two changes to be made and write the suggestions on the food record. Explain the reasons for the changes.

6. Give the client the food record with changes, suggesting that it be hung in the kitchen for frequent reference.

7. A copy of the food record with recommended changes should be filed with the medical chart or if there is none, in the nutritionist's file.

8. When there are subsequent visits, check each time on how the plan is progressing. As the client completes one change, suggest further changes as needed.

9. When changes have been accomplished, take another food record that will show whether further counseling is needed.

Counseling should continue until the client has made the recommended changes or until it is clear the changes will not be made. Successful change should be commended. The unsuccessful client may be invited to return at a later date when the possibilities of change are greater.

Sometimes the food record shows that a good diet is consumed; then the client should be congratulated or praised and apprised of the importance of continuing this as a good health practice. Johnson suggests that when there is no health crisis the client should be counseled on starting and managing a preventive care program. (15) The nutritionist should help the client to define health goals and plan the preventive program.

Group Counseling.   This is a midway point between individual counseling and teaching a class. It works best for a group of three to five who have similar needs (e.g., pregnant women, obese teenagers). The counselor should first read the medical records when individuals have been referred by a physician or nurse. The food records should be taken before the first meeting when possible; otherwise, they should be taken at that time. (26)

There are several advantages of group counseling. Group members may learn from each other or may make a joint decision for action. Group teaching materials and activities can be used (e.g., a tasting party). These are effective methods of teaching and motivation.

The general process for group counseling is similar to the process for individuals, with the group identifying their problems and planning what to do. The steps are the same as for individual counseling. First, the group members and teacher must get acquainted and establish a friendly relationship. Problems are identified from the food records. The group considers how to apply the food guide in the family setting and group members suggest foods to change or add to improve their diets. Finally, the group members, individually or together, decide on changes to be made.

Group members should be encouraged to discuss their similar problems, to contribute their experiences, and their recipes for favorite dishes. For groups where weight control is a problem, a good shared activity is for members to devise ways to reduce fat and sugar content in their favorite recipes. It should be remembered that generalizations may not apply to all members of the group and that one who does not concur in the group decision needs special attention to devise another change that is acceptable.

Methods for Large Groups

Group programs of greater formality and more elaborate arrangements are used for community education and nutrition education as well as for staff development to cover broad areas of knowledge rather than a specific problem or question. Sometimes they are used for combined groups of professionals and the public, such as parents and teachers.

A good way to prepare this kind of educational program is to plan with a small committee from the group the approach and methods to be used. Group education is especially suitable for covering specific subjects. With professionals this might be an update on nutrition for maternal health, or on changes in recommended dietary allowances, or on new labeling laws. In community education it might be to inform community leaders about a new program that is planned or needed. In nutrition education the purpose is to change food practices for improvement of nutrition.

For professionals, the presentation often includes both subject matter and method, such as a symposium on how to conduct the nutrition education of diabetic patients. It may include a demonstration of counseling with real clinic patients as participants or role playing by group members. The nutritionist may use films, posters, exhibits, food models, or foods to illustrate the talk. Real food, especially when sampling can be included, makes an effective way to encourage consumption of specific foods. It is important that those who hold the pursestrings realize that making a presentation vital and exciting takes a major effort and much time along with expenditure of funds for food, display materials, art work, and other resources. The amount of showmanship and flair that is appropriate will have to be decided in an individual situation.

Kinds of Large-Group Meetings.   The nutritionist will need to decide on a suitable type of meeting. The best kind to use depends on the nature of the group and the purpose of the program. The various terms for group meetings are often used interchangeably but they will be distinguished here in specific ways.

An *institute* is a short teaching program for people in the same field of work. The purpose may be to present nutrition subject matter, or to describe methods or motivate to action, or do all three.

A *symposium* is a program in which a particular subject is discussed. It offers a good way to present specific subject matter in depth. An all-day symposium for nutritionists and dietitians on "Everything You've Always Wanted to Know About Weight Control" included four speakers on (1) the role of exercise in weight control, (2) exercise in preventive medicine, (3) testing for fitness, and (4) community resources for exercise. (12) A two-hour symposium for the public on diet and heart disease included three well-known speakers on the problem of heart disease, diet for prevention, and other methods of prevention.

A *workshop* is an action-oriented meeting to help the participants acquire specific skills. Twenty-five public health nutritionists held a workshop to study the 1974 RDA and determine necessary modifications of their food guides. There was a keynote speech in which a member of the committee that prepared the RDA reported some of the more significant changes and the reasons for them. Then the nutritionists were divided into six workshop groups to consider the RDA for the various age groups and the specific changes needed in food guides. All groups met at the end of the day to report their findings.

A *conference* is a formal meeting in which members of the audience discuss a particular topic. Twelve members representing local weight control groups met with two public health nutritionists to discuss the possibility of a series of educational meetings for leaders from groups in the area. The nutritionists, who had requested the meeting, presented a training plan that was discussed and modified as suggested by the group.

A *panel discussion* is a discussion carried on among a selected group of speakers before an audience, sometimes in response to questions posed by a panel leader. A panel discussion was one part of an all-day institute for nurses. A health educator was the panel moderator and the participants were a pharmacist, a nutritionist, and a physician. The topic was "What should we do about the present fad for megavitamins?" The moderator had talked with panel members ahead of time to get their ideas and had prepared a list of ten questions to be used as a structure for the discussion. She sent each panel member a copy of the outline and questions. The program began with a two-minute discussion of the title question by each panel member.

Then the moderator posed the questions to specific members of the panel, letting the other members also speak on a question if they wished. Some questions were posed for discussion by all panel members. There was a thirty-minute audience question-and-answer period. Fifteen minutes before closing time, the moderator closed the discussion with a brief summary, then asked each panel member to state the most important point that had been made.

A *lecture* is an informative talk presented to an audience. It may include a question-and-answer period. The lecturer may use many kinds of audio-visual materials to illustrate the talk. Probably the best use for a lecture is to present specific information in a relatively short time to a group that is already motivated to make use of the information presented. Though the method is often considered to be ineffective, many groups like this kind of presentation. Example: A nutritionist was asked to lecture to a group of 85 parents and teachers on "Preventing Obesity in Children."

The Nutritionist as Participant. Each of the methods has application to particular situations. Sometimes several of the methods are combined in a single program. The nutritionist may be either a *participant* or a *planner*; the methods and responsibilities are somewhat different depending on the role. The steps for the participant are similar whether the nutritionist is the only participant or one of several.

When the initial contact is made, the nutritionist needs to get information to determine whether or not the invitation should be accepted. Before accepting, the nutritionist should know the objectives of the group for this particular meeting, who the members are and their particular interests, the date, hour and place for the meeting, the time allowed for the presentation and for audience participation, and whether there is only one speaker or several. If the nutritionist accepts the invitation, additional information should be obtained, such as: the maximum and minimum numbers expected, how the audience will be seated (classroom-style, in a circle, at tables, in auditorium, and so forth), the facilities and equipment available, such as projector (kind) and projectionist, chalkboard, stage, podium, table for printed matter. A tentative structure for the meeting should be selected (e.g., lecture or workshop).

The second step is planning on the basis of the above information. The nutritionist should decide on an objective for the presentation, such as a change desired. For example, the objective might be to correct misinformation or to improve undesirable child-feeding practices such as urging the consumption of too much food. Then the nutritionist should list points to be included, outlining content and sequence, and following this, decide on some attention-getting devices, plan the illustrative materials to be used, and plan the printed materials to be distributed.

The nutritionist should prepare for the meeting as early as possible, ordering printed materials for distribution, studying resources, developing content, and practicing the program to fit it into the allotted time.

Evaluation may be done formally by means of a questionnaire or reaction sheet, or informally from comments of the group and subjective observations by the nutritionist or by conference with the planning group.

The Nutritionist as Planner. The Nutritionist may carry all or much of the responsibility for planning some group educational events or may be the chairman or a member of a planning committee. The steps are similar for any audience, consisting of a series of decisions. Meticulous attention to detail is necessary to achieve a smooth-running, productive meeting.

Deciding on objectives for the event. For the exercise symposium mentioned on page 167, the objective was to present subject matter on (1) the relationship of exercise to weight control, especially as a preventive measure, (2) starting an exercise program, and (3) the kinds of programs available in the area and the characteristics of each kind.

Deciding the kind of program. Consider the available facilities and the best structure with timing, rest breaks, and a lunch period if it is an all-day meeting. Decide on a presider or chairman to conduct the program.

Deciding on a date with a possible alternative. Check for possible conflicts with other meetings for the same group.

Developing a list of possible participants. This was done in the exercise program by the committee members asking other persons for names, including those of several nutritionists, an exercise physiologist, and the heads of the women's athletic departments at the various universities and colleges.

Investigating facilities. Make sure that the facilities and equipment are adequate and appropriate. Plan refreshments or meals if they are to be included.

Screening possible speakers and making decision. Unless speakers are already well known to committee members, a personal contact should be made when possible. In the first telephone contact for the exercise symposium, plans were explained, the interest of the potential speaker was ascertained and suggestions were requested for other persons who might fit into the program. Then the committee visited each speaker and discussed the plans. This resulted in decision as to the speakers and program content.

Preparing the program and announcements. Include a registration blank if there is to be a preliminary reservation (necessary when attendance is limited, when food is to be served, or when printed material is to be prepared for distribution; not necessary when the meeting is to be held in a large auditorium and the supply of materials is not limited.) At the proper time send announcements and take reservations. Also be sure overnight accommodations are arranged for speakers or participants coming from a distance.

Confirming speakers and arrangements. A week before the date of the program, the committee should contact each speaker to find out if there are questions or if requirements for equipment have changed. This also serves to assure that the speaker has the date in mind. The manager of the facilities should be contacted to be sure plans there are in order. In one case, it was found after the announcements had gone out that the event was not on the calendar at the place that had been reserved.

On day of event. Arrange to greet individuals as they come. Check off reservations or have each sign an attendance sheet. Have someone at the door to answer questions.

After the program. Evaluate as suggested on page 169.

SKILLS IN COMMUNITY NUTRITION

The list of skills in Figure 10.1 was adapted from a list initiated by three public health nutrition program directors* to identify the components of the field of community nutrition and the staff level at which they could be used. The list was later expanded and developed by the author. Additional skills are needed by the director of a program with a large staff. These may include planning and coordinating components of a large program, interviewing and selecting staff, orienting, supervising and evaluating performance, preparing the annual budget, preparing a project proposal for grant funding, planning surveys or research projects, training a staff in survey methods, supervising the collection and processing of the data, and interpreting the results. Some of these skills, such as preparing an annual budget, may also be needed by the community nutritionist or other nutrition team members.

In the agency where this list was developed, the skills of each new nutritionist were appraised with the identification of those that were adequate and those that needed to be enhanced or acquired. This helped the nutritionist to gain an early broad view of the practice of community nutrition and to develop the individual's potential. A broad concept of practice is necessary to visualize and develop the possibilities in a program and to minimize some of the frustrations experienced by community nutritionists due to a lack of ideas and skills with which to attack problems.

Though each of these skills becomes a part of the activities of nutrition personnel, performance is facilitated and enhanced if it is recognized that they are skills and that the ability to use them easily and well depends on knowledge, training, and practice. Few individuals will master all of these skills because they require a very wide variety of knowledge and experience and because few jobs will need all of them or provide experience in all; however, the scope of a program determines

---

* Helen E. Walsh, California Department of Health; Elsie W. Russell, Los Angeles City Health Department; and Jessie C. Obert, County of Los Angeles Health Department.

Skill and Use	Has Skill	Needs Practice	Must Learn
Skills in Nutrition Education			
Obtain the food record			
Evaluate food records, meal plans, or food patterns for individual and family and adjust to specific needs			
Instruct and counsel individuals and groups on normal diet			
Instruct and counsel on standard modified diets			
Instruct and counsel individuals and groups on therapeutic diets			
Instruct and counsel individuals and groups on home management			
Teach large groups			
Review and evaluate printed materials for nutrition education			
Prepare teaching materials for nutrition education			
Skills in Professional and Paraprofessional Education			
Provide consultation to individuals and small groups			
Review and evaluate resource materials			
Prepare educational materials for professional persons			
Demonstrate teaching method			
Skill in Community Education			
Promote community interest in good nutrition			
Skills in Preparing and Using Teaching Media			
Conduct food demonstration			
Collect information for survey of food prices or food practices			
Calculate cost of individual or family foods and meals			
Calculate nutrient content of intakes and dietary patterns			
Use food composition tables			
Adapt materials and methods to cultural practices			
Use audiovisual equipment and media			
Skills for Anthropometric Measures			
Take accurate weights			
Make accurate measurements			
Record precise measurements			

Source: County of Los Angeles Health Department Division of Public Health Nutrition.

Figure 10.1 Skills in Community Nutrition—Appraisal Form.

the variety of skills needed and most nutritionists will need to learn some of them near the time they will be required. The director of a large nutrition program needs some understanding of all of the skills because it may be necessary to arrange for others to learn some skills that are minimal with the director.

Many community nutrition programs are relatively uncomplicated and need only a few skills; for example, a small nutrition program for the elderly requires only a minimal knowledge of food service and of individual and group teaching, including a need to adjust to the food practices of one cultural group. In a large health agency with a number of staff working in different locations under several supervisors, there may be a need to prepare teaching materials based on the food patterns of several ethnic groups and to conduct education for professionals, paraprofessionals, and many publics.

The need and use for each skill will be discussed briefly with special note of how it may be acquired and who is expected to have it. The number of skills needed by a specific employee will vary with the position. An aide may have only a few skills, spending full time in one or two activities such as small-group teaching. A clinic nutritionist who spends full time counseling patients needs a high degree of that skill. It is expected that a well-qualified community nutritionist will be responsible for the program and the others will work under direction, but sometimes in actual practice the only source of counseling is a lesser-qualified individual and regular supervision is not available.

The skills in each group are arranged in order of difficulty with those that require less training listed first. The nutritionist who supervises the other team members needs to evaluate competence, decide which skills the aide or other person can acquire, and train and supervise. In the discussion of each skill that follows, there will be suggestions about other nutrition personnel who may be expected to learn the skill. The positions of nutrition aide, nutrition technician, and nutrition counselor were discussed on p. 51–54.

SKILLS IN NUTRITION EDUCATION

The skills include those for individual or small group teaching and those for teaching large groups.

Obtaining the Food Record

The food record is completed first. This may be done by the client either in the office as a 24-hour recall or at home by keeping a record.

The method must be explained when the form is given to the client. This is sometimes done by a social worker or other person who handles intake. The client needs to know how the food record will be used (i.e., as the basis for helping with the prescribed diet and how to record the information including servings and measures). It may be well to have someone available to give individual help as the records are completed, answering questions, checking the record for completeness and asking about apparent omissions or discrepancies. When the record is completed at home it must be checked when it is returned, usually at the time of the interview.

Sometimes the nutritionist or nurse may wish to complete the record as a 24-hour recall by interview rather than have the client complete it, to get additional information for a particular reason. In the case of an underweight child, the counselor wanted to assess whether the problem was with the family diet or with the child's own likes and dislikes. The counselor first discussed the child's food intake for the previous 24 hours, asking what the child had eaten that day, and as that information was obtained, asking what the rest of the family had eaten. Questions were phrased to avoid "yes" and "no" answers, for example, rather than asking if the child had milk at noon, asking what the child drank at the noon meal. The counselor used food models and pictures to help get information about portion sizes.

Nutrition aides and technicians can be trained to obtain these records as can nurses and other nutrition counselors.

An example of a completed food record is given in Figure 10.2. Ms. Watkin, age 28, was referred by her physician because of obesity and high blood cholesterol, with recommendation for a 30-pound weight loss and a diet to reduce the cholesterol level. The nutritionist weighed and measured her and established her ideal weight, which indicated the loss of 30 pounds. She instructed her in how to keep the food record, which was returned a few days later. When the nutritionist evaluated the record, she obtained additional information. The morning and evening meals were eaten at home, while lunch was eaten at a restaurant. Soft drinks were used frequently at meals and between them. Ms. W. was already highly motivated for weight loss, so the nutritionist advised her to eat three meals a day, reduce the size of the meat serving, drink nonfat milk, use dietetic salad dressing, have a fruit snack instead of the candy bar, and use diet soda or tea without sugar instead of other soft drinks. Ms. W. agreed to make these changes, but said that instead of drinking milk at lunch she would have nonfat milk with cereal at breakfast.

The food record provides information about current food practices to be used for counseling, so being able to obtain a good record is a very

INSTRUCTIONS:

Write down everything you eat and drink in one day.
Give name of every food you eat.
  Examples: not just SANDWICH, but BOLOGNA SANDWICH
             not just SALAD, but LETTUCE and TOMATO SALAD.
Tell how much you eat of each kind of food and beverage.
  Examples: 2 SLICES rye bread with 2 SLICES bologna
            and 1 TABLESPOON of mayonnaise.
            1 CUP black coffee with 2 TEASPOONS sugar.
Tell if food was raw or cooked; if cooked, tell how.
  Examples: 2 FRIED eggs, 2 slices ROAST pork with GRAVY.

BREAKFAST

1. _Black Coffee_   4. _____
2. _____   5. _____
3. _____   6. _____

Between Breakfast and Noon

1. _Black Coffee_   2. _____

NOON MEAL

1. _Small bowl white rice_   4. _Pickled cabbage 1 tsp. relish_
2. _Japanese beef and vegetables_ 5. _Tea - no sugar_
3. _Cooked in tomato sauce_   6. _____
       _4-5 oz._

Between Noon and Evening Meals

1. _Candy bar_   2. _____

EVENING MEAL

1. _6 oz broiled sirloin_   4. _Small tossed salad_
2. _1 large baked potato_   5. _Russian dressing_
3. _2 tsp. butter_   6. _12 oz. whole milk_

Between Evening Meal and Bedtime

1. _2 Cinnamon_   2. _6 oz. soft drink_
   graham crackers

Name _Margene Watkin_ Day of Week _Tues._ Date _7/21/76_ Case No. ____

Figure 10.2 Record of Foods Eaten in One Day by a Female Clinic Patient.

important skill. The ability to complete records accurately without immediate guidance or to complete records at home after instruction depends on motivation and educational level. Sometimes it is necessary to provide the form in another language (perhaps on the reverse side) or to have the instruction given by a person who speaks that language. Often in a group some members will interpret for others or will help by explaining what is to be done. If necessary, the ingenious nutritionist will find even further ways to bridge these gaps with the clients, as using sign language, models, or pictures.

Evaluating Food Records and Adjusting Food Plans

The food record is evaluated by comparison with the four food groups or by estimation or calculation of calories and nutrients. The evaluation is used as the basis for counseling. The food served to small groups such as a day care center or a home for the aged may be evaluated by a menu pattern. In some states food served in these facilities must meet specific state or local requirements, which should be used for the evaluation. Available information such as menus, meals, market orders or information from other sources can be used to identify problems such as high cost, cultural taboos, unsuitable foods for age, inadequate calories or nutrients, excessive fat or calories, or unsatisfactory distribution of fatty acids. The plan or menu is adjusted to remove the problems. A menu that contains a porterhouse steak can be altered to a chuck steak to reduce cost, or one that includes no protein-rich food may be improved by adding cheese or eggs, or the fatty acids in a day's menu can be altered by using vegetable oil instead of animal fat. Technicians and many aides can learn this skill.

Instructing and Counseling Individuals and Groups on Normal Diet

The dual verb form is used to indicate that the diet counselor furnishes knowledge in a systematic manner while engaging with the client in an interchange of ideas about possible courses of action. Once analysis of the food record has shown the changes in food consumption that are needed, the counselor selects changes for discussion to elicit information about purchasing and cooking practices. In the counseling process, ways are suggested to improve the diet, their acceptability is evaluated by the response, and the individual or group is led to a decision to make changes. The mother, whose child refuses to drink milk may be ignoring the issue, hoping for a change without taking any action. The teacher must get the mother to think about the problem and help her understand why the child needs milk and what the alternatives are. In one maternity program where most of the patients are teenagers, the nutritionists are encouraging breast-feeding. The girls are resisting, apparently because of modesty. They live at home and their mothers are not concerned because breast-feeding was not emphasized when they had their children. The education must be with both mother and daughter so that the mother will help motivate the girl and support her in breast-feeding.

Instructing and Counseling on Standard Modified Diets

These include modified diets such as low calorie, bland, and normal pregnancy. The only adjustments necessary are in the selection of the individual foods and in the quantity and the consistency of the food. The main help needed is with alterations to accommodate personal preferences, cultural practices, appropriate budgets, and available facilities. The food record provides the basic information for helping the individual fit the modified diet into the family food pattern.

Counseling includes discussing the diet and the way it differs from the normal diet, reviewing the likes and dislikes of the individual, indicating the amounts to be consumed, and discussing preparation and cooking methods. Thus there is education for change that is then monitored. There must be discussion with the client or group to be sure the diet is understood and to find out what changes clients are willing to make. It is especially helpful when this can be done by a person familiar with the practices of the particular ethnic group involved. With suitable training, aides and technicians can learn to counsel on standard modified diets. (19, 23)

The *diet history* is an indepth inquiry about the food practices of a specific individual, used mainly in research. It is an expensive method because the interviewers need special training that must be provided for the particular research project and because it takes considerable time. The method was developed by Burke (3) for the Harvard prenatal studies. Beal described the method as a one-hour home interview that included a detailed nutritional history about food consumption and related practices. The interview was supplemented by a 24-hour recall and a three-day food record, which were used as a crosscheck on the history. (1)

Though this method is not often used in community nutrition programs, the nutritionist may use some of the techniques in interviewing and counseling, for example, crosschecking to get additional information about specific foods or food groups.

Ways to Handle Some Common Problems.   The nutritionist will have to devise ways to deal with many problems. Some of those most frequently encountered will be discussed.

Too small a breakfast.   Discuss the importance of this meal and suggest a meal plan using well-liked foods from the food guide, which need not be the traditional breakfast foods.

Lack of dark-green or deep-yellow vegetables or citrus fruits.   Explain the unique contributions made by these foods as sources of vitamin A, vitamin C, and folic acid.

Low milk consumption.   Explain the need for calcium. Stress the use of milk in cooking and discuss the use of dry or evaporated milk, showing the amount of money that can be saved in a week. Point out that in a year this saving could buy new shoes for the children or other appropriate items.

Low iron.   Explain the importance of iron, and the prevalence of anemia, especially among children, teenage girls, and pregnant women. Suggest foods rich in iron.

Too many calories.   Discuss the excess calories contributed by fat-and-sugar meals and snacks. Suggest use of basic foods instead of foods high in fat and sugar. Explain the need to consider snacks as part of the day's intake of food.

Buying expensive foods.   Suggest the use of less expensive foods such as lower-cost meat cuts and evaporated or nonfat milk.

Overuse of convenience foods.   Suggest more home preparation of foods with emphasis on those low in fat and sugar.

Lack of planning.   Suggest planning menus that include the Four Food Groups, making a shopping list, and taking advantage of sales.

Instructing and Counseling Individuals on Therapeutic Diets

The steps are the same as those just described above, but the special background of the nutritionist or dietitian is needed to understand the principles involved in the diet and the effect it is expected to produce. The counselor must also be aware of the problems that may arise with the specific diet, recognize them as they occur, and know which are related to the diet and which should be referred to the physician. In some programs, nurses who have had special training from the nutritionist can counsel on some therapeutic diets that are used constantly. In other situations, the patient receives the initial instruction from the dietitian at the time of discharge from the hospital and the nurse follows up by monitoring the diet in the home, consulting the nutritionist for further advice as needed.

Instructing and Counseling Individuals and Groups on Home Management

This can often be done by an aide or technician familiar with the community. Some aspects of home management are covered in almost every nutrition counseling contact to give help on practices that interfere with following a good diet. Sometimes lack of homemaking skills interferes with individual or family nutrition and instruction is needed on home practices such as food purchasing, food preparation, dish-washing, use of equipment, child care, or eating problems. For example, a young homemaker mentioned that she used ready-to-eat dinners and other convenience foods almost every night and seldom served vegetables because caring for her three small children took all of her time. While counseling, the nutritionist learned that she spent an hour or two a day baking cakes and cookies, so she suggested that this time could be used to prepare main dishes and that frozen or canned vegetables could be prepared quickly. The homemaker decided to try making her own main dishes, making fewer cakes and cookies and limiting the ready-to-eat dinners to once a week. At the next visit she reported that the family liked the changed meals and did not seem to miss the cakes as much as she had expected.

Teaching Large Groups

The lecture is often used for nutrition education in a large group meeting, but other formats can be used (page 166). The nutritionist should try to use teaching media or devices that will hold the attention of the audience.

A free nutrition education symposium was held in a community in New York City with two physicians and a dietitian. (22) A pretest and post-test were given to those who attended. A return of 64 percent of the questionnaires indicated a high rate of interest. The questionnaires also showed a high rate of learning.

In some communities the local dietetic association maintains a speaker's bureau to supply speakers for community groups. Most requests for programs come from parent-teacher groups and weight control clubs. Senior citizens and service clubs are other groups who make use of the service.

Most nutritionists find that they have many requests for talks to groups. The results and values should be carefully considered for decision as to whether these meetings make the best use of time.

Reviewing and Evaluating Printed Materials for Nutrition Education

Many printed materials are available free of charge or for purchase, but before use, each needs to be evaluated for scientific accuracy, suitability for specific use, emphasis, and other points. Usually the nutritionist will perform this task, but it can be done by another staff member who has enough background to identify inaccurate and misleading statements, information based on out-of-date resources, and overemphasis of specific foods, sometimes found in materials prepared to promote a particular food or product. Besides evaluating new materials, periodic review and evaluation must also be applied to the agency's own materials to assure their continuing accuracy, value, and suitability.

Evaluation should cover the accuracy and suitability of the content and the probable use and influence of the particular item. It is important that evaluation be objective, be made for a specific purpose, and cover all important points. Evaluation definitely should *not* be made after a cursory examination, which results in a decision that "I like it" or "I don't like it."

The *purpose* of evaluation should be decided before the review takes place. Materials may be reviewed for one of two purposes: to see whether they have possible uses in the program, or to determine which of several items is best for a specific purpose. One nutritionist in the Los Angeles County Health Department devised a checksheet for materials for both nutrition education and resource use, with the following items:

Possible uses: general distribution, teaching aid, illustrative aid, subject-matter resource for self, subject-matter resource for staff, teaching method resource for self or staff.

Possible audience: Anyone interested, children (age), teenagers, expectant mothers, parents, senior adults, teachers, nurses, physicians, dentists, nutritionists. Income level of audience.

Points for Judging

Purpose: to arouse interest, give information, develop attitude, guide discussion, stir to action.

Appearance: cover (attractive, pertinent title, easy to read).

Shape and size: appropriate, easy to handle, pleasing proportions.

Layout: print easy to read, suitable for reader group.

Content: information authentic, up-to-date, positive approach, suitable scope, relevant material, well organized, emphasizes important points, author and organization have credibility.

Readability: easy-to-read style, interesting approach, words and structure suitable for intended reader.

These details may appear to make the review a time-consuming task, but the nutritionist who has the skill that comes from necessary basic knowledge and from practicing review by objective methods will find it fast and useful. Technicians and aides may conduct preliminary reviews, but most of the evaluation must be done by the nutritionist.

Preparing Teaching Materials for Nutrition Education

The decision to prepare a teaching leaflet should be made to fill a definite need when there is no material available that suits a given purpose or when it is the policy of the agency to prepare its own materials. The nutritionist must know the food practices of the people with whom the leaflet will be used. This includes the kinds and amounts of different foods and how they are prepared and seasoned. The use of milk and cheese or other calcium sources is of special concern. This information may be obtained from food records of regular clinic patients or by taking some records for the purpose. Additional information can be found in the data from the food consumption studies of the USDA, which cover the country (p. 21). Other information should be obtained locally from observations or interviews with leaders who know the community.

For one study of ethnic food practices, a nutritionist got information from a minister who had worked in the community for many years and from two female community leaders who were known in the community as persons who could help families with their problems. There are other values of interviewing the leaders, as shown in one program for which a nutritionist from a particular Asian ethnic group prepared a food guide in the native language for use with clinic patients. The guide was used by nutritionists and nurses and was well received by the patients. However, it was later reported by a physician from the same cultural group that the community leader among the women had criticized the leaflet, apparently because of her resentment at not having been asked to assist in its development.

The community nutritionist should keep in mind the method and desired outcome when deciding what teaching materials to use and how to use them, and whether to prepare special materials for the specific situation or to use material already available from another source. In some states, the state health department prepares all materials for use in local health departments; in others, local departments prepare their own. Community nutritionists in other agencies will find it helpful to know materials the public agencies use before preparing their own. Often it will be advantageous to make sure new materials concur with others already in use in the community. Sometimes a cooperative effort of the public health nutritionist, other nutritionists, and hospital dietitians can result in more effective education by using the same teaching leaflets and consistent instruction for patients in hospital and home. This is especially useful for a diet that will have wide use, such as a diet for normal pregnancy.

A leaflet for a specific, immediate use may be quickly prepared by a nutritionist or by auxiliary personnel. However, it takes a high degree of skill to make an attractive, appealing leaflet, based on proper nutritional values and suited to the specific socioeconomic situation, that can be used as a teaching tool over a long period of time. In either case the steps are to define the need, decide the use, develop the content, decide the format (size, shape, illustrations, type, and so forth), prepare a preliminary copy, pretest, revise, test, prepare final copy, and print. The preliminary copy and pretesting steps can be omitted for an item for single-occasion or short-term use. Other factors that determine what can be done are the resources available—budget, personnel, methods of reproduction, and facilities for artwork. Often technicians and aides can assist with many of these steps and nurses can provide much useful information about food practices and management in the community.

Pretesting a teaching tool before it goes into final quantity production is an important step. An example of questions used for this purpose is shown in Figure 10.3. The pamphlet was prepared to the preliminary copy stage, then the nutritionist had several mothers read it after

1. What are the two important foods for a small baby?
2. Why is cereal important for the baby?
3. What is the least expensive kind of milk you might feed your baby?
4. What kind of juice can the baby drink?
5. How can you give the baby fluoride?
6. Why is fluoride important?
7. Should you give the baby water to drink?
8. Was there any part of the leaflet that was confusing? Tell me the words that were confusing.
9. Would you lend the leaflet to a friend with a new baby?
10. Do you have any suggestions about the leaflet?

Figure 10.3 Questions Used to Pretest Pamphlet on Infant Feeding.

explaining that it was new and she wanted to find out if other mothers would understand it. After each woman had read it, the nutritionist asked these simple key questions. The pamphlet was then revised as indicated.

SKILLS IN PROFESSIONAL AND PARAPROFESSIONAL EDUCATION

This section includes the skills used only with professionals and paraprofessionals. Skills used also with clients such as methods for teaching large groups were covered under Education in Community Nutrition, (p. 158).

Providing Consultation to Individuals and Small Groups

Consultation is considered here as an educational method. It is defined as a process in which a specialist (the *consultant*) makes professional knowledge and skill available to help another professional (the *consultee*) solve a problem. (2, 7, 17) It is also an art that requires knowledge of both materials and skills for the area involved. It is the responsibility of the consultee to adapt suggestions to specific situations. The consultant has no authority and no direct responsibility for implementing action. The consultee has the responsibility only to use what can be used and the freedom to use only what seems appropriate.

The title of consultant is also used by persons who represent an official controlling agency such as a state health department. Their responsibility is to explore, review, make recommendations, and monitor for correction of problems. The role of the community nutritionist as consultant is most often in the first sense. The nutritionist may provide technical information, identify a problem, motivate change, act as a mediator between two factions or points of view, help in evaluation, or do all of these or several in turn while giving information, stating an opinion, teaching, or counseling.

Consultants are consulted because they are knowledgeable and have proved able to help others solve their problems. The effectiveness of the consultation depends on the value of the consultant's ideas, skill in transmitting them, and, probably, the professional prestige of the consultant, which also seems to be a factor in motivating change.

The process of consultation takes place in a specific interaction with the objective of a change in knowledge, skill, or awareness on the part of the consultee. It is focused on a problem that the consultee has encountered in practice, hence is limited in scope. A problem in seeking and giving consultation is that the consultee may not be able to identify the exact need. Then the skill of the consultant must help in defining the problem, by a judicious use of nonjudgmental, nonthreatening questions and comments, encouraging discussion until the problem has been clearly identified. Only then can the consultant provide information that will really help to solve the problem. Consultation usually proceeds in a series of actions.

Request for Assistance. The consultee makes a preliminary statement of the problem; the consultant restates it and makes sure the problem is within the area of expertise.

Development of Rapport. Rapport is a process of getting acquainted, the consultant learning about the broader aspects of the consultee's work and the consultee learning more about the consultant's experiences.

Identification of the Problem. The consultant helps the consultee explore the problem and clarify basic ideas about the source. The consultant restates or summarizes what both have said.

Consideration of the Problem in Different Ways. Possible solutions are considered, including solutions already tried. The consultant reacts, summarizes, and suggests solutions.

Conclusion of the Process. This may be a decision by the consultee for a specific action, or occasionally a mutual agreement that there is no solution to the problem. There may also be a need for further consultation at a later date, or for the consultant or the consultee both to study the problem or obtain more information and then to consult further.

When the consultant and consultee are regular members of the same staff and well acquainted with each other, the consultation process may proceed in an informal way, omitting some of the steps.

There are a number of problems that may arise to block progress during the consultation. The consultee may start discussing other problems, especially personal ones not directly related to the subject, or asking personal questions about the consultant. Then the consultant should bring the discussion back to the problem by summarizing the course and present state of the consultation, by asking a question, or by a comment on some phase of the problem not yet discussed.

In any consultation, the consultee may feel threatened by having to ask for help, may dislike to admit a problem, or be afraid of being asked to do unwanted things, or of possible loss of status with superiors or staff who might report problems to higher authority.

Consultation may also take place in a small-group situation with two or three persons who have similar problems as in the second example that follows.

Example of Consultation to Film Script Writer. A film company producer telephoned the health department nutritionist for help in the initial stages of planning an educational film on the subject of teenage obesity. The purpose was to get an opinion about the need and possible demand for the film, to obtain information about community resources, and to learn sources of technical information. This was in an area where the nutritionist had considerable experience and felt qualified to advise, so an appointment was made with the script writer.

At the time of the conference rapport was quickly established by mutual interest in the subject. Then the consultant reviewed the problem as seen from the previous conversation. The producer discussed the ideas and the plans in greater detail. The company intended to make a film on prevention of obesity for teenagers and young adults and wanted (1) assurance that there was need for the film, (2) to find a nutritionist who was working with a group of obese teenagers, and (3) names of references for use in acquiring a background and in getting information such as the calorie value of foods, energy use in the body, value of exercise, and so forth.

The nutritionist named the films currently available, outlined the kind of requests regularly received, and said the film was needed. She told the script writer there was only one such group of obese teenagers in the area, and it did not quite meet the specifications outlined. However, he decided to contact that nutritionist and took her phone number and address. The consultant called the other nutritionist and explained the need and the nutritionist agreed to see the writer. The consultant also suggested names of three researchers in local universities and colleges who had done research in fields related to obesity, and provided some books and pamphlets, and names of other references. She further suggested the most useful sources of nutrition subject matter and food composition values and advised where these books could be purchased.

Together the nutritionist and the writer summed up the results of the consultation, decided that the next steps were for him to talk with the researchers and visit the teenage group.

Both the consultee and consultant expressed the feeling that the consultation had been very productive. The consultant expressed approval that the writer was getting information from authentic professional sources and agreed to give further help as necessary. This terminated the contact.

Example of Consultation to a Small Group. The small-group consultation is illustrated in this report of three health educators who requested the nutritionist to advise them about food misinformation problems that had recently come to their attention. They reported the problems and the nature of the misinformation: (1) a school nurse was trying to get the school lunch to stop serving all products made with white flour and to use honey instead of sugar because "white flour has no food value" and "honey has special nutritional values"; (2) a former chemistry teacher was lecturing on nutrition in an adult education program, teaching that saccharin causes birth defects, that bleached flour is poison, and that arthritis is caused by too many carbohydrates; and (3) a local radio station was carrying lectures by a person who claimed to be a nutritionist but who advocated only "natural" foods.

The health educators wanted the correct facts, information about these problems, and suggestions about how to combat the misinformation.

The nutritionist answered their questions about food and nutrition and provided them with literature giving some additional information.

Then the four discussed approaches that might be used to get rid of the problems. The health educator decided that it would be well to talk first with the school principal about the nurse's misinformation, to find out the district's policies about misinformation and whether an official request could be made that the nurse desist. A second approach was to find out from the school lunch manager how much harm the nurse was doing to the children's attitudes about lunch. Another suggestion was to discuss the problem with the chairman of the health committee of the parent-teacher group.

The nutritionist reviewed the requirements for the Type A lunch and suggested that the nurse be advised that she handicaps the lunch program and the children by giving them information that conflicts with the official policies.

The problems of the lecturer and the radio program were discussed in a similar manner, with the nutritionist in the role of nutrition expert, consultant, and advisor. On each problem there was an interchange of information and suggestions among all four present, and the nutritionist gave much more information than would probably be used, leaving it to each health educator to decide which approach would be most likely to succeed in the particular situation.

Reviewing and Evaluating Resource Materials

Resource materials include teaching media of all kinds such as films, publications, and posters, which are used for staff education and references. The method and points are the same as those given under nutrition education on pages 173–183, but evaluating content may take longer because of the need to verify statements or data with standard reference sources. The credibility of the author and the agency are more critical than with materials for nutrition education because the professional audience has more knowledge than the general public.

Preparing Educational Materials for Professional Persons

These include resource materials such as those mentioned above and devices for using them in nutrition education. Printed materials such as monographs on pertinent topics, for example, food practices of a specific ethnic group or the nutrient content of vegetarian diets, are the most common kind, but nutritionists may also use and make films, videotapes, and other items. It is sometimes necessary to make a guide for staff to show how to use leaflets or other teaching materials. An adviser or advisory committee can be of great help in determining what should be included in the content, how members of the group will use the resource, and how much background they have. Collecting information from nutritionists who have conducted similar projects, who work with the same ethnic groups, or who have had similar experiences is also helpful.

The method used in one health department for preparing resource materials includes part or all of these steps: (1) defining the need, (2) review of available materials on the subject (books, periodicals, pamphlets, and leaflets), (3) assembling available data in the local area or from nutritionists in other areas, (4) collecting new data as necessary, (5) analyzing the data, (6) synthesizing the data for the specific use, and (7) preparing the publication. The nutritionist should present the finished publication to the staff who will use it and make suggestions for use.

Demonstrating Teaching Method

The nutritionist can demonstrate for nurses or aides a method of conducting nutrition education by means of a conference in office or home, showing how the nutritionist approaches the family and establishes rapport, how questions are phrased and asked, and other ways in which the nutritionist gets and gives information, how the nutritionist notes what is important to the client, how the best motivation is selected, and, finally, how changes to improve practices are suggested. The use of visual aids can also be demonstrated.

SKILL IN COMMUNITY EDUCATION

Promoting Community Interest in Good Nutrition

Individuals and groups, especially community leaders and persons in influential positions, need to be convinced of the importance of good nutrition and its value in enhancing the quality of life for the residents. This must be done by collecting evidence, learning the channels, and presenting the evidence in a convincing way. One community nutritionist learned from teachers at the school that at least one-third of the children came to school without breakfast. She found that "The Tranquillizers," a group of well-to-do young wives, were interested in a community project for their group. The nutritionist had just acquired a dynamic retired home economist volunteer to assist in the nutrition program and the latter suggested that they see if "The Tranquillizers" would develop a Better Breakfast campaign. The nutritionist and the home economist spoke at a meeting of the group, presenting the information about the school children and information from surveys as evidence of need. "The Tranquillizers" decided to conduct a year-long campaign for better breakfasts. They surveyed the needs for training and teaching materials, cooperated with the school to finance and arrange training in methods of nutrition education, and interested the parents in the project. In addition, they developed a system of rewards for the children who improved their breakfasts. At the end of the year, the teachers reported that fewer children came to school without breakfast.

In a New York City community, a workshop was held to organize the community for prevention of heart disease. This was done after an initial symposium on prevention of heart disease. The group organized, forming committees to investigate various resources such as reading materials in the libraries and health education in the high school. One of them was organized for political action. (22)

SKILLS IN PREPARING AND USING TEACHING MEDIA

Though excellent media can be purchased, the only way to have personalized kinds that illustrate a point the nutritionist wants to make at a particular time on a specific topic is to prepare them at the time and for the purpose. Often a special leaflet on prices in the neighborhood stores or a recipe for a seasonal food can be used together with a commercial leaflet on the four food groups. Sometimes a poster, chart, or exhibit will provide just the right emphasis or teach a particular point in the best and strongest way. Food used as a teaching device offers some of the most graphic and persuasive opportunities to illustrate points and to change practices.

Conducting Food Demonstrations

Though demonstrations may range from the very simple to a whole meal, the most useful ones in community nutrition education are simple ones, for example, use of nonfat dry milk, or preparing raw vegetable snacks. Having clients participate in preparation and sample the food makes this more effective. Showmanship and persuasiveness help to achieve the objective of getting the individual or family to change food practices.

Collecting Information for Survey of Food Prices or Food Practices

A questionnaire on food practices or a list of foods to be priced is prepared and tested by the nutritionist, who instructs others helping with the project in the methods of obtaining uniform data. It is important in obtaining data for comparative pricing that the same items are compared, for example, the same size loaf and same kind of bread, the same size and quality of canned tomatoes, and the same size and grade of eggs. Again, the purpose must be kept in mind, that it is for practical information to be used in practical ways.

Calculating Cost of Individual or Family Foods and Meals

This is needed to determine how costs can be reduced by using alternative foods or different quantities, or how nutritional values can be increased at the same cost. Information about alternative foods and food composition will show changes that can be made in kinds and quantities of foods without endangering the nutrient content. Background information includes facts about fat and bone in meat to use in estimating number of servings, characteristics of a cereal to estimate servings from a box, and preparation and cooking changes to estimate the number of servings from a market unit of vegetable. This must be a practical estimation to make good use of foods.

Calculating Nutrient Content of Intakes and Dietary Patterns

Estimation or calculation is used to check the adequacy of the nutrient content of food intake as shown by food records or dietary patterns. Checking for the Four Food Groups provides a rough method of estimation, but calculation is desirable for a more definitive determination. At the same time it must be remembered that this is only an indication since intakes are not precisely measured. Checking the food values of dietary patterns and menus used in teaching materials is necessary to be sure that meals planned accordingly are adequate. The actual calculations can be made by a nutrition aide, clerk, or secretary after the nutritionist has interpreted food records or other data sources.

Data from food composition tables are now available for purchase as computer programs; however, there are few community nutrition programs which have sufficient volume to make their use practical. But this possibility should always be kept in mind when there is a large volume of data. (30)

Using Food Composition Tables

In using food composition tables, many values may be taken directly from the tables. When ingredients or portions are different, calculation will be necessary. It should be remembered that the value in a table does not necessarily represent the value of a specific food under consideration, a point that needs to be interpreted in teaching professionals and the public.

The nutritionist should be aware of the proximate nature of food values as given in the tables rather than regarding them as exact amounts. They should be used in practical ways, for example, in comparing the ascorbic acid values of one-half cup of fresh, frozen, and canned orange juice, which are respectively 62, 60, and 50 milligrams (27) it should be recognized that the portion size in the home is usually guessed, not measured. If the amounts vary by one-half tablespoon low for fresh or frozen or one-half tablespoon high for canned, the values for one-half cup would be almost equal. It should also be remembered that there is much natural variation, for example, in the ascorbic acid content of tomatoes and citrus fruits. To avoid confusing professionals as well as homemakers, a practical rather than rigid approach is desirable in teaching food composition and the use of tables.

There may also be a need to calculate values from recipes used in a specific home since ingredients may vary a great deal, for example, amounts of fat and sugar in quick breads. When exchange lists are used, the family or patient may be denied the use of its favorite foods unless the actual recipe is considered. One nutritionist who asked a group of nurses "How much fat do you use when you fry potatoes?" received answers from one tablespoon to one-half cup, with the comment from one nurse "I guess I just cook lean, no wonder I don't have a weight problem!"

In calculating values for a group of people, the largest possible value from the table should be used because the rounded figures for smaller amounts when multiplied by the number of persons will also multiply the inaccuracies. For example, when each of 12 persons eat one 25-gram slice of bread, the *total* weight of bread consumed should be determined in pounds and that weight used with the amount of nutrients in one pound rather than taking direct calculation from the figures for one 25-gram slice.

Adapting Materials and Methods to Cultural Practices

Sometimes a good teaching leaflet is available but some changes are needed in order to use it with a local cultural group. This task is best performed by a person from the specific cultural group or one familiar with its customs and practices who can advise about foods, cooking methods, and serving practices, and help adapt materials prepared for other groups to the current customs of the specific group. The nutritionist may need to take time to get acquainted with the cultural group before a piece of material can be successfully adapted.

One community nutritionist was revising a pamphlet on food practices of Latin-Americans because many new foods had recently appeared in the local markets. A nurse who worked in the area where many Latin-American families lived suggested the names of several residents who had recently immigrated from Central America and Mexico and were familiar with the foods. The nutritionist interviewed several of these persons and was able to enlarge the list of foods and to learn changes that had taken place in food practices since the pamphlet was originally prepared.

Using Audiovisual Equipment and Media

Skill in the preparation and use of projection equipment is important. The nutritionist or other staff member in charge of the preparation or showing of films or other visual materials must have skill in using the equipment. This includes knowing how to thread or load the projector, how to turn on and adjust the sound, testing to be sure the material can be seen and read when projected, and how to set up the screen. It is also important to know how dark the room should be and how to identify problems that are likely to occur. The author was once told by a projectionist that most materials used in the opaque projector have such small or dim print that it cannot be seen beyond the first row. He was much pleased when he saw the copy for use was handwritten in large, very black script that showed clearly on the screen. It had taken some experimentation ahead of time to achieve the desired effect, but training had taught the facts and several trials had produced the result. Some artistic ability is desirable to prepare an exhibit or a bulletin board or a chart, but in its absence, knowledge, training, and practice can develop the desired skill.

SKILLS FOR ANTHROPOMETRIC MEASURES

Many poor practices have been noted in weighing and measuring, such as use of the wrong kind of equipment, carelessness in maintaining uniformity of amount of clothing worn during weighing, letting the child slump when measuring height, and not stretching a baby to full length when doing recumbent lengths. The nutritionist needs to acquire skill in weighing and measuring and to teach these skills to other staff members who actually take the measures. (4, 5, 21, 24)

Taking Accurate Weights

Weight is taken for individuals of all ages. Beam balance platform scales are used. They should be calibrated several times a year. Children should be weighed in light clothing (underpants or cotton gown), adults nude if possible, otherwise in street clothes without shoes. The individual stands on the platform facing the scale while the operator adjusts weights to balance. Weight is taken to nearest $\frac{1}{4}$ pound or $\frac{1}{10}$ kilogram.

Making Accurate Measurements

Measurements and method depend on age. Those commonly taken for infants are recumbent height and head circumference. Measurements often used for children over two years of age and for adults include chest circumference, arm circumference, and skinfolds of triceps and subscapular area. Measurements are taken to nearest ⅛ inch or 1 millimeter.

Recumbent Length of Infant.   This is always used for a child under 24 months and may be used for a child 24 to 36 months. Two operators are necessary to use the required special equipment. This equipment has a measuring scale on a frame, a fixed headboard, and a movable footboard. With the child lying on its back, one operator holds the child's head in alignment with the body so it contacts the headboard. The other operator holds the feet with the toes straight up, applies pressure to the knees so the legs contact the base, and brings the footboard against the child's heels (Figure 10.4).

Standing Height After 36 Months of Age.   The best equipment is a measuring stick or tape attached to a wall or other vertical flat surface, and a block squared to a right angle with a wall. The movable

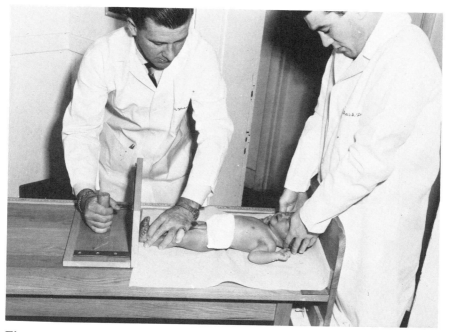

Figure 10.4   Measuring Recumbent Length of Infant. (*Source.* Jelliffe, Derrick B., *The Assessment of the Nutritional Status of the Community,* World Health Organization Monograph Series No. 53, Geneva, 1966.)

measuring rod of a platform scale is not recommended because of the difficulty in getting an accurate measurement (Figure 10.5).

The individual stands on the floor or other flat, bare surface and is directed to stand as tall as possible with the head, shoulders, buttocks, and heels touching wall. The operator brings the square to the crown of the individual's head and takes a measurement at that point to the nearest ⅛ inch or 1 millimeter.

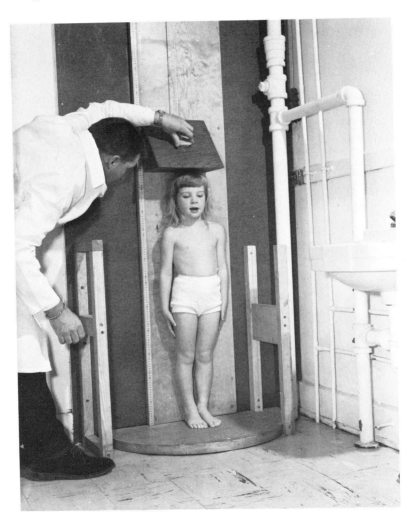

Figure 10.5 Measuring Standing Height. (*Source.* Jelliffe, Derrick B., *The Assessment of the Nutritional Status of the Community,* World Health Organization Monograph Series No. 53, Geneva, 1966.)

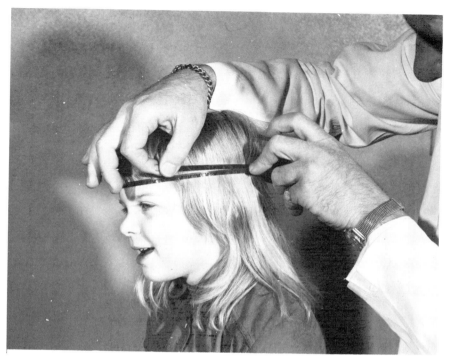

Figure 10.6   Measuring Head Circumference. (*Source.* Jelliffe, Derrick B., *The Assessment of the Nutritional Status of the Community,* World Health Organization Monograph Series No. 53, Geneva, 1966.)

Head Circumference.   This measurement is required for infants in the WIC program. The head may be measured up to 36 months of age using a nonstretchable flexible tape to conform to the head. A special tape with a slotted end and visible measuring point is available. The measurement is recorded to nearest ⅛ inch or 1 millimeter (Figure 10.6).

Recording Measurements Precisely

Precautions should be taken to record accurately, since, as it has been noted, many errors occur in recording. Special forms with spaces for the various measurements to be taken will facilitate recording. The growth charts available from the Center for Disease Control provide a convenient way to record data for children and for keeping a graph that will show unusual body size.

SUMMARY

The community nutritionist uses many skills that must be mastered so they can be done quickly and well. The nutritionist must also teach some of the same skills to other professionals and paraprofessionals.

The educational process is the basis for all teaching. It includes establishing rapport and changing practices and habits. The skill of interviewing is used with both public and professionals, in both education and information gathering. Individual and small-group counseling are widely used skills in nutrition education.

Large-group education is used with both professionals and public for nutrition education and technical education. The nutritionist may be a participant or a planner. The success of this method depends on careful planning and meticulous attention to detail.

The nutritionist also uses skills in making anthropometric measurements in nutritional assessment and surveillance and teaches the method to other staff and volunteers.

The skills used in various kinds of education and programs have been described and suggestions have been made for acquiring and using them.

REFERENCES CITED

1. Beal, Virginia A., The Nutritional History in Longitudinal Research, *J. Am. Diet. Assoc.,* 51 11/67 426.
2. Boehm, Werner M., The Use of the Consultant: 3. The Professional Relation between the Consultant and the Consultee, *Am. J. Orthopsychiatry,* 26 4/56 241.
3. Burke, Bertha S., The Dietary History as a Tool in Research, *J. Am. Diet. Assoc.,* 23 12/47 1041.
4. Center for Disease Control, Evaluation of Body Size and Physical Growth of Children, U.S. Dept. of Health, Education, and Welfare, leaflet, n.d.
5. Christakis, George, ed. *Nutritional Assessment in Health Programs, Am. J. Pub. Health,* 63 11/73 Supplement.
6. Craig, David G., Guiding the Change Process in People, *J. Am. Diet. Assoc.,* 58 1/71 22.
7. *Encyclopedia of Social Work,* 16th issue, Vol. 1, National Association of Social Workers, New York, 1971, 156.
8. Frankle, Reva T., Betsy McGregor, Judy Wylie, and Mary B. McCann, Nutrition and Life Style: I. The Door, A Center of Alternatives—the Nutritionist in a Free Clinic for Adolescents, *J. Am. Diet. Assoc.,* 63 9/73 273.
9. Garrett, Annette, *Interviewing: Its Principles and Methods,* 2nd ed., Family Service Association of America, New York, 1972.
10. Gifft, Helen H., Marjorie B. Washbon, and Gail G. Harrison, *Nutrition, Behavior, and Change,* Prentice-Hall, Englewood Cliffs NJ, 1972 258.

11. *Ibid.*, 264.
12. Greater Los Angeles Nutrition Council Symposium, Los Angeles, 2/26/76.
13. Guidelines for Diet Counseling, *J. Am. Diet. Assoc.* 66 6/75 571.
14. Guidelines for Developing Dietary Counseling Services in the Community, *J. Am. Diet. Assoc.* 55 10/69 343.
15. Johnson, Clair Agriesti, The Need for Better Nutritional Care, *J. Am. Diet. Assoc.* 67 9/75 219.
16. Kadushin, Alfred, *The Social Work Interview,* Columbia University Press, 1972, 1.
17. Koch, William H., A Stance Toward Helping: Reflections on the Role of a Consultant, *Adult Leadership,* 15-16 12/67 202.
18. Leypolt, Martha M., The Teaching Learning Process With Adults, *Adult Leadership,* 15-16 12/67 212.
19. Lumsden, James E., Kathleen Zolber, Peter Strutz, Shirley T. Moore, Albert Sanchez, and David Abbey, Delegation of Functions by Dietitians to Dietetic Technicians, *J. Am. Diet. Assoc.,* 69 8/76 143.
20. National Research Council, Food and Nutrition Board, *Recommended Dietary Allowances,* 8th ed., Washington DC, 1974.
21. NCHS Growth Charts, 1976, National Center for Health Statistics, *Monthly Vital Statistics Report* (HRA) 76-1/20, 25, 6/22/76, Supplement, U.S. Dept. of Health, Education, and Welfare, Rockville MD.
22. Podell, Richard N., Louis R. Gary, Kathryn Keller, and Michael Mulvihill, The Public Seminar as a Nutrition Education Approach, *J. Am. Diet. Assoc.,* 67 11/75 460.
23. Position Paper on the Dietetic Technician, *J. Am. Diet. Assoc.,* 67 9/75 246.
24. Public Health Service, *Growth Charts with Reference Percentiles,* four leaflets, n.d., U.S. Dept. of Health, Education, and Welfare, 1976.
25. Reed, Leni C., Patients Learn from Recording of Diet Counseling, *J. Am. Diet. Assoc.,* 66 6/75 615.
26. Robinson, Corinne, *Normal and Therapeutic Nutrition,* 14th ed., Macmillan Co., New York, 1972, 393.
27. United States Dept. of Agriculture, *Nutritive Value of Foods,* Home and Garden Bulletin No. 72, Government Printing Office, Washington DC, rev., Jan. 1971.
28. Vargas, Julie S., Teaching as Changing Behavior, *J. Am. Diet. Assoc.,* 58 6/71 512.
29. Vaughn, M. Elizabeth, Nutrition Consultation for Public Health Nurses, *J. Am. Diet. Assoc.,* 49 12/66 505.
30. Watt, Bernice K., Susan W. Gebhardt, Elizabeth W. Murphy, and Ritva R. Butrum, Food Composition Tables for the 70's. *J. Am. Diet. Assoc.,* 64 3/74 257.

ADDITIONAL REFERENCES

Andrew, Barbara J., Interviewing and Counseling Skills, *J. Am. Diet. Assoc.,* 66 6/75 576.

Hunerlach, Carol L., Private Practice: Nutrition Counseling, I. Some

Considerations In Establishing a Private Practice, *J. Am. Diet. Assoc.*, 67 11/75 470.

Kunis, Beila S., Family Nutritionist on the Primary Health Care Team, *J. Nutr. Educ.*, 8 4–6/76 77.

Nutrition in Medical Education, *J. Am. Diet. Assoc.*, 63 7/73 13.

Ohlson, Margaret A., The Philosophy of Dietary Counseling, *J. Am. Diet. Assoc.*, 63 7/73 13.

Schwartz, Nancy E., Nutrition Knowledge, Attitudes, and Practices of Canadian Public Health Nurses, *J. Nutr. Educ.*, 8 1–3/76.

PART 4

THE TECHNIQUES

The tools and skills discussed in Part III are applied in broad techniques that are used in developing and conducting a nutrition program. The techniques are those of community organization, management, professional education, and public education.

Community organization shows the nutritionist how to develop the resources and talents of the community and its citizens, providing leadership and services so they can solve their own problems and enrich their lives.

The nutritionist uses the technique of management to make the most of the resources of money, time, and energy. Management is decision making to determine the best use of available resources. Management also shows how to develop routines that reduce the time needed for everyday activities and allow more time for special programs.

The nutritionist provides or arranges education in subject matter and methods for professionals in the health field. There is currently renewed emphasis on education of other professionals to enable them to participate in nutrition programs.

Public education includes the programs and activities designed to change personal practices necessary to improve the nutrition of individuals. It includes community education and nutrition education.

11 COMMUNITY ORGANIZATION

In a simple society each family looks out for itself, making its own personal decisions on a basis of family needs and wishes that are relatively unsophisticated and uncomplicated. As society has become more complex and government more structured, more needs have been met through public services and the individual has lost contact with those who determine the functions of government. The town meeting, which functioned in simpler days as a place where the citizen could participate in decision-making, has been replaced by the process of community organization. (6)

The community nutritionist needs to use community organization for mobilization of community forces to bring about solutions to social problems that can be solved only by community action. Community organization should be considered as a possible technique when there is need for modification in social structures, especially government, to make them represent the values of the citizens and work to fulfill their needs. Community planning for nutrition and coordination of programs can be accomplished by using the process of community organization.

THE PROCESS

Community organization is a process by which individuals, groups, or organizations find solutions to social problems by planned action in which forces, people, and resources are organized and used to meet needs. (1)

Community organization developed as a field of social work but, coupled with social planning, is now used by city and regional planners, public administrators, public health, adult education, and other applied fields. One of its purposes in the solution of health problems is to make it easier for the poor to engage in planning and decision-making; however, the community organizer must work with all economic and cultural groups. (2) There has been much emphasis recently on poverty and minority groups, but it should be remembered that the employed middle class, including self-supporting older citizens, sets the pace and pays the bill, has health problems, and gets diseases, and that successful community organization will include all segments of the community.

THE PURPOSE

The purpose of community organization is to provide a democratic way for individuals, groups, and organizations to participate in planned action to change or develop social institutions or to correct social problems. Our present complicated governmental structure has produced an environment in which decisions are usually made by elected officials who are not very responsive to a single vote.

In the present political society, one person (e.g., the governor or mayor) or a group (e.g., union, school board or legislature) makes the decisions. Citizens, either individually or collectively, can have a voice in such decisions only in an indirect way by participating in the political decision-making process, that is, by voting for officials who will be the decision-makers or for issues which will set the policies and standards for decision-making. Community organization provides a way in which people can modify social structures so they are responsive to their needs and in harmony with their values. (1)

HOW COMMUNITY ORGANIZATION WORKS

The principles of community organization are the same for all population groups, regardless of cultural origin, income, and other factors. There may, however, be great differences in the sophistication of the group about the process of community organization and how to identify, develop, and utilize power to accomplish its objectives.

Any community action must consider politics, which involves popular concerns and the powers and values of political units, along with the information and motivations of the public and of groups that have special interests. Political action is usually the result of negotiation and compromise by the interested individuals and groups even when it seems to occur spontaneously, as when with no discussion a city council votes on a motion. The only true control the public or professionals have over the actions of politicians is the ballot; however, politicians can be kept informed of the needs and wishes of their constituents and can be influenced in this way.

In their turn, politicians have to identify the concerns of their constituents, estimate the power distribution in the population, educate the public and special interest groups, and negotiate possible solutions for action and use of resources. (7)

The basis of the community organization process rests on several assumptions, first, that this is a way in which social effects can be influenced by conscious effort, second, that it depends on deliberate efforts to establish ways to influence people, and third, that there are always some altruistic persons who want to develop a better community life and who will work to accomplish this end. The nutritionist who would use the process must identify the channels of influence, make deliberate efforts to influence people and to motivate others to similar action, and find the altruistic persons to serve as leaders to develop and implement the action.

Though community organization is used for larger issues, it is most effective when used to attack problems of limited scope based on issues that are larger than the range of the individual. Problems of personal nature such as inadequate money for food should be solved on an individual basis, although it may sometimes be possible to transpose the problems of individuals to public issues, as when many welfare families have inadequate money for food, an attempt might be made to augment the welfare food allowances rather than try to find additional resources for each family.

Seder (7) points out that most individuals and groups are so preoccupied with their personal problems and interests that they do not recognize the possibility that others have the same problem and that a community effort at solution may be in order. An example of this occurred when a neighborhood health center was built on top of a hill, four blocks from public transportation. At first the individual patients who came to the health center complained about the distance they had to walk, or they borrowed cars or used taxis, each handling the problem on an individual basis. Later, when they were brought together by community leaders, they decided to ask the city to re-route the bus line so it would go past the center. Eventually this was done. The process involved recognition that many people had the same problem, that individual solutions were expensive and difficult, and that the city, which placed the center in this inaccessible location, should provide transportation to it.

THE STEPS

The steps that constitute the process of community organization are analysis of problems, identification of resources, definition of program objectives, development of program with strategy, and interpretation of the needs to be met and the problems to be solved. The community nutritionist needs to use the process of community organization to identify and solve the nutrition problems of the community. The process must involve all cultural groups, both poor and rich, both disenfranchised and powerful. The leaders must get the support of community groups that have the power to influence those who make the decisions and allocate the money. These groups include established institutions, groups organized to support specific causes, community planning agencies, and many others.

Planning and decision making begin with the information provided by the people who are directly affected by a problem. The first plans and decisions are modified at the lowest level of government and final decisions are made and priorities set at the highest level. (6) In the case just cited, of getting bus service for the health center, the community leaders decided that there should be a bus. They discussed the need with their city councilman and asked for a new bus line. The councilman suggested that existing bus service could be changed to meet the need by rerouting buses, and agreed to present this proposal to the entire city council. The council decided that the request was justified and reasonable, and after study proposed that the need be met by adding more buses during clinic hours and rerouting others to provide the extra service. The council approved the proposal and directed the city-owned bus company to develop a plan and budget. The plan was presented, the council made further modifications, and allocated the necessary funds in the next year's budget.

Generally the community organization process takes considerable time and is characterized by gradual development. The planning stage may take a dozen or more meetings of a committee over a period of time, but it is very important that enough time be allowed. Haynes has commented that developing rapport between professional leaders and the community demands much time and energy. (5) Though in recent years much change has been accomplished with considerable speed, these changes have often been accomplished by other methods than community organization, usually with action produced by pressure, which is more likely to bring about a later reversal action than when change is accomplished through a gradual process.

Since community organization offers the most promising approach to solving community nutrition problems, the community nutritionist needs to know the process and how to use it. However, the nutritionist's primary function is that of nutrition specialist; community organization should be used as a technique for the solution of problems rather than become the main activity of the nutritionist. The nutritionist may assume the role of community organizer to start the process, but should actively seek other leadership and then revert to the primary role of nutrition specialist.

LEADERSHIP

Leadership is important. The job of the leader is to see that things get done, that groups get together, that facts are collected, that funds are raised, that plans are made, and that the program has continuity and direction. The leader must also see that the group considers all points of view and reaches a concensus rather than being dominated by the most vocal, passionate, or opinionated members. It is important that the leader facilitate the group development in such a way that all voices are heard, all opinions are aired, and all members share in the development of the final plan of action. One experienced community nutritionist says that the key to accomplishing any community project lies in finding the right community leader who recognizes the need and value of the project, who can identify the sources of help and support, and who knows how to interest others and overcome the obstacles.

As a community becomes sophisticated in its use of the community organization process, it can eventually depend on its own resources to achieve its goals, with many informed citizens working under indigenous leadership on a variety of problems. The community leaders must have training, which can be one of the contributions of health professionals.

Cohen has said that health practioners carry out community organization tasks when they seek to solve community problems, to enhance and improve community life, and to eliminate social injustice and inequities. The problem-solving focus is organization and planning, including strategies for change. (3)

The nutritionist's skill in functioning effectively in community organization comes from the ability to utilize the knowledge, skills, tools and techniques of community nutrition, putting them into a framework where they are accessible when needed. For example, the nutritionist should know that there is a model for community organization and should understand the general community health structure as a basis for developing and implementing nutrition programs.

Thus it can be seen that the community nutritionist needs to know the community organization process and have a practical view of the way it operates in the community. The nutritionist needs to determine how and by whom the decisions are made (especially those governing allocation of funds), how new programs are initiated, and who supports them. For acceptance in the community, the nutritionist must have a deep appreciation for the existing life of that community and must understand the functions performed by various individuals and institutions, even when they perform these functions inadequately. An understanding of the *role* a person plays in the community is of greater value than merely a direct acquaintance with the person who currently fills the role. The community organization process may work in the "community" of an agency as well as in the broader community.

HOW THE COMMUNITY NUTRITIONIST
USES COMMUNITY ORGANIZATION

The community nutritionist needs to identify the persons in the community who assume leadership roles. They are usually found in clubs and other local organizations. Social action used to be one of the prime objectives of service clubs, social organizations, and civic groups, and in some places they still play a prominent role, although in poverty areas this function has often been assumed by action groups from the community that needs the service.

In most programs the nutritionist will not be the community organizer or will assume this role only temporarily until another leader appears. In some communities there will be existing leadership either from the community itself or from a health educator or other person in a health agency; in others the nutritionist may need to provide or participate in leadership during the initial stages of the program.

Leaders may be found in churches, senior citizen centers, parent-teacher organizations, labor unions, neighborhood houses, women's organizations, voluntary health agencies, and economic opportunity groups.

Development of leadership from the community is important because it establishes a power base for change important to the group. Professional leadership can prevail only for a limited period before returning to other activities, and it is often interpreted as imposing a program upon the community.

Once the group has been organized with a leader, it may organize a number of task forces or committees, each working on a specific problem under the leader. These task forces or committees gather data, explore problems, attack problems that can be solved with available resources, and seek resources and methods for other problems.

In establishing a nutrition committee or council of individuals representing various agencies or interests, nutritionists should keep in mind that there will be a natural tendency for each representative to put agency or individual interests before overall nutrition goals. Only skillful leadership can unite the group for planning for the entire community.

The nutritionist may act in one or more roles as (1) *enabler* or catalytic agent to help the community describe its nutrition problems, such as difficulty in getting food stamps, (2) *advocate* to promote nutrition activities for the solution of problems, such as getting a WIC program as a source of additional food, (3) *planner* to help the community plan ways to deal with its nutrition problems, such as developing an emergency food supply, and (4) *adviser* or consultant to the community leaders by suggesting possible resources or activities for handling a problem. Other possible roles are those of *partisan* who takes sides in a social conflict, and *activist,* who makes judgments and acts on a professional appraisal of the community needs. These may sometimes be appropriate for the nutritionist, depending on the purpose and policies of the agency where the nutritionist works. (2, 4) Some relationships of nutritionist and nutrition committee with the community are shown in Figure 11.1.

Grosser points out (4) that the community organizer interacts with three systems: the *general public* with whom the contact may be indirect through the leaders, the *participants* who are directly engaged in activities with the organizer, that is, the committee or other group involved, and the *target* for change, which may be a bad state of affairs (e.g., hungry children), an agency (e.g., the welfare department), or a category of persons (e.g., parents who neglect children). The organizer may act as a *mediator* between public and target, as a *negotiator* to help the two groups reach agreement, or as an *adviser* or consultant to the leaders when there is no direct communication with the public.

OBTAINING INFORMATION

In the process of identifying community needs and resources, the nutritionist will want to collect information about the various local agencies that have or may have nutrition programs. This is usually done by a

Group	Role of Community Nutritionist	Role of Nutrition Committee
1. Citizens as voters	enabler advocate	enabler advocate
2. Community leaders	enabler advocate planner	planner adviser
3. Politicians	planner adviser	planner adviser advocate
4. Professional and volunteer leaders of official and voluntary agencies	planner adviser	planner advocate
5. Managers of business and industry	advocate adviser	advocate adviser
6. Communications media	advocate planner	enabler advocate
7. School officials and teachers	planner adviser	adviser advocate

Figure 11.1   Role of Community Nutritionist and Nutrition Committee in Public Education.

direct contact in which information is exchanged about agencies and programs. The first contact is usually initiated by a telephone call to the director or to the agency nutritionist if there is one. When there are no nutrition activities in the agency, telephone contact with the director may suffice to obtain all pertinent information; however, if the director has definite ideas about nutrition problems, or contemplates a program, or has information about other programs, a personal contact should be arranged.

In the Cooperative Extension program described on page 58, the nutritionist asked one question to open the conversation: What activities or programs are there in your organization that are designed for health improvement through food and nutrition? If the agency has nutrition-related programs, there should be a discussion of how that program and the one in which the community nutritionist works can relate to each other, how the two agencies can cooperate on programs, and how referrals can be made between the two agencies. During a visit, the nutritionist can answer questions about the agency nutrition program, show materials, and explain services and program plans.

Some questions to be answered in this analysis of each agency are the following: What is the overall goal? What are the specific objectives of current programs? What services are provided to the public? What services to professionals? What nutrition problems are seen in the community? What nutrition or related programs are conducted? Is there a nutrition staff? What are their functions? Do other staff members or volunteers conduct nutrition activities? What media are used for nutrition programs? Are any nutrition-related surveys or research currently under way? Are there reports of past activities?

This information from public and voluntary agencies and other organizations with related programs will give the nutritionist a good picture of the programs in the area and will help to show program gaps as well as possible overlapping or duplication.

A MODEL FOR COMMUNITY ORGANIZATION

The following model that may be used by the community nutritionist is adapted from one suggested by Cohen (2) The steps in the process are:

1. Identify the problem to be solved or the need to be met.
2. Identify the resources.
3. Arrange facts and information to show the relationships.
4. Provide for inputs from all involved in the problem, especially the persons to be served, the group to be changed, and the related agencies.
5. Consider existing policy and the need for policy changes.
6. Prepare several plans for possible solution of the problem, with the probable consequences of each; one alternative should always be "no action."
7. Provide for appropriate structure to carry out the plan selected.

Cohen emphasizes the need to adapt the model to a specific situation at the time it is to be used. Related benefits should be considered; for example, when a citizen-based community project is solving a problem, an additional important goal is to help the community develop its ability to deal with its own problems. Many times some of the information is not available so one or more steps are omitted; however, consciously following the steps helps to assure that no important matter is overlooked.

Though development of the following example did not follow the order of the steps of the model, all elements of it entered into the process. The soundness of the process and its result are shown by the quality and endurance of the service that was developed.

HOW ONE PROGRAM DEVELOPED

This example reports the development of a Meals-on-Wheels service in the city of W—. The local public health nutritionist learned from nurses and senior citizens that there were 30 or 40 elderly persons living in their own homes who were unable to market or prepare adequate meals for themselves. At a Coordinating Council meeting, the nutritionist described the need for 30 to 50 hot meals appropriate for seniors to be delivered to homes in the area daily. The group moved to explore the need and the possibility of meeting it and asked that a meeting be called to consider it further. One of the most interested persons was a dietitian, wife of a local physician who had a large number of chronically ill patients. The dietitian suggested that the local Women's Club of which she was a member might be willing to sponsor the service. The nutritionist invited the dietitian, the president of the Club, and the health department's health educator to a conference to discuss the project. The president thought the group would be interested and invited the nutritionist to talk to the Club about the project and how it could be developed. They also invited a prominent senior citizen to speak about the need and resources of the persons who could benefit from the service.

The Club members were very enthusiastic and voted to start the service, appointing the dietitian as chairman of the M-O-W Committee. The group, accompanied by the nutritionist, visited a similar service that had been operating in a nearby city for several years. They invited the chairman of that project to give an illustrated talk to the Coordinating Council about the meals, funding, delivery, use of volunteers, and reception in the community. The Council voted to allocate money from the previous year's Walk for Hunger to start the program. It was also decided that because modified diets were needed the food should be prepared by a hospital.

Two local hospitals were approached about providing the food, but at first they were not willing because of insurance problems as they would be responsible if the recipients became ill from eating the food. The hospital's insurance covered them as long as the food was on their own premises but ceased at the door. With some support from physicians on the hospital staff, the hospital agreed to provide the food, with its responsibility to cease when the food was taken from the hospital. The Women's Club obtained volunteer legal assistance for help on obtaining insurance to protect the Club when it assumed responsibility for the food. This was done by the Club incorporating on a nonprofit basis and purchasing their own insurance. This solved the problem of the food. Office space was provided by the Health Department. The donated money was used to pay for a telephone, and to purchase equipment. Bookkeeping service was provided by a volunteer. At first the project was entirely a volunteer service, but later a part-time director was hired to take the orders and schedule the volunteers who delivered the food.

Five years later, the project is still in operation. They have an annual recognition dinner for the volunteers to which the nutritionist is always invited even though she was transferred to another area several years ago.

SUMMARY

Community organization is a way to bridge the gap between the individual and social forces that must be changed to correct some nutrition problems of individuals. The community nutritionist can help the community to organize and develop leadership for social action.

Leaders are often found in organized groups in the community such as women's organizations, labor unions, and voluntary health agencies. The nutritionist may act in the capacity of enabler, advocate, planner, or adviser, but should relinquish leadership as soon as it can be developed within the group.

REFERENCES CITED

1. Brager, George and Harry Specht, *Community Organizing,* Columbia University Press, New York, 1973, 27.
2. Cohen, Morris H., Community Organization in Social Work, Ch. 18, edited by Arthur E. Fink, 6th ed., *The Field of Social Work,* Holt, Rinehart and Winston, New York, 309.
3. Ibid., 333.
4. Grosser, Charles F., *New Directions in Community Organization,* Praeger, New York, 1973, 190.
5. Haynes, Alfred, A New Medical Center, in *The University Medical Center and the Metropolis,* edited by Eli Ginzberg and Alice M. Yohalem, Josiah Macy, Jr. Foundation, New York, 1974, 45.
6. Schwebel, Andrew I., Richard Kershaw, Susan Reeve, John H. Hartung, and William Reeve, A Community Organization Approach to Implementation of Comprehensive Health Planning, *Am. J. Pub. Health,* 63 8/73 675.
7. Seder, Richard H., Planning and Politics in the Allocation of Health Resources, *Am. J. Pub. Health,* 63 9/73 774.

ADDITIONAL REFERENCES

Bruhn, John G., Planning for Social Change, *Am. J. Pub. Health,* 63 7/73 602.

Jay, A., How To Run a Meeting, *Harvard Bus. Rev.,* 54 3-4/76 43.

Kane, Robert L. ed., *The Challenges of Community Medicine,* Springer Publishing Co., New York, 1974.

Level, Dale A., Committees: Functional or Fancy, *Adult Leadership,* 16 12/67 214.

Mattison, Berwyn F., Community Health Planning and the Health Profession, *Am. J. Pub. Health,* 58 6/68 1015.

Melvin, Ernest E., The Community in Concept and in Development, *Adult Leadership,* 24 10/75 53.

Springer, Ninfa, and Robert M. Segal, Dietitians' Attitudes Toward Advocacy, *J. Am. Diet. Assoc.,* 67 11/75 445.

Wang, Virginia Li, Using Cooperative Extension Programs for Health Education, *Am. Jour. Pub. Health,* 64 2/74 107.

Wang, Virginia Li, Arlene Fonaroff, and John Dawson, Problem Solving for Common Goals in Two Types of Community Agencies, *Am. Jour. Pub. Health,* 65 8/75 809.

Wang, Virginia L., *Planning for Community Health Services: Challenges to Extension,* MEP 285, Cooperative Extension Service, University of Maryland, College Park MD, April 1969.

12 MANAGEMENT AND PLANNING

Management is accomplishing a purpose by the use and control of time, energy, money, and other resources. This is done by making a series of decisions about the use of the resources and about the action to be taken. Community nutritionists need to understand the technique of management because most of them are responsible for managing a program, or some part of a program. Sometimes it encompasses only their own activities and sometimes the work of a staff. Management duties include planning, budgeting, directing personnel, keeping records, and procuring supplies. The methods of management to be described will be applicable in all programs, although the nutritionist-director of a large program will need to acquire additional training in organization theory, personnel practices, data systems, cost analysis, and operation in the agency power structure.

The purpose of using management technique is to make the most of resources. One of the keys in its use is to save time by reducing to a routine as many functions as possible, thus releasing time for other activities. Acquiring the skills discussed in Chapter 10 is one way; for example, a nutritionist can reduce the time needed to evaluate printed materials by acquiring skill in the procedure described (p. 180).

Management cannot perform miracles, but it can make the most of limited resources although in itself it cannot increase the resources available. For example, good management of food money can enable a family to get the best possible diet for its money, but it cannot increase the amount of money available for food, although better management may be able to free some from other parts of the budget.

DECISION-MAKING AND PROBLEM-SOLVING

One element of management used in every step is *decision-making,* which consists of choices about use of time, energy, money and the desires of people. It is an integral part of all personal and professional planning. Decision-making can be a very sophisticated process although in community nutrition practice this is not often possible. At the other extreme is conceiving one plan and putting it into effect without consideration of alternatives. It is good practice to base a decision on the best available data also considering the outcomes of previous similar decisions by the planner or by others.

Decisions should be based on facts, and should avoid bias although they are sometimes reinforced by emotion. Decisions need imagination and originality to induce a constant flow of new thought. Wise decision-making takes flexibility of thought, as in adapting various ways to look at a problem and to express it. The decision-maker must recognize that some decisions will be wrong and must accept the limitations imposed by position, time, energy, education, knowledge, and ability of both self and others.

A good decision-maker recognizes when the time is right, makes small decisions quickly, but faces difficult decisions with equanimity, keeping alternative plans in mind. Occasionally there should be a review of long-standing decisions to see if they are still valid.

Problem-Solving

Drucker considers minor or everyday decisions as problem-solving or operational, reserving the term decision-making for important decisions that determine policy. (2) Problem-solving involves these steps:

1. Statement of the problem with the pertinent facts.
2. Identification of the main problem and the reason it exists.
3. Analyzing and listing the cause.
4. Imagining various solutions and recording the probable consequences.
5. Weighing and listing the relative merits of each solution.
6. Deciding the action to be taken and listing the steps needed to implement the solution.
7. Planning how and when to evaluate the results.
8. After a suitable lapse of time, evaluating the results.

Example of Problem-Solving. Problem-solving often occurs in a crisis as in the example which follows.

Problem. At 9:15 a.m. ten nurses are waiting for a nutritionist due at 9:00 to conduct a two-hour workshop on food money management. The chairman telephones to ask if someone else can come. The main problem is failure of the nutritionist to appear because of an accident. The chairman suggested that she could hold the afternoon session in the morning if a nutritionist could come to the afternoon session.

Possible solutions. *Solution 1:* Staff Nutritionist Ms. A. could take the program. She could do it with a minimum of preparation since she has done the same program several times with other groups and has an outline and materials ready. However, she is supposed to attend an important meeting of a health planning group that afternoon, but is in the office until 12 o'clock. *Solution 2:* Nutrition Director might take the program, but she is due at Executive Staff meeting. *Solution 3:* Staff Nutritionist Mrs. B. could come from her health center 15 miles away to conduct the program, but she would have to miss a regularly scheduled clinic, and reschedule appointments to another date. *Solution 4:* Staff Nutritionist Ms. C. is free but started on the job only three days before. She has never conducted this type of meeting but is willing, provided Ms. A. will help her plan and prepare. *Solution 5:* Tell the chairman that it is not possible to send anyone in the afternoon. Solution 5 was immediately rejected because this was the first time that this particular group had requested staff education, and since the nutritionists had noted that the nurses used considerable misinformation, they wanted to develop a good relationship and have other educational meetings for them. Any one of the other solutions was acceptable to the staff.

Steps to implement. *Solution 4* was selected as the best. The necessary steps were for Ms. A. to show Ms. C. the outline for the session, the available teaching tools, and printed materials. After these were selected, resource materials were given to Ms. C. She looked over the materials, and studied the map to avoid delay. She was well accepted by the nurses who had particularly wanted the subject matter, so the decision was considered to have been a good one. The staff members were especially gratified when the group later requested a second session on another topic. It is unlikely that they would have done so had a way not been found to keep this commitment.

Decision-Making

The basic steps in making a specific decision (2) should be stated in writing so that the nutritionist considers the entire process, and the statement can be used to explain the reasons for the decision to persons who will be involved in the implementation.

1. State a concrete goal.
2. Identify the policies and premises that relate to the goal.
3. Develop a list of alternative solutions including "no action."
4. Consider each alternative with special attention to the strategic or limiting factors, visualizing the implementation and possible results.
5. Evaluate the various possibilities, considering the benefits and results of each.
6. Select the best plan. Sometimes this may be done on the basis of past experience, sometimes testing or further investigation may be indicated.

Example of Decision-Making. The goal of this activity is to identify children with signs of retarded growth and obesity and to correct these problems in early life.

Policies and premises that relate to the goal:

1. There are no special funds to budget for this activity.
2. The plan must be accomplished with existing personnel, which includes nurses, nutritionist, and secretary.
3. The method should be one that can be continued at least six years.

Alternative solutions, related factors, implementation:

Plan A. The nutritionist could use figures on height, weight, and hematocrit available from charts of all children known to the health care center, with the secretary keeping the records. There are a number of limiting factors. Height and weight are taken by inaccurate methods. It would be difficult or impossible to get children to come to the health center regularly for weighing and measuring. There will be changes of personnel that will make it difficult to maintain continuity. An impending change in the record system at the center could mean records might be kept elsewhere after one year. One advantage would be that the nutritionist would have control over the activity.

Plan B. This is similar to Plan A but would use only data from the EPSDT program at the health center. This plan would include most five-year-olds known to the health center. The nutritionist could teach accurate weighing and measuring to the personnel. The number of children would be small enough for the secretary to handle the record keeping. The limiting factor is that there might be changes in agency personnel and record keeping that could terminate the project.

Plan C. Establish the program in the public school when children enter the first grade. Weighing and measuring are routinely done every four months by teachers with help from the school nurse. The nutritionist could teach accurate measuring methods and provide growth charts for recording the data. The specific objective is to identify children whose growth records show that they are deviating from the limits of normal growth. The growth record could be kept until the end of the sixth grade. When there is evidence of retarded growth or obesity, the need would be discussed with the parent and care arranged. The limiting factors are that some children will move, so monitoring will end for them, and that the nutritionist will be an adviser rather than the director of the activity, therefore lacking authority to see that the activity is correctly implemented.

Plan D. This is a no action plan so it has no success and leaves the situation where it now is, with no solution to the problem.

Evaluation. Plan A has some chance of success but the number of children would be limited and coverage incomplete, and there is no assurance of continuity. The nutritionist might spend considerable time starting the plan and the plan may be discontinued after a short time. Plan B may have a good chance of immediate success for children covered, but there is no assurance that they can be followed as this would depend on their returning to clinic at regular intervals and experience has shown that they do not come in for preventive care. Plan C provides a way to follow the children for six years. Children who move could take their records with them to a new school and this might result in the initiation of a similar program there. The possibility of accurate measurement is good because nurses and teachers are interested and would like for the nutritionist to arrange a workshop on how to weigh and measure. Children who have problems can be referred to the health center for care. Surveillance by growth chart provides a graphic way to show children and parents the progress of each child. This will require considerable attention from the nutritionist in the initial stage but minimum attention afterwards. Plan D will not, of course, achieve the goal. Plan C is selected as having the best possibility of success.

The listing or recording of choices, ideas, and other factors is an important technique of both decision-making and problem-solving. It forces intense thinking and clear observations and eliminates extraneous matters. A quick glance over the records and lists shows where the thinking has been, how it evolved, and where it is going. Many decisions are made quickly without considering all the factors involved or more than one alternative; however, many turn out to be poor decisions that have a profound influence over long periods of time on staffing, patient care, employee relations, permanent facilities, and other important matters. Carefully conceived decision-making is more likely to result in long-range operations that give better service to the clientele and more satisfactory working conditions for employees than when it is a hasty, haphazard process.

STEPS IN THE MANAGEMENT PROCESS

Management proceeds in a series of steps that includes:

1. Planning
2. Organizing and coordinating
3. Putting the plan into action
4. Controlling the plan in action
5. Evaluation

Planning as used in this context means identifying needs and potential threats to the population, analyzing the possible ways of allocating resources in ways that will best handle needs and threats and determine the costs and benefits of the various alternatives. This kind of planning is not for the purpose of supporting any one course of action but to project the effect of various courses on the specific measures selected. (9)

The major planning in community nutrition is program planning, one of the most important activities of the community nutritionist.

Program Planning

A *program* is the combination of personnel, facilities, money, equipment, supplies, and other items directed to accomplish specific objectives. Program planning is putting the problems and resources into a framework to provide the best use of the resources to solve the problems. The process has nine steps.

Determining the Problems. This is done from already known statistics, from data collected for the purpose, or from information supplied by other community agencies or leaders.

Setting a Baseline from the Data. This is the point from which the progress will be measured, as in a community dental clinic where 80 percent of the children have four or more cavities.

Stating Goals, Objectives, and Methods of Evaluation. A *goal* is the concrete end toward which action will be directed. Goal is sometimes equated with *mission;* however, it is better to use "mission" to denote the more general level, such as "optimal nutrition for everyone in the community." The lack of a precise definition of optimal nutrition, the impossibility of reaching it, and the impracticability of defining the point when it is reached make this an unsatisfactory landmark for a program.

A goal should be a point that can be clearly defined and recognized on arrival. The goal might be "to improve the nutritional status of preschool children." This meets the criteria as we can assess nutritional status by specific measures, provide treatment designed to correct the problems, and assess again. A broad goal such as this is best handled by division into a number of specific objectives, for example,

1. by June 30, 1977, 50 percent of the children with iron deficiency anemia will be eating an adequate diet.
2. by December 31, 1977, 75 percent of the children will have hemoglobin levels standard for their age and all other identified cases of anemia will be under treatment.

The objective is stated in terms of a result expected rather than in terms of operation or action. The objective should be concrete, measurable, and attainable. An action as operating goal or objective may sometimes be appropriate, especially for the community nutritionist whose work is administration rather than directly executing programs; for example, in setting up a project or program, operating goals may be: (1) by June 30, to have all staff on the job, and (2) by July 15, to start nutrition classes.

Developing Plans for Various Interventions. Include all that can accomplish the goals. Decide the feasibility of each according to available resources of time, personnel and money. Usually, after defining overall goals, the planning of specific objectives must proceed concurrently with planning the use of resources to meet the goals. In actual practice, the planning does not proceed in a straight line but deviates to consider the various possibilities, then a decision is made to select the best. Figure 12.1 illustrates the process of program planning.

The feasibility of each approach and the probability of success must be considered. The consideration of various alternatives should be done in a very practical way, basing the decision on the best available data, with a consideration of successes achieved in previous programs by the planner or by others as found from personal inquiry or literature search. It is unfortunate when one plan is conceived and put into effect without consideration of alternatives that might produce a better result.

Method The Preschool Anemia Project	Intervention: Various Ways to Achieve Objective	Educate mother to provide proper food Provide an iron supplement Provide breakfast and lunch at child care center Establish a WIC program for supplementary food	Consider Probable Results of Each Intervention and Select the Most Promising	Result-Objective In one year reduce the number of anemic children by 50 percent

Figure 12.1   Deciding on the Best Way to Achieve Objective.

Selecting the Best Plan of Evaluation.   Evaluation is the process of ascertaining the value of the program or activity. It must be planned before the program is started or it cannot be done. The evaluation plan must include:

1. What is to be evaluated. This may be change in food practices, such as increasing the amount of citrus fruit consumed by the family.
2. What will be measured. This might be amount of citrus fruit before and after an educational program.
3. Method of measuring the change. This must be a way to determine how much citrus fruit was used before and after the program.
4. How the data will be collected. This includes a way to obtain an accurate record of the kind and amount of citrus fruit used.

Organizing and Coordinating

This is the preparation stage. If there are other staff involved besides the nutritionist, they must be directed and their work coordinated. Sometimes there are one or more other nutritionists or dietitians, a home economist, and a nutrition technician or nutrition aide, along with a clerical staff. The kind and extent of resources must also be considered. There may be only the nutritionist's time and a few hours from a clerical worker, or there may be the substantial interest and time of a nurse who visits the family in the home. In some areas an EFNEP worker may be available to assist the family. Often the key resource is the amount of money available and the specific uses for which it is intended, as for purchase or repair of equipment. For example, in the school measuring program, scales are available but need to be calibrated, and measuring tapes need to be purchased and mounted on the walls where measuring will take place. A workshop must be arranged so teachers and nurses can learn measuring methods, and a letter sent to parents to explain the project and obtain consent for their children to participate.

Putting the Plan into Action

This is when the program actually begins. The staff have been trained, space and equipment are ready, and consents have been obtained. The nutritionist attends the measuring and helps the nurse enter the data on the graphs. The date for the second measuring is set. The nurse talks with parents about the children who are underweight or overweight or who show retarded growth, and checks later to see that necessary care has been provided.

After the program is under way, there is a periodic review to control the direction and extent of progress and to make sure that the program is moving along to accomplish the stated objectives. Since this is a long-range program, the periodic review is especially important.

Evaluation

Evaluation is the process of determining whether an activity or a program has accomplished its purpose or how much of the purpose has been accomplished. The decision to continue or to discontinue, to repeat, or to modify an activity should be based on what the program has accomplished. The evaluation method should be objective if possible, although subjective evaluation can also be valuable.

When the stated goal has been achieved, or the alloted time has elapsed, the action and results should be evaluated. Sometimes this takes place while the program is still in operation, sometimes after it has been terminated. In the school program, the first major evaluation will be made at the end of the first year, with attention given to the progress of individual children within normal growth patterns. By that time, this surveillance will have become a regular feature of the school program.

The children whose growth patterns are not within the normal range will be identified and the parents counseled about action needed. These children will be weighed and measured at regular intervals as a high-risk population, at least until they are back in the normal range.

The intervention that is used should also be evaluated. The effect of nutrition education may be evaluated by change in food practices as shown by food records taken before and after the education. The effect of teaching a nurse how to counsel on normal diet can be evaluated by observing the counseling before and after the educational program. The effect of counseling on the individual can be evaluated by measuring adherence to the diet before and after the counseling. The effect of a known increase in iron intake may be evaluated by hemoglobin values before and after the increase. Sometimes it has been proposed that the physiological change in the patient (hemoglobin in anemia) can serve as a direct measure of the value of counseling, but the intermediate step of determining the change in food intake seems to be necessary since some other factor may have been at work.

Controlling the Plan in Action

The school staff have learned the proper methods of weighing, measuring, and recording. The nutritionist supervises the first measurements, which become the baseline. Before the second measuring, the nutritionist meets with the staff to review the methods. They are responsible for the entire process, but the nutritionist drops in to answer questions and discuss the progress of the children.

DISCUSSION

How much planning can take place in a specific community nutrition program depends largely on the policies and practices of the nutritionist's agency. In some there is extensive scientific planning with an agency program that includes all elements. Sometimes the nutrition program is already ongoing and has been structured. Management may want it to continue as is, it may want specific changes, or it may expect the nutritionist to manage the program under general direction from higher authority, often expecting the nutritionist to survey needs, plan the program, suggest activities, and implement the program.

The program manager-community nutritionist must learn to operate within the framework that exists, working toward changes that will enhance nutrition and health, while learning how to manage the nutrition program even if there is little overall agency planning, or when the major interest is in another area such as social counseling. Though the prevailing medical model gives first priority to the sick patient, with the physician making a diagnosis, prescribing treatment, and referring patients for nutritional guidance when indicated, the nutritionist must assume responsibility for using nutritional care to prevent disease and promote health, and for making judgments about the nutritional needs of individual, family, and community.

In the neighborhood health center, which is the current base for primary medical care, the nutritionist should extend the nutrition component of the program into the community rather than limit activities to consultation to the primary care team or attempt to counsel all patients, because many nutrition problems must be solved by prevention.

The nutrition needs of the community will be best served when the program is managed by a nutritionist whose primary background is firm grounding in the application of the science of nutrition to the community, and who adds to this the ability to use management technique.

SUMMARY

Every community nutritionist manages some part of a program and should know the principles, processes, and steps in management and how to apply them in community nutrition.

Decision-making is an important part of management while problem-solving, a similar but lower level process, occurs frequently. A written statement of the action in each management decision clarifies the process, helps in thinking about it, and explains the reasons to others. In decision-making, it is important that the possible alternatives be considered and evaluated by probable results, and the best decision selected from the alternatives.

Program planning is a management process which occurs in nine steps. Each is accompanied by the necessity of making decisions and solving problems.

REFERENCES

1. Day, Mary Lou, and Gertrude Blaker, Management Attitudes and Personality Characteristics of Dietitians, *J. Am. Diet. Assoc.,* 65 10/74 403–409.
2. Drucker, Peter F., *The Effective Executive,* Harper and Row, New York, 1967.
3. Gordon, John E., and Nevin S. Scrimshaw, Evaluating Nutrition Intervention Programs, *Nutr. Rev.,* 30 12/72 263.
4. Make Decisions You Can Live With, *Supervisory Mgt.,* 19 12/74 28–31, condensed from *Christopher News Notes,* 10/74.
5. Making Changes That Stick, *Supervisory Mgt.,* 18 12/73 14.
6. Mattison, Berwyn F., Community Health Planning and the Health Professions, *Am. J. Pub. Health,* 58 6/68 1015.
7. Neumann, Alfred K., Charlotte G. Neumann, and Aaron E. Ifekwunigive, Evaluation of Small-Scale Nutrition Programs, *Am. J. Clin. Nutr.,* 26 4/73 446.

8. Oppenheim, Irene, *Management of the Modern Home,* Macmillan Publishing Co., New York, 1972, 51–74.

9. Seder, Richard H., Planning and Politics in the Allocation of Health Resources, *Am. J. Pub. Health,* 63 9/73 774.

10. Walsh, Helen, The Changing Nature of Public Health, *J. Am. Diet. Assoc.,* 49 12/66 93.

11. Williams, Flora L., The 15 Golden Rules for Success as a Manager. *J. Home Econ.,* 66 9/74 30.

13 PROFESSIONAL EDUCATION

Professional education is used here to mean all the activities of the community nutritionist in training other professionals and paraprofessionals in nutrition subject matter and methods of conducting programs. Community nutritionists have always depended on other health personnel such as nurses, physicians, dentists, home economists, social workers, health educators, and teachers, whose regular work puts them in direct contact with people, to carry much of the nutrition message. For this reason, professional education is one of the most important and productive phases of the nutritionist's work. Inservice education can increase competency and give nurses and other health personnel confidence in their ability to deal with nutritional care as a part of their own fields of practice.

With the growth of many new health professions and paraprofessions, this education needs to be at both professional and paraprofessional levels, the latter referring to nutrition technicians and nutrition aides. In addition to the employed health professionals and paraprofessionals, there is need for community nutritionists to participate in professional education for students from a number of disciplines during their field work or internships in health agencies and to plan educational events to increase their own knowledge and capabilities.

In many health settings, the nurse has been responsible for most of the family health education, including nutrition. Though there has been a considerable increase in the number of nutritionists working directly with patients, most of them are in specially funded projects for mothers and children, many functioning as clinical dietitians with little or no community involvement.

The purpose of professional education is to add to the knowledge of nutrition, (e.g., nutrients of new importance), to increase the understanding of clients (e.g., food practices of vegetarians), to encourage use of new teaching methods (e.g., a series of new leaflets for teaching mothers to feed children during the early years), to present methods of nutrition education (e.g., demonstrate counseling on controlled-fat diet using food exchanges), or to develop a favorable attitude (e.g., to get a physician to use the agency diet for pregnancy rather than one from a commercial source).

In order to teach other health professionals, the community nutritionist needs, first, an extensive knowledge of subject matter to establish and maintain credibility; second, knowledge of the clientele; third, knowledge of educational methods and their application in community nutrition programs; and fourth understanding of the educational background and function of other professionals, both as a discipline and in the agency.

Various professional persons will already have some of the skills, for example, public health nurses have counseling skills, teachers know how to teach, and home economists are knowledgeable about helping families with homemaking and management, while health educators know how to help the community organize for the solution of problems.

The physician, nurse and home economist receive some formal education in nutrition as part of their training. Others who conduct nutrition education or support nutrition programs may not have had formal nutrition training, for example, writers of popular publications on nutrition, paraprofessionals in allied health fields, food editors, radio, film and television scriptwriters and advertising copywriters.

In addition to giving professional persons the necessary information about nutrition and methods, the nutritionist needs to motivate them to conduct nutrition education. This is done by emphasizing nutrition as an important part of health care, which can make their work more effective by helping families solve immediate problems that interfere with their following good health practices or a medical care plan.

Professional education may be conducted in a variety of ways. The knowledge needed by practitioners of other disciplines depends on how they will relate to the community group. Generally everyone who does nutrition education should know the nutrient needs of the various age groups, the basic foods that make up a good diet, the amounts of foods needed, food sources of nutrients, (especially whether a nutrient is widely distributed or needs to come from a few foods), the effect of cooking and storage on food values, alternate foods, cultural food practices, kinds and uses of equipment, food costs and how to plan within specific cost levels, place of vitamin, mineral, and other food supplements and factors that influence family spending and buying. They must also know how to identify the persons who can profit from nutrition education and how to recognize their problems.

The nutritionist needs to give other professionals a perception of how the nutrition education process works, emphasizing that it starts with a review of family food practices, and the factors that determine them and how members of the family feel about them. Good family food practices must be identified and reinforced while the counselor leads the family into a decision to change poor practices. The counselor also needs specific information on the conditions most often encountered in specific programs, such as obesity, underweight, diabetes, hyperlipidemias, hypertension, dental caries, constipation, and diarrhea. Community nutritionists need to maintain their own perception and skills in patient counseling by seeing at least a few patients from time to time, and where there is a staff of clinical nutritionists, to maintain community liaisons for them. Each member of the health team can contribute to the nutritional care of the individual or family; likewise, the nutritionist should contribute to their activities.

PHYSICIANS

Flynn suggests that the physician needs to know how to find out what the individual eats, (i.e., by food record or diet history), how to use the RDA as a standard for assessing the diet, how to make a rough estimate of the adequacy of calories, protein, calcium, and iron, and how to identify possible future vitamin problems by comparing intakes with the recommended allowances. (9)

Flynn believes that because there are inadequate numbers of clinical dietitians, the family physician or nurse-practitioner who is initially involved in care of the patient should handle the less complicated nutrition problems rather than refer them to the dietitian. She points out that the physician's greater knowledge of the family background may make the physician more effective than the dietitian could be.

Frankle (10) suggests that the physician should know the sources of nutrition information that are available and act as a consumer-advisor to the patient. The National Nutrition Consortium suggests that the physician know the effect of nutrition on health, how to apply nutrition principles in patient care, and when to use nutrition specialists. (15) Hegsted sees the physician's role as knowing enough about nutrition to diagnose the nutrition problems and prescribe the proper diets. (11)

Though the establishment of nutrition course work in the curriculum at some medical schools has been accomplished, there are still many physicians with little nutrition knowledge, some of whom become food enthusiasts, even faddists.

The community nutritionist in an agency where there are physicians needs to work with the physicians to help them understand what they need to know, to identify their deficiencies in nutrition information and practice, and to participate with them in developing ways to correct these deficiencies. Some of the common needs are (1) to develop an appreciation that good nutrition enhances patient care and makes treatment more effective and that improving food practices and related health practices (e.g. exercise) makes a lifelong contribution to health, (2) to suggest practical ways for nutrition education, and (3) to develop the understanding that patients with complicated diets or multiple socioeconomic problems that interfere with nutrition should be referred to the nutritionist, who is qualified to help with their problems.

When working with physicians, the nutritionist should recognize that there are inherent, fundamental differences in the way nutritionists and physicians look at the individual and initiate treatment. Many physicians have been trained to think in terms of an individual with a problem that must be immediately diagnosed and a treatment prescribed because this is what the patient expects. The nutritionist, who is not under this constraint of immediacy, can see that all significant facts are marshalled and considered in planning a care program, with special attention to identifying and putting under care the persons most likely to become malnourished.

Examples of Education for Physicians

Gives oral report to clinicians on problems of 20 diabetic patients and their families as identified from food records.

Prepares a written report for clinicians on food intake of families of obese infants.

Sends reprint of article on prenatal nutrition from a nutrition journal to director of maternal health.

Gives consultation to internist in private practice on methods of assessing adult obesity.

Sends regular newsletter reporting current nutrition highlights to professionals.

Prepares exhibit with handout leaflet on medications that interfere with nutrition and recommended solutions.

Advises physician in alcohol program about management of food service in a halfway house.

Prepares exhibit on new Exchange Lists for physicians' symposium on heart disease, and answers questions of persons who visit the exhibit.

NURSES

Most nurses working in health agencies, hospitals, physician's offices, industry, and schools have many opportunities to influence food practices. The community nutritionist should encourage them to incorporate nutrition education into their regular work. Nurses have the closest and most continuous contact with patients, hence great influence, and they carry out nutrition education in many settings in both planned and unplanned ways, thereby supporting or negating the teaching done by others. (19)

According to Tinkham and Voorhies, the community health nurse's role includes being the health teacher and coordinator of services provided by other members of the health team. (19) They describe the function of the community health nurse as collaborating with families and groups in identifying their health problems and needs and in finding community resources to help in meeting their needs. In a home visit, the community nurse may interpret the physician's recommendations, answer questions about nutrition information heard on the radio, or counsel the homemaker on family meal planning. The nutritionist must give the nurse the necessary background so that the nurse can help the family solve its nutrition problems. There is much variation in nurses' knowledge and attitudes about nutrition, believed to be determined by the content of their education. (13, 20)

The extent of the nurse's information about nutrition may vary from little to much, depending on the nursing school, the interest that has led to further education, and previous contacts with nutritionists and dietitians. In most cases, more emphasis has been placed on diet therapy for the acutely ill patient than on normal nutrition for the family. The nurse needs to know sex-age adaptations for family members and other modifications for persons in the family circle, such as the pregnant or lactating woman, a diabetic adult or child, or an adult on a weight-losing, restricted sodium, or controlled fat diet.

In a study by Vickstrom and Fox, it was found that older nurses had less nutrition knowledge than younger nurses, but they tended to have more positive attitudes towards nutrition education. (20) The study also showed that nurses' knowledge of normal and therapeutic nutrition was about 50 percent accurate; however, there was considerable uncertainty in their feelings about what they knew and their ability to apply it.

In discussing the relationship between nutritionist and nurse, Anderson and Browe say (1) ". . . the nurse by virtue of her close and continuous contact with families or individuals, is the appraiser of needs, and the counselor or teacher; and the nutritionist, by virtue of her specialized preparation, is the resource person for appraisal and planning and when circumstances demand her special content in this area, the advisor or counselor."

Examples of Education for Community Nurses

Regularly provides education by lecture, discussion, or workshop for groups of community nurses. Topics may include: new information on nutrition in pregnancy, nutrients receiving current emphasis, accurate methods of weighing and measuring, using new resource materials, current food prices and their effect on family food costs.

Routinely acquaints new nurses with agency policies, methods, and materials by conference and consultation.

Arranges food demonstration by a home economist from the electric company on new convenience foods showing cost and nutrient content.

Demonstrates use of patient records to identify possible nutrition problems.

Explains how nurse can monitor diabetic diet of man recently discharged from hospital.

TEACHERS

Teachers in lower grades should have preparation in nutrition and methods so they can influence the food and other health practices of children and parents and recognize problems of nutrition or diet for referral to nutritionists. Because of their close continuing contact with the children, they are in a strategic position to carry on nutrition education effectively when their own background gives them confidence.

Some community nutritionists are in positions where they can influence the preparation or provide inservice education or consultation to teachers. If this can be a priority for the nutritionist's time, the nutritionist should get acquainted with key personnel in the schools. The principal, nursing director, curriculum director, home economics teacher, and others may be in a position to influence nutrition education. This will often result in requests for the nutritionist to talk to groups of teachers, parents, or children, or to participate in curriculum planning or preparation or revision of teaching materials, or to conduct a workshop to help individual teachers plan how to teach nutrition.

Many teachers need to be shown how to incorporate nutrition teaching into their classroom work. Once, when a nutritionist was talking with a group of high school teachers about how they might improve poor food habits among their students, she suggested that each incorporate some nutrition concepts into their regular classroom work. One teacher laughed and said, "You can't do that with Latin!" The nutritionist suggested that the students find out what the Romans ate and what diseases they had and analyze the information for possible relationships. Calculation of the nutrient content and cost of food eaten by students offers a way to incorporate nutrition teaching into mathematics.

Nutritionists in some public agencies have responsibilities for the public schools; in others they do not, and few school systems have nutrition specialists on their staffs. Some school systems are funded for outside consultants, and in one agency where policies did not permit staff nutritionists to work in the public schools, the nutritionists were able to conduct workshops and institutes on their own time for regular school consultant fees. One five-day institute covered nutrition subject matter and food money management. Nutritionists may fill another important role by helping teachers plan inservice education for themselves.

In Massachusetts, 6- to 12-hour workshops in several sessions were held for teachers. (4) When possible, groups were held on released time; attendance was limited to 15 and teachers divided into primary (K–3) and intermediate (4–6) sections. The workshops were informal and action-oriented. They were initiated by contacts of the state Department of Education, Bureau of Nutrition Education and School Food Services, with administrators, curriculum coordinators, health educator, school nurses, and school food service personnel.

A project in five southern states to study team teaching by classroom teachers and school food service personnel identified nutrition competencies needed by personnel to participate in the team-teaching. (12) These were the top four:

1. Identify the major nutrients, their sources in foods, and relate the main nutrients to the basic four food groups.
2. Describe the characteristics of normal growth and development processes for the age group of children with whom they are working and relate proper nutrition to the process.

3. Demonstrate the relationship between nutrition and personal health of the individual, including the concepts of nutritional deficiencies, weight control, empty calories, and so forth.

4. Distinguish among a wide variety of foods and demonstrate a selection from this variety that meets individual nutrition needs and is personally satisfying.

Physical education teachers and athletic coaches seem especially likely to have misinformation on food and nutrition. Cho and Fryer gave a nutritional knowledge test to 138 physical education majors and 81 non-nutrition majors who were completing a course in basic nutrition. They found that the physical education students who got most of their information in college courses (health and sciences, physical education, and home economics) had significantly higher scores than those who got their information from coaches or parents. The basic nutrition students scored higher on the tests than the physical education students. (5)

A test of the two groups in application of their knowledge to foods for athletes showed that both groups "made recommendations that have no scientific basis and emphasized use of such supplements as protein, iron, and multivitamins, although PE students were more prone to recommend honey, wheat germ, gelatin, and Gatorade." (6)

An inservice education program for home economics teachers was reported by Cowell and Sobelsohn. (7) It was requested by the schools to provide new nutrition information and help with their special problems due to a variety of cultural groups. Specific objectives were (1) to provide knowledge, (2) to demonstrate teaching techniques on how to use the new knowledge, keeping in mind the cultural patterns of students and families, (3) to use consumer information to improve individual and family food practices, and (4) to provide opportunity for teachers from K–12 to share experiences. They held three 2-hour sessions using several techniques: (1) presenting nutrition information in a dialog between a public health nutritionist and a physician, (2) displaying various media—exhibits, slides, bulletin boards, resource materials, snack foods—and having a demonstration of a good food shopper and a poor food shopper, and (3) developing lesson plans that adapted ideas about the meaning of food, and nutrition theory to cultural food patterns.

The author's recipe for enabling home economics teachers to keep up to date and be able to act as a resource in nutrition can be applied as well to other professionals. It recommends that the teacher keep two college nutrition textbooks and one popular nutrition book, replenishing each every five years on a staggered schedule so that one book is always up to date. The teacher also needs a nutritionist, dietitian, or college nutrition teacher as a consultant when further advice is needed, and should take a refresher course in nutrition at least every five years. The five-year period is set because of the rapid development in the field that necessitates updating at least this often.

Examples of Education for Teachers

Provides information for a sixth grade teacher on nutrient content of foods used by East Asians and suggests markets where the foods are sold.

Provides list of recent references on how to teach nutrition to a home economics teacher.

Participates in arranging a symposium for physical education teachers, nutritionists, and dietitians on nutrition for athletes.

OTHER PROFESSIONALS

Nutritionists conduct education by providing teaching and resource materials, arranging large and small group activities, and giving individual conference and consultation to other professionals such as dentists, dental hygienists, social workers, health educators, counselors, food editors, and radio and television personnel.

Examples of Education for Other Professionals

Gives lecture and discussion for social workers on food money management and welfare food allowances.

Sends an article on dental nutrition that appeared in a nutrition journal to the health center dentist and dental hygienist.

On request sends summary and references on fluorine from recent nutrition journals to health center dentist.

Gives lecture and discussion on nutrition of the aging for a group of senior citizen counselors.

Provides information and references to food editor on sources of zinc, folic acid, and vitamin B_{12} in vegetarian diets.

Presents information of general interest to professionals and other agency staff, such as results of food price survey and impact on family food expenditures. Group may include physicians, nurses, social worker, health educator, office manager, clerical staff, sanitarian, custodian, and other personnel.

PARAPROFESSIONALS

In the last few years, there has been a great increase in the number and classes of paraprofessionals who work in nutrition programs. These include nutrition aides and nutrition technicians. There has also been a tendency to combine training and avoid specialization in allied health groups and to provide both vertical and horizontal career mobility. Nutrition personnel will need to have additional training for this specialty. This may mean that the nutrition aide who comes from a general background must devote more time to preparation for a generalized position such as community worker than to preparation for the nutrition aide position.

The nutritionist will need to train staff for the specific job, in some cases being able to build on formal training received in junior college, nursing curriculum, or community worker courses, in others starting with an individual who has no concept of the health field, and providing orientation and training about the health field as well as about the agency. Specific subject matter must also be taught. This may require a long training period with the aide assuming one task at a time while training takes place. Some agencies have a standard training program for all employees; in others the nutritionist will need to plan and arrange the training and conduct much of it. Sometimes a local school can add such a training course to the curriculum, but only if there appears to be a need for enough of this class of personnel to provide jobs for all the persons who complete the course. Considerable misinformation is found in this group, so it is well to explore factual knowledge and attitudes and correct this problem early; often it is harder to train such a person than to train one with little information on nutrition.

The kind of training provided for EFNEP program aides would provide an excellent background for nutrition aides who need some knowledge of food, nutrition, other areas of homemaking, methods for teaching, motivation, and community resoources. (18)

Since the curriculum for the dietetic technician is determined by the American Dietetic Association (16) and conducted in a two-year associate degree college program, technicians have a more uniform background than most other classes for whom the community nutritionist may plan inservice education; however, most of the field experiences are in hospitals and nursing homes and may lack a community component.

An inservice educational program for dietetic technicians working with older persons has been described by Caliendo. (3) The clientele were geriatric patients who lived in a center that provided care in different settings from apartment living to skilled nursing homes. The technicians worked as members of the resident care team; however, the elements of training could be adapted to training of technicians to work with older persons living in their own homes. Classes covered six broad topics: (1) interpreting the medical records, (2) getting a record of food intake and other pertinent data, (3) interpreting the intake data and calculating nutrient intake, (4) planning nutrition care, (5) monitoring nutrition care, and (6) assessment, counseling, and followup.

Examples of Education for Para-professionals

Teaches home health aides the diet for the patient and special preparation methods and seasoning.

Trains nutrition aides in how to take food records, and how to monitor the patient's diet.

Provides field experiences for students in the dietetic technician course.

NUTRITIONISTS, DIETITIANS, STUDENTS, AND TRAINEES

The community nutritionist must be aware of the educational needs of practicing nutritionists and dietitians, and of students and trainees in the profession, identifying needs, participating in arrangements for group sessions through professional associations, community groups, or educational institutions, and giving education directly in the area of specialization by consultation, conference, or group methods. Identification of the nutritionist's own educational needs and arranging to meet them are other important activities.

Examples of Education for Nutritionists, Dietitians, Students, and Trainees

Orients dietetic student to the community nutrition program, arranges field work, and helps the student evaluate the experiences.

Arranges a symposium on current topics in nutrition, with talks on fiber in the diet, nutrition and cancer, and new knowledge of trace elements.

Arranges a workshop in which nutritionists hear a lecture on hypertension, receive training in use of the sphygmomanometer, and practice taking blood pressures.

MOTIVATION FOR CHANGE IN PROFESSIONALS

This is one of the major problems for the nutritionist, who usually works as one person among many from a variety of other disciplines, each of whom has special problems, concerns, and interests. The best motivation is showing them how nutrition teaching will help achieve their own objectives and provide better service for their clientele.

One technique that has often proved of value is to get the proposal for change to come from a member of the group, such as one of the nurses or a physician. This can sometimes be accomplished by advance notification that a change is pending, would be in order, or would be valuable. The nutritionist suggests the new idea, new program, or a change a number of times in different ways in different settings.

One example occurred when a nutritionist identified a need for staff training in a uniform method of weighing and measuring, which was being done in a health center by hastily trained volunteers. The first reactions to the idea were that the equipment was not available, it would take too much time, the volunteers would not be willing to participate in so much training, and the small differences were not important.

Instead of participating in an overt struggle to accomplish this immediately, the nutritionist engaged in a subtle campaign over a period of several months, mentioning the matter to each of the persons directly involved as well as to the physician in charge of the health center. The approach was from a very tentative level, suggesting the training as a possibility in the future, asking advice, seeking opinions and information, mentioning the procedures used elsewhere, and showing pictures of the equipment and pointing out its simplicity.

After a period of time, a physician brought up the matter in a staff meeting as a new idea. At that time, several members of the staff with whom the nutritionist had talked supported the idea. A way was found to calibrate the scales and to purchase the necessary measure for attachment to the wall near the scale. The nutritionist was asked to teach the method to the volunteers and interested nurses. Fortunately the new growth charts had just arrived and were available for recording, so the nutritionist also showed the volunteers how to keep the growth records. When the idea became a shared concern to members of the staff, the action became a reality.

A promising way to motivate professionals and the public to study nutrition is found in a plan under consideration at the national level, sponsored by the National University Extension Association, the American Association of Collegiate Registrars and Admissions Officers, the United States Civil Service Commission, and the United States

Office of Education. (13) It is based on the establishment of a Continuing Education Unit (CEU), which is a means for recording completion of programs in adult and continuing education in a framework for lifelong learning comparable to credit measurement for college courses. The program could include any post-secondary school level learning experiences for which no diploma or degree credit is earned.

METHODS

The examples that have been given illustrate the variety of methods used by the nutritionist for professional education. These are:

1. Consultation for individuals or small groups.
2. Conferences with individuals or small groups.
3. Group education, such as institutes, symposia, workshops, and lectures.
4. Preparation of resource materials.
5. Demonstration of teaching.
6. Advice on self-education and referral to other resources.

Consultation

Perhaps the education method mentioned most often is consultation. This was discussed on pages 183–187. The community nutritionist usually functions as a consultant to help the consultee solve a current work problem for the benefit of clients. Most often the consultation provided by the community nutritionist will be on request of another professional person, usually a nurse. Most times the nutritionist has no authority and is present only to answer the request.

Most of the community nutritionist's consultant activities to other professionals will skip one or more of the steps given on page 184. The same persons will probably consult the nutritionist many times so that the establishment of rapport is a minimal process. The nutritionist and staff already know each other, and the nutritionist is familiar with the kinds of problems that occur. Thus the role of the nutritionist is mainly providing consultation in an informal situation.

Just as the community nutritionist acts as a consultant to other professionals, the nutritionist will often use the consulting process to get help on problems. The nutritionist may get consultation from a physician, a nurse, a social worker, health educator, or teacher on matters within their areas of expertise on some question to which the nutritionist must find a solution. Often the nutritionist will have a partly formed plan to handle the matter but needs information, advice, and help with testing a variety of solutions. Examples: consulting the leader of an Indian community for advice on planning the best way to develop an education program about the use of WIC foods; consulting a health educator about a food fair being planned by a committee. In some agencies much consultation takes place between the members of the nutrition staff with those who have expertise in special areas, such as maternal health or programs for older persons, consulting each other. Seeing consulting as a *process* rather than just the consultant as a person, facilitates finding sources of help on many problems.

The consultation process may also be used with a group of several people who have the same problem; for example, a committee of three nutritionists is planning inservice education for nutritionists and dietitians on the treatment of hypertension. The committee may consult a social worker and a physician to help them weigh the merits of several plans for the meetings and to suggest teachers for the event.

A conference or informal discussion between nutritionist and an individual or a small group provides a fast, easy way in which the nutritionist answers questions about nutrient content of mixed dishes, suggests a leaflet to use as a teaching tool, or gives other general or specific information.

Group Education

A group may be composed of persons in the same kind of work, such as nutritionists or nurses or social workers, or the general cross-section of personnel found in a health center or similar work situations. Then the group might include physicians, nurses, a social worker, a health educator, an administrator, an office supervisor and some community workers. The group method used must be adapted to the needs and characteristics of the persons in the group.

Referral to Other Resources

For professionals or paraprofessionals who are interested in courses that provide more nutrition background than can be given in inservice education, the nutritionist may take leadership in locating available resources. There may be courses at local universities or colleges, or workshops, institutes, or symposia at the same institutions. These are available in most areas but if no suitable ones are being scheduled, the nutritionist may take leadership in developing them. They can be developed at all levels to fit the needs of nurses, teachers, aides, and others.

Another channel is through special professional meetings on the subject of nutrition. The present requirements of several professional organizations for inservice education have created a new interest in such programs.

Preparation of Resource Materials

This is an indirect method of education that will conserve the nutritionist's time and can provide a readily available resource for the nurse and other professionals. Carefully prepared resource materials, for example, on food money management and cultural food practices, can be used over long periods of time by periodic updating on food costs, recommended dietary allowances, and food laws.

Regular publications in the newsletter format are a way of reaching many people. A Georgia nutrition consultant published a monthly release, "For Your Patient's Nutrition Problems—Have You Tried This?" It was mailed to professional persons in health, especially public health nurses, but also teachers, health department nutritionists, medical centers, and so forth. One issue told how to explain to the mother of a three-year old child the difference between sickle cell anemia and iron deficiency anemia, and how to answer the mother who asked whether she should change her baby's formula to skim milk. (17)

Team Action

This is another channel for inservice education among professionals. It is a concept that is frequently mentioned; perhaps this gives the impression that team action occurs more often than it actually does occur. In other working patterns, professionals often have limited and incorrect concepts of each other's roles. The nutritionist needs to learn the background of the nurse, the social worker, the health educator, and other professionals, and help others become well informed about the background of a nutritionist. If no provision is made for this interchange of information, the nutritionist should promote the development of interdisciplinary training sessions for this purpose.

The objective of team care is to make the skills of varied professionals available to provide the best health care for the family. It is important that all team members understand the function of each member and what that person can contribute to health care. The nutritionist's function is to help other team members understand nutritional care and how they can contribute to it as well as know the role and contribution of the nutritionist.

In the team concept, one or more members are designated as the primary members for a case with other team members contributing in case conferences. In some programs, there is a specific team, often the physician and nurse, which is responsible for the case; in others the responsibility for most of the contact is assumed by one team member, for example, physician, nurse, nutritionist, or community worker. (2)

Members of the team should meet regularly for discussion and planning of care for individual families, usually those with severe or multiple health and socioeconomic problems. Thus the different team members contribute their varied skills to health care. The nutritionist must act as the specialist who has a specific contribution to make to the health care team, assuming responsibility to see that adequate nutritional care is provided. This responsibility includes seeing that accurate weights and measures are taken and recorded, that a nutritional assessment is made, that the diet is adequate, and that nutritional health is maintained by preventive measures. The nutritionist should also plan and conduct studies or surveys to determine food costs or nutrition practices or the effect of various factors. Nutritionists and dietitians must assume the role of nutrition specialists also by reviewing records of patient care, screening to search for evidence about whether nutritional care is adequate, and supplementing the physician's knowledge about nutrition. (8)

SUMMARY

The community nutritionist conducts education of other professionals and paraprofessionals in nutrition subject matter and program methods so that they can help their clients with nutrition problems. The community nutritionist must be well grounded in both subject matter and methodology to have credibility and to be able to motivate others for nutrition activities.

Everyone who conducts nutrition education needs to know how to find out what the individual eats and how to evaluate the food intake by comparing foods eaten with a food guide, or by comparing nutrients ingested with the RDA. Also needed is a knowledge of nutrition education methods, including how to motivate change.

Physicians conduct nutrition education with patients, community nurses help the family in their own home, and teachers can influence school children to improve their diets. Dentists, social workers, health educators, and others have opportunities to conduct nutrition education with their clientele.

Specific ways for the nutritionist to work with physicians, nurses, teachers, other professionals, and paraprofessionals have been presented with examples. Suggestions were made for planning by the nutritionist and dietitian for their own needs and those of students. Some ways to motivate professionals to conduct nutrition activities were suggested. Use of the CEU as a possible motivating factor was discussed.

REFERENCES CITED

1. Anderson, Linnea, and John H. Browe, *Nutrition and Family Health Services,* W. B. Saunders Co., Philadelphia, 1960, 126.
2. Barney, Helen S., and Mary C. Egan, Home Economists as Members of Health Teams, *J. Home Econ.,* 60 6/68 427.
3. Caliendo, Mary Alice, In-Service Educational Program for Dietetic Technicians Involved in Geriatric Nutrition, *J. Am. Diet. Assoc.,* 69 8/76 164.
4. Callahan, Dorothy L., Inservice Teacher Workshops, *J. Nutr. Educ.,* 5 10–12/73 233.
5. Cho, Marjorie, and Beth A. Fryer, Nutritional Knowledge of Collegeiate Physical Education Majors, *J. Am. Diet. Assoc.,* 65 7/74 30.
6. Cho, Marjorie, and Beth A. Fryer, What Foods Do Physical Education Majors and Basic Nutrition Students Recommend for Athletes?, *J. Am. Diet. Assoc.,* 65 11/74 541.
7. Cowell, Catherine, and Olga E. Sobelsohn, Stirring the Cultural Melting Pot, *J. Home Econ.,* 65 10/73 20.
8. Downs, Sr. R. G., Dietitians' Inertia Lends Validity to Butterworth's Charges, *Hospital Progress,* 55 12/74 11.
9. Flynn, Margaret, Dennis Keithly, and Jack M. Colwill, Nutrition in the Education of the Family Physician, *J. Am. Diet. Assoc.,* 65 9/74 272.
10. Frankle, Reva T., Nutrition Education for Medical Students, I. What Is It? *J. Am. Diet. Assoc.,* 68 6/76 515.
11. Hegsted, D. Mark, The Development of a National Nutrition Policy, *J. Am. Diet. Assoc.,* 62 4/73 394.
12. Lee, E. D., and T. L. Covington, Team Teaching Nutrition: What It Takes, *School Foodservice J.,* 29 4/75 39.
13. Meskill, Victor P., and Marlyne E. Hynds, Measuring Adult Educational Experiences: The Continuing Education Unit, *Adult Leadership,* 23 5/75 323.
14. Newton, M. E., M. E. Beal, and A. L. Strauss, Nutritional Aspects of Nursing Care, *Nurs. Res.,* 16 1967 46.
15. Nutrition in Medical Education, *J. Am. Diet. Assoc.,* 65 9/74 259.
16. Position Paper on the Dietetic Technician and the Dietetic Assistant, *J. Am. Diet. Assoc.,* 67 9/75 246.
17. Problem-Solving Approach to Nutrition Education, *J. Am. Diet. Assoc.,* 65 7/74 49.

18. Spindler, Evelyn B., "Program Aides" for Work with Low-Income Families, I. Use of a Home Economics Aide, *J. Am. Diet. Assoc.,* 50 6/67 478.

19. Tinkham, Catherine W., and Eleanor F. Voorhies, *Community Health Nursing,* Appleton-Century-Crofts, New York, 1972, 177.

20. Vickstrom, Janet A., and Hazel M. Fox., Nutritional Knowledge and Attitudes of Registered Nurses, *J. Am. Diet. Assoc.,* 68 5/76 453.

ADDITIONAL REFERENCES

Food and Nutrition Seminars for Health Professionals, series of videotapes, U.S. Department of Health, Education, and Welfare, Rockville MD, 1975.

Mase, Darrel J., Health Manpower Vs. Mindpower, *J. Am. Diet. Assoc.,* 69 12/76 613.

O'Connell, Shirley, The Nutrition Consultant for Visiting Nurses, *J. Am. Diet. Assoc.,* 68 3/76 247.

Schwartz, Nancy E., Nutrition Knowledge, Attitudes, and Practices of Canadian Public Health Nurses, *J. Nutr. Educ.,* 68 1–3/76 247.

14 PUBLIC EDUCATION

Public education is the application of the educational process to various publics. It is divided in this book under *community education,* to produce changes in the forces that control community action, and *nutrition education,* to effect changes in individual and family food practices. The two major publics to be considered are (1) those who can produce change in the community, and (2) those whose food practices are in need of improvement.

The action in community education should focus on the establishment and protection of nutritional health rather than on crisis intervention. This means emphasis on the development of preventive programs rather than on treatment or handling of problems after they arise. For example, with present concepts about nutrition in the etiology of heart disease and cancer, community education should try to get the public to modify dietary fat content and to maintain normal weight to prevent these diseases.

Sometimes nutrition education has been considered to constitute the whole job of the community nutritionist; however, changes in the community are frequently needed before individual food practices can be changed. Sometimes the activities here called community education are included under nutrition education, and the term nutrition education is sometimes used to refer to nutrition courses or subject matter in the curriculum of professional schools, such as medical schools. The division into community education and nutrition education is used here to define the two areas.

COMMUNITY EDUCATION

The term *community education* is used in this book to designate activities planned to change the knowledge, attitudes, and actions of the publics who influence the màking of the policies and decisions that affect nutrition. Community education must include changes in legislation, technology, production, merchandising, and research as means to solving nutrition problems.

The purpose of community education is to develop recognition of the importance of food and nutrition as a primary factor in the health and well-being of the community, and of community characteristics as they affect nutrition. Navarro suggests (27) that it is more important to study factors in the environment that determine individual behavior than to study individual behavior itself.

Nutritionists in the community need to take several kinds of overall action to initiate solutions to nutrition problems, especially the following:

1. Organize professionals concerned with motivation for leadership in solving nutrition problems.
2. Mobilize other community leaders into an action group that is broadly representative of the entire population.
3. Inform politicians, officials, and others who make policies and decisions of action needed and move them to such action.
4. Promote the idea of personal responsibility for health and nutrition stressing individual and parental responsibility for good nutrition.

Developing Professional Leadership

One of the first steps is the organization of food and nutrition professionals for leadership in community education. Those who have a particular stake in this endeavor include nutritionists, dietitians, home economists, and others with a nutrition background whose work is hampered by community situations that affect nutrition. In this discussion, this group will be called a "nutrition council."

Such a council can identify the problems and the barriers that interfere with their solution and serve as a coordinating body. Its functions should be planning and leadership rather than executing programs. Examples of appropriate activities are (1) making a community nutritional assessment by determining how the social and environmental factors in the community impact on nutritional status; and (2) making a comprehensive nutrition plan for the community as part of the overall health plans. The council should not duplicate the work of agencies or organizations that conduct nutrition programs but should strive to help them fulfill their functions.

The first action needs to be putting available data, both from the community and from other places, into a framework which applies to the community. Data from other sources will need to be projected to local application. It is best to be able to state local figures, for example, the number of children showing a tendency toward obesity in the specific community and who are thereby at risk in later life of certain chronic diseases. If such figures are not available, a projection may be made on the basis of figures that are available. A nutrition profile of the community may be prepared using data from HANES, the Ten-State Survey, the USDA Food Consumption Studies, or reports about food practices, nutrition knowledge and attitudes, and other studies that can be found in the literature.

In the interpretation of data, the importance of good food practices in the prevention and treatment of all health problems should be emphasized. Crisis intervention can cure summer diarrhea in a young child, but changing sanitation practices in food preparation and storage and improving personal hygiene in one apartment building may prevent it in fifty children. Likewise, emphasis should be placed on the importance of good nutritional status in prevention and treatment of all health problems; for example, poor nutritional status makes the individual more vulnerable to other health problems such as contracting infectious diseases.

Developing an Action Group

The second step in community education may be to organize an action group of community leaders and professionals, here called a "nutrition committee." The purpose of this group is to develop a receptiveness in people to action about food and nutrition problems, and show them how to take action. This group can use the profile on nutritional status, food consumption, and other evidence of nutrition problems in the community to develop an action program needed to correct the problems. The committee needs to have professional members who can serve as enablers, advocates, planners, and advisors to help the group verbalize and present their food and nutrition problems.

The function of this group is to arouse interest in nutrition problems and educate the public to understand the kind of public health programs needed. The public in turn must promote programs and overcome the opposition of vested private interests. They must see that competent, qualified health officials and personnel are appointed, that they are educated and qualified in public health, not just in treatment of disease, and that they are supportive rather than antagonistic to public health as a way of solving community health problems.

Some of the programs that have the potential of relieving or solving nutrition problems are community health planning, government programs, federal food stamp programs, food distribution programs, and food service programs for children and senior citizens. (28)

The structure and membership of this group should be planned to provide channels to six groups who wield .power to change policies and programs. These groups are:

1. Citizens as voters.
2. Community groups whose purpose is the improvement of society.
3. Politicians who lead governments and professional and volunteer leaders who determine policies of official and voluntary health agencies and facilities.
4. Managers of business and industry who are responsible for advertising, labeling, and marketing food.
5. Persons who are responsible for the communications media—newspapers, television, and-radio.
6. School officials and teachers who determine how children are taught.

Each citizen has the power of the vote as a way to influence government action; however, most persons do not consider the ballot as a very powerful way to exert such influence. Nutritionists need to help them see ways to use power.

The kind of action a community nutritionist takes must be in accordance with the policies of the agency or organization in which the nutritionist works. The nutritionist will act in various capacities, especially those of enabler, advocate, planner and adviser (page 207).

Roles of Nutritionist

The community nutritionist's influence on the individual voter will be mainly as enabler or advocate, through a community group such as the nutrition committee or through the media. In the *enabler* role, the nutritionist or committee might work with representatives of community groups, for example, churches, ethnic groups, or action groups, to describe the problems of the people in the community or neighborhood. A specific neighborhood problem may be a lack of supermarkets within the shopping area; a specific community problem in a housing project may be inadequate refrigerators in the apartments.

Help may be given to describe the supermarket problem by describing the boundaries of the area, the number of families, the number and kinds of markets in the area and adjacent to it, their limitations, and the possible patronage for a supermarket in the area.

As an *advocate,* the nutritionist or committee might promote the establishment of a supermarket in the area using information previously gathered. As a *planner,* the nutritionist or council might help the group plan ways to deal with the problem of lack of supermarkets, considering various solutions such as getting one of the chains to establish a supermarket in the area, or organizing a cooperative market or organizing a buying group that would shop for all members at the central wholesale market twice weekly. As an *adviser,* the nutritionist or another council representative might meet with leaders of the group to suggest ways for them to deal with the lack of supermarkets.

Community groups such as service clubs, women's auxiliaries to professional organizations, and civic groups exist largely for the purpose of community betterment. They conduct programs to support their projects, raising money, providing volunteer service, and getting support from influential persons in the community. The nutritionist's relation to these groups may be as advocate, to obtain their support for a project such as a free dental clinic for children, or planner, to help the group plan ways to deal with a problem they have selected, or adviser, to provide technical advice on nutrition-related matters.

Politicians, professional and volunteer leadership, and health agency administrative and program personnel are important as policy-makers and decision-makers. Community nutritionists or professional nutrition groups may deal with them (1) as advocates to obtain their support for nutrition legislation or policy changes on allocation of funds, or to have a nutrition component in their programs or to add a staff nutritionist; (2) as planners to help the decision-makers plan programs through which they can solve nutrition problems or develop preventive measures; and (3) as advisers on ways the leadership can solve some of the nutrition problems of the community or assist them in planning how to implement their programs.

The nutritionist may want to contact advertisers as advocate to obtain their support for correct nutrition information in their copy, to request that easily comprehended nutrition information be included in advertisements, or to recommend changes in labeling and marketing. A business that makes its profit in the community should have some concern about alleviating social problems.

Newspaper food editors and radio and television producers may request an adviser for assistance in their programs or may want technical advice, while they will in turn publicize various kinds of information that the nutritionist can provide.

The community nutritionist sometimes has an official function in the schools and will then be ready to act in all capacities as needed. When there is no official function, the major roles will be enabler, planner, and adviser.

Sometimes one community nutrition program stimulates many others. A seminar program was started in Massachusetts by Kraus to train members of medical auxiliaries for service as nutrition advocates. A package program was developed and presented in workshops in four locations in the United States. This resulted in groups in 27 states organizing in 1973-74 to call attention to nutrition needs. Many activities were included such as preparation of book lists, a cooking class for elderly men, development of a meals-on-wheels program, and consumer education. (6) In San Francisco, members of the Medical Women's Auxiliary participated in a training course so they could serve as nutrition advocates in the community. (24)

Participation of the Community

Participation in community action can result in needed changes in the health care system. Federal requirements assure consumer participation in health planning; however, improvements in an individual's nutrition practices are brought about only through personal involvement. (22)

Participation can lead to involvement when members of the group learn about possible action by considering various solutions, expressing their thoughts freely, and deciding on action with an equal voice. Participation becomes active involvement when group members are led to understanding by a progressive set of situations in which learning may occur.

Some of the factors that have prevented low income persons from participating on policy-making boards and committees were a lack of understanding of the professional's technical language, conditioning within a cultural group, and inconvenient meeting times in unfamiliar places. Considerable progress has been made in getting low-income persons to participate in policy-making and planning for their communities by election or appointment to membership on policy-making bodies (e.g. board of a voluntary health agency), by having bilingual meetings, and by holding meetings at times they can attend and in locations where they can feel at ease.

Decisions as to how resources should be used for promotion and protection of health depend on community opinion about what is desirable as well as on professional judgment about what is effective and safe.

NUTRITION EDUCATION

In this book the term *nutrition education* is used to mean the process of changing food practices. Here is the author's definition: "Nutrition education is the process of applying a knowledge of nutrition, related scientific information, and social and behavioral sciences in ways designed to influence individuals and groups to eat the kinds and amounts of foods that will make a maximum contribution to health and social satisfaction."

The American Dietetic Association has defined nutrition education as "the process by which beliefs, attitudes, environmental influences, and understandings about food lead to practices that are scientifically sound, practical, and consistent with individual needs and available food resources." (30)

Leverton has added that it "is a multidisciplinary process that involves the transfer of information, the development of motivation, and the modification of food habits where needed." (20)

Gifft and coauthors characterize nutrition education as planned change and say that nutrition education tries to change knowledge about nutritional needs and food values into "eating practices that will promote health and well-being" using both nutritional and behavioral sciences. (8)

The *purpose* of nutrition education is (1) to change food practices when needed so that each individual eats the right kinds and amounts of foods; and (2) to help the individual acquire significant information and put it into a frame of reference so it can be used later. The latter purpose includes giving anticipatory guidance to new parents about eating habits, for example, to make them aware that after the first year the child may be expected to reduce its food intake. Another example is to make teenagers of normal weight aware of the need to recognize and avoid the beginning of weight gain that often accompanies early adulthood because of a decrease in activity without a corresponding decrease in food intake. In these cases, knowledge is acquired and attitudes affected, but there is no immediate change in practice.

Need for Nutrition Education

Nutrition education plays an important role in community nutrition. It is one of the primary ways through which nutrition and health problems can be attacked. The community nutritionist uses nutrition education in the prevention and treatment of conditions such as dental caries, diabetes, heart disease, hypertension, iron deficiency, nutritional disorders of pregnancy and infancy, obesity and undernutrition. Nutrition education for prevention of these specific problems is concerned with the people of all ages who are most likely to develop them. Education for the general public is also indicated because if each person could be persuaded to eat a proper diet there would be less need for corrective measures.

Education may be conducted with individuals, small groups, large groups, and through the media and other mass methods. Nutrition education is indicated when improvement in diet is important to nutritional health, when it is requested by an individual or group, or when there are harmful practices that should be corrected.

Nutrition education for individuals aims to instill appropriate practices such as lower caloric intake and more activity in the overweight person, proper balance of fatty acids for adults at risk of heart disease, increase in nutrients for the pregnant woman, adherence to the modified diet for a child with an inborn metabolic disease, and food for children that will support growth, avoid excessive weight gain, and provide for good dental health.

Three groups of people are special targets for nutrition education. First is any community of individuals for the establishment of good food habits and practices. Second are the persons responsible for the family food so they will feed their families properly. Third are the persons who provide food for people away from home, such as those responsible for food service in boarding homes, hospitals, extended care facilities, school cafeterias, restaurants and other group-feeding facilities.

Selection of individuals, groups or communities for nutrition programs is sometimes made on the basis of subjective judgment about the group that needs it. Targets may also be selected on the basis of the vulnerable or high risk groups that usually include pregnant women, infants, adolescents and older persons; however, this omits adult males who constitute a high risk group on the basis of the death rate from coronary heart disease.

Even among the vulnerable groups, the individuals who need nutrition services should be identified in terms of existing nutrition problems as shown by anthropometric measurements, biochemical assays, or nutrient intake of less than the recommended dietary allowances. Substandard growth rates, malnutrition with either underweight or obesity, and low biochemical values show an imbalance of nutrients in the past.

A diet that is currently low in nutrients should be corrected to avoid future problems.

Nutrition Educators

Nutrition education is conducted by many persons. Some nutrition counselors and teachers have had academic training in nutrition, but many have not, and limited knowledge of a complex subject sometimes results in teaching based on inaccurate information, and in the promotion of unbalanced meals or fad diets.

The educators include:

1. The nutrition team of nutritionist, dietitian, nutrition technician, nutrition aide, and home economist.
2. Nutrition counselors whose primary work is in another discipline— physician, nurse, dentist, dental hygienist, and others.
3. The teachers and other personnel responsible for nutrition education in the schools.
4. The writers and producers who prepare copy for newspapers, magazines, television, radio, and advertisements, and authors of books on nutrition.

The nutritionist and other educators share the responsibility for good food practices even though the individual is ultimately responsible for the food consumed and for other health habits that affect nutrition. The community nutritionist has the particular responsibility of helping other educators by providing authentic nutrition information through consultation, group education, and resource materials.

Often the various audiences for nutrition education need help with other related topics that affect food practices, so these topics need to be incorporated into nutrition education. Three topics, discussed below, are especially important because they are involved in providing adequate food at minimum cost, managing the household, and accomplishing housework. These related topics should be the responsibility of the home economist when there is one on the nutrition team; otherwise the nutrition counselor may help the homemaker with these problems or find other resources to correct practices that interfere with nutrition before nutrition education itself can become effective.

Consumer Information. This provides help with purchasing practices so that purchases will be suitable for intended use and will represent good value. Nutritionists may need to mobilize community resources for education in subjects that affect the ability of the family to have a good diet, for example, food purchasing, family budgeting, and the metric system.

Household Skills.   Many women who have never learned to keep house need help in developing ability to handle household tasks. The help may be given by referral to a community resource for learning the skills of child care, housecleaning, and other tasks. Aides from the Expanded Food and Nutrition Program (page 99) have been successful with many such families. Other community resources include adult education programs, radio and television programs, printed media, and demonstration and instruction during visits by a nurse or nutritionist, or a homemaker from a welfare agency.

Home Management Tasks.   These are concerned with the wise use of money, time, and energy. The nutrition counselor may help the family make better use of these resources, for example, purchasing bread at a discount bakery, finding a source of free food as extra income, and learning ways to perform household tasks that save time and energy.

Subject   Matter

Previous chapters have covered the knowledge and skills needed by community nutritionists and the tools used in their work. Attention here will be directed to the subject matter and how it is used by the community nutritionist in the process of changing food practices. The nutritionist must develop ways to do this that will work in the particular programs involved.

Three methods of presentation will be reviewed. Using the same method for all nutrition education in a particular program or area helps to avoid the confusion that occurs when a person with very limited information about nutrition is confronted with what appears to be conflicting information, for example, being told (1) that bread is a low protein food, and (2) that bread is a good source of protein. The confusion arises from noting that one slice of bread supplies only 2 to 3 grams of protein while one small serving of meat supplies about 24 grams. The individual must understand that six or eight slices of bread consumed in one day provide as much protein as the meat, so that its status as a good source of protein is understood.

The three following methods use the same base of information and all work toward development of similar concepts. The differences are in the approach that may emphasize foods or nutrients, or both, and in the amount of subject matter taught.

Basic Concepts Method. These concepts were developed in 1964 by the Interagency Committee on Nutrition Education (14) and have been widely used by nutrition educators of all backgrounds. They are intended to be used as background rather than taught as stated. The concepts, which can be used in any method of teaching, are:

1. Nutrition is the food you eat and how the body uses it.

   We eat food to live, to grow, to keep healthy and well, and to get energy for work and play.

2. Food is made up of different nutrients needed for growth and health.

   All nutrients needed by the body are available through food.
   Many kinds and combinations of food can lead to a well-balanced diet.
   No food by itself has all the nutrients needed for full growth and health.
   Each nutrient has specific uses in the body.
   Most nutrients do their best work in the body when teamed with other nutrients.

3. All persons throughout life have need for the same nutrients, but in varying amounts.

   The amounts of nutrients needed are influenced by age, sex, size, activity, and state of health.
   Suggestions for the kinds and amounts of food needed are made by trained scientists.

4. The way food is handled influences the amount of nutrients in food, its safety, appearance, and taste.

   Handling means everything that happens to food while it is being grown, processed, stored, and prepared for eating.

Any nutrition educator can use these concepts as a way to help individuals make decisions about food. The concepts may be used for planning any program of nutrition education, with the educator selecting the content that will help develop the concept. The educator also selects the experiences and materials to be used in the specific learning situation— individual, classroom, large group, publication, or radio or television program.

The concept framework includes the establishment of the existence and importance of nutrients, but the amount of information to be given about them can be adjusted to the needs of specific situations. That is, the facts taught may cover only part of the concepts, or may cover all.

All concepts can be taught over a period of time, or one may be used in individual counseling.

Key Nutrient Method. A manual based on this method was developed by two public health nutritionists in one public health agency for teaching leaders from weight control groups. Later they adapted it for teaching nutrition aides in the poverty programs, for teaching students in several local schools of nursing, and for participants in a coronary prevention program. In each case the necessary adaptations were made by modifications in parts of the manual but the basic teaching remained the same. (21) The Key Nutrient method can be adapted for use with any sex-age group, for most modified diets, or for individual teaching.

This method starts with the idea that there are fifty to sixty nutrients used by the body and that everybody uses these nutrients but also that different people need different amounts. The concepts on which this teaching is based is that nutrients are called KEY Nutrients because if the foods eaten supply enough of them the rest of the nutrients will also be supplied.

The KEY Nutrients used in the courses cited here were carbohydrates, protein, vitamin A, thiamin, riboflavin, vitamin C, calcium, and iron. The teaching was developed around the function of these nutrients and use of the foods that supply them.

Food Guide Method. Hill suggested a way to use a food guide as the basis for nutrition education. The illustration is based on the USDA Daily Food Guide. Hill presents the Food Groups and suggests nutrition information to use about each Food Group. (13)

For example, fruits and vegetables are divided into sources of vitamin A and vitamin C. Examples of serving size are given and a few simply stated facts about the two vitamins, that vitamin C helps hold body cells together, build healthy gums and body tissues, heal wounds and resist infection, while vitamin A helps eyes adjust to dim light, helps keep linings of mouth, nose, throat, and digestive tract healthy and resistant to infection, and keeps skin healthy and promotes growth. Sources of vitamin A are discussed as is the use of carotene and the occurrence of vitamin A in liver and other foods. The discussion of fiber starts with this group, which is one source, and continues with the bread and cereal group. Similar information is given about the other three Groups.

Hill also discusses how to put the Food Guide to work, making the point that once Food Guide specifications have been met, other foods can be added for more nutrients and/or energy. The supply of energy can be checked by watching weight, reducing calories when necessary by limiting amounts of foods, and increasing physical activity. Undue emphasis on minimum number of servings may result in meals that are not satisfying; the use of extra foods from the Groups adds interest, variety, and more food value.

The ingredients of commercially prepared mixed dishes must be assigned to the appropriate groups. Hill points out that occasionally measuring the amount of meat or vegetable in a mixed dish will help in future estimations. The subject matter about the groups is enough information for 15 to 20 ninety-minute lessons, but only small amounts of the supporting information can be used at one time. The long series of classes was intended for school use, but the approach and ideas are adaptable to other less-structured nutrition education where the contact is shorter. Hill stresses that the learners should be involved in experiences about food, letting them make menus, evaluate their own food intakes, prepare and sample some of the foods suggested, or make a field visit to a supermarket for a study of labels.

In using the Food Guide method, emphasis should be placed on the need for variety within each Group, with frequent use of the foods that are especially nutritious. The nutritionist will also need to check the nutrients provided by the foods used in meals and meal patterns to be sure they provide the RDA.

Some Points for Nutrition Educators

One of the questions in nutrition education is how much nutrition subject matter to include. Some educators emphasize teaching about foods, with concentration on selecting and preparing meals that are palatable and attractive and that meet accepted nutrition standards, with facts about nutrition used mainly for motivation. Others teach the subject matter of nutrition first, with the need for nutrients and their functions in the body, going from this approach to the food sources of nutrients and their uses in the diet.

Nutrition labeling has stimulated interest in nutrients and has caused many persons to request more information. The amount taught must be determined by the readiness of the learner.

Hill discusses (13) two major difficulties in teaching food selection in terms of nutrients:

1. There are many gaps in information about nutrients in foods, especially in relation to ready-prepared mixed dishes, which offer a special problem because the formulas are frequently changed and companies do not make their recipes known. [Author's note: Additional information is now available from labels that conform to the new labeling law and from the Nutrient Data Research Center, but there are still many gaps in information about nutrient content.)

2. The teacher must assess the kind of information the client is ready to receive. Though people recognize some of the words from advertising and the mass media, many do not understand how to utilize them in concepts. Hill stresses the advantages of using an approach based on eating and enjoying food, which is an appealing approach to most individuals.

There are other problems in teaching from the Four Food Groups. One is that the foods in each Group (e.g., apple and potato) are not equivalent in food values, so that some knowledge about food values is necessary to make the selection. Some nutritionists are now modifying the Food Groups for greater emphasis of raw dark-green leafy vegetables as a source of folic acid. Others question the advisability of teaching different facts at the local level than are taught in materials distributed nationally, which requires ongoing explanation and is likely to confuse the public.

Each nutrition educator will need to develop a style and method of operation and find out which means of presentation and motivation produce the best results. Different methods are necessary when the community nutritionist meets an individual in one or two brief contacts than are used in a series of counseling sessions or in school where the teacher will see the pupils several days a week for several months.

It is possible to eat a proper diet by following a good food pattern with a minimum of information about nutrition; however, it will be easier for the individual who is well informed on nutrition to plan meals, market, and evaluate information in advertisements and in the media.

Nutrition subject matter should be used mainly for *motivation*, that is, to get the individual to get a good diet, or to get the mother to serve one to the family, and may be included only in a minimal way. As Leverton says, "People vary greatly in how much they want to know about nutrition and food composition. In a recent study of the knowledge, practices, and opinions of homemakers regarding food and nutrition, we found that 30 percent was not interested in having more information." (20)

Gussow states it this way: "If people eat a good diet, it really doesn't matter what they 'know' about nutrition. It follows from this that whoever teaches a person which *foods* to like (because they're fun; because they taste good; because they'll make him happy, healthy, strong, popular) is teaching him nutrition." (10) Gussow furthermore believes that good nutrition must be sold to people in the same way that popular food items are sold, that is, with a hard-sell approach: "If we use television merely as another route for talking people to death about vitamins, minerals and protein, there is not the remotest chance that we shall ever interrupt the downward trend of American diet."

Manoff proposes the use of advertising techniques for changing food habits, suggesting the use in radio and television of a short message inserted into a program, designed "to make its point, to achieve maximum memorability, to be emotionally appealing and capable of repetition many times a day, many times a week and for many weeks and months." It demands neither interest nor motivation. The success of this method in selling a product suggests that it would be effective in changing food practices. (23) Manoff characterizes much of the information people need to know as "nonoptional education" because some foods (e.g., dark-green leafy vegetables) are so important that they must be included in the diet. He believes that advertising techniques would be successful in changing the eating habits of Americans if they could hear the messages for individual foods that are of special importance because of their unique nutrient contribution.

Using a similar idea, the American Broadcasting Company recently developed some announcements to promote the use of nutritious foods among children with a nutritionist as consultant. The consultant believes that children from the age of five can learn good food practices. The short animated spot announcements are shown along with children's programs on the network, and emphasize basic foods. (25)

It is a common practice in nutrition education to emphasize a food for its most abundant nutrient, for example, orange for vitamin C and milk for calcium. It is important to stress also that almost all foods supply varying amounts of many nutrients and that the day's allowance of some nutrients (e.g., iron, thiamin) is usually obtained from a number of foods. Harker and Kupsinel (11) suggest that emphasizing a food for its contribution of one specific nutrient may lead to the impression that this is the only food source of the nutrient or that this food has no other merit, and even to the impression that a synthetic source of that one nutrient can replace the food. It would be well when using such information to make sure by feedback and testing that the individual understands the value of getting nutrients from food rather than from a synthetic source and that most foods supply many nutrients.

Nutrition education is intended to help the individual improve meals for self or family when the need is shown by a food record or other method. Individualized teaching concentrates on one or two changes and presents the reasons the changes are needed. It is the task of the nutritionist to decide how much information about food and nutrition the individual needs and to teach it in ways that will motivate the individual to make the change, but it is the individual's right to decide how much information is wanted or will be used.

The nutrition educator has the responsibility to decide in specific teaching situations how much of the subject matter is really basic to the development and maintenance of good food practices. In community nutrition, most opportunities for teaching are short, often with distractions such as the presence of small children or anxiety about seeing the physician. The educator should select one or two practices that it is most important to change and concentrate teaching on these until the desired change has been achieved.

Sometimes when changes in food practices are needed for prevention or treatment, an individual is not willing to change. Some writers consider that, since the individual has the right to decide whether to change or not, efforts to change an uninterested person are unethical. They consider such an attempt as placing the educator's values above those of the individual, and furthermore, one forced change often produces other changes which may not be desirable. However, in the framework and philosophy of community nutrition and public health, there is a mandate to help with problems that cannot be handled by the individual, so it appears that the community nutritionist has an obligation to try to effect change for prevention or treatment. Moreover, in community nutrition the educator cannot force changes but must act by presenting the reasons for a change in terms of the benefits to the individual. Such a presentation can hardly be seen as forcing change since the individual can choose whether to accept or reject efforts for change or simply not cooperate in the attempt. This should not be assumed to mean that coercion is condoned or should be used.

Why Food Practices Change

There are many ways of viewing the process of nutrition education, but there seems to be general agreement that it is difficult to get people to change their food habits. This emphasizes the importance of carefully identifying the individual or group, assessing need, surveying the possible methods and approaches, planning the method and sequence, carrying out the program, and evaluating the result.

Food practices, even in adults, do change, sometimes very quickly and drastically. The reasons may be physical, as when there is a change in cooking facilities (e.g., a gift of a small, easily cleaned electric broiler may reduce the use of fried foods, or the purchase of a new range may increase the use of roast meats and home-baked bread), or a move to another area with different kinds of markets, or a change in life-style by marriage or by moving into a commune. People change for physiological reasons, as one who decides to lose weight, or who is diagnosed as having diabetes, or who has had a coronary heart attack. People change for psychological reasons such as becoming a vegetarian or adopting a different religion. They change by adapting to a less expensive diet when income is reduced or to a more expensive one when it is increased. There are also social reasons for change, for example, the man who retires and eats lunch at home instead of having a full meal with cock-tails, or the woman who is left alone by the sudden death of her husband.

Some people change their food practices because they consider it sophisticated to eat a greater variety, especially of unusual or expensive foods, some have a zest for trying new foods and over a period of time add some of them to their regular diet. One of the frequent types of change seen by the community nutritionist is that in the family from another country which comes to the United States and can no longer get the foods they have usually eaten. Often the changes are undesirable ones; the family adopt foods of lower nutrient content than were pre-viously eaten, as in changing from whole grain bread to sweet rolls or from fruit for dessert to fat-and-sugar-rich pastry. Sometimes the reasons given for change have no basis in fact, as in the case of the woman who urged her friend to eat meat instead of beans or eggs at lunch, saying that meat "does something for you that those substitutes cannot do, even though they have the same nutrients."

Some people change because they hear about new scientific informa-tion. An example of a desirable change for such a reason is that many people have heard about the relationship between saturated fats and cholesterol and heart disease and are using lean meats, nonfat milk, and other products that make up the diet for prevention.

Another reason for change, especially among lower economic groups and young people, is to imitate the practices of the upper and middle classes who set the tone for the American way of life. Though some deviation from this influence has taken place in the last ten years, this is probably still true. There is also a tendency to follow the eating practice of persons high in government or prominent in society or the entertainment world. Publicity given to nutritionally good meals eaten by such people would help to create a desire among others to eat in similar patterns. Too often the foods featured in such publicity are limited, bizarre, or faddish. Improvement in the diets of such prominent people would help make nutrition education of others more effective.

Some information about past changes in eating patterns is available from The National Menu Census taken by the Market Research Cor-poration of America, as reported by Creasy. (4)

These points are of particular significance:

1. There was a marked trend toward more casual eating with fewer items, foods easier to prepare, and meals served informally.

2. There was increased meal-skipping, especially in the 18 to 24 age group, and more frequent eating, with the average person taking some kind of food (a "food contact") six or seven times a day and some persons as many as 20 times.

3. Snacking was most frequent among children under 12 and women 25 to 44. Coffee, soft drinks, and fresh fruit were the snacks used most often.

4. Ice cream, cake, and pie were served more often as evening snacks than as part of meals.

5. There had been a large increase in use of potato chips and soft drinks at meals.

It appears probable that these trends have accompanied the change to the television-oriented life now followed by many families, characterized by inactivity, irregular mealtimes, snacking, and eating the foods advertised.

Obviously there are many reasons for changes in food habits, and many ways in which nutritionists who wish to change them can do so. The problem is to find the right method that will produce the desired change in the existing situation. Knowing the skills and tools will help the nutritionist do this.

Meaning of Food

The food practices of humans are determined by values, attitudes, and beliefs, which are the products of tradition, culture, and contacts. Food values represent the standards or principles that the individual or group holds about the desirability of food, for example, preferring high grade beef with a high fat content. Food beliefs represent the ideas about food and nutrition that the individual or group accepts as true. Some people use only the "real thing," cream and butter; others place great emphasis on "protein foods" and eat no bread or cereal products.

Food attitudes define the manner in which people act, feel, or think about food, such as the woman who considers white bread as greatly inferior food so does not feed it to her family, and the current popularity of raw spinach salad, which may be related to publicity about its value as a source of folic acid.

Food has important meanings to everyone from birth to death and changes take place throughout the life span. Providing food for oneself or for a group involves a series of decisions about what to buy, how to prepare it, whether to eat it, and how much to eat. The goal of nutrition educators is to motivate people to make decisions about food that will lead to consumption of a nutritious diet. They will do this only if health is desirable by their values, beneficial by their beliefs, and reasonable and possible in their perceptions. Often the individual has different ideas, placing a low value on health as a goal, or holding beliefs which have no basis in fact, taking the attitude that it is too much trouble to change practices.

Food may mean comfort, security, prestige, indulgence, denial, company, or health. It has emotional connotations and is often a status symbol or a means of expression. It follows that the community, especially the cultural group, affects the food of individuals within it. Every community has its own patterns and practices, with ideas as to which foods are good for people at different ages and which are not really food at all.

What people think about food is also affected by what is available. In the present era, although most food comes from the supermarket, there has been a resurgence of interest in gardens, health store foods, and home preparation, especially of breads. This is partly a revolt against middleman profits and partly nostalgia for a return to a simpler, more independent life.

How Food Practices Develop

Attempts at nutrition education must start with the knowledge and practices of the persons to whom the education will be directed and an understanding of how individuals and groups get their food practices.

Food habits develop early in life and undergo modification throughout the life span, some to a considerable degree, some only as necessary to conform to external forces. Gussow's discussion (10) of the message carried by television to preschool children suggests that new influences are at work. She discusses the way preschool children learn about eating from television, finding in this study that time at the set averaged 35 hours a week. Most of the commercials were about sweetened cereals, pastry, cookies, candy and other snacks, and sweetened beverages. Thus children learn early that sweet and fatty foods are desirable and hear little about other foods. Recently there has been a small improvement with some advertising devoted to basic foods, and with some television specials using a nutrition consultant in their planning. Nutrition educators still need to find ways to make better use of this impact for the development of good food habits in small children and for the improvement of the nutritional quality of diets of older children and adults.

The mother is the most influential person in early life, when food practices are formed. It appears that mothers are concerned about what babies should eat and that they seek advice from physician, nurse, nutritionist, or friends. They follow the advice during the first year, deviating most often by giving foods earlier than advised. Once the baby is on table food, this interest wanes and during the preschool years they seek advice only when there are problems.

During the school years, the mother seeks advice mainly when the child is obese or ill. When adolescents rebel, many parents accept the action as a part of life and assume they can no longer influence them. At this period the young person may recognize that food is related to problems concerned with skin, weight, and strength, and may seek help.

Low income mothers usually get advice from friends, or from a community clinic, or do without, while the middle class mother relies on books, magazines, and advice from friends. The affluent seek paid advice from physicians or nutritionists, or follow the ideas of movie stars or other prominent persons.

Children learn their food practices and their attitudes and values about food and health from their parents or other adults with whom they associate, or from advertisements on television. Most persons responsible for children know fairly well what foods should be eaten but do not know how to get the children to eat those foods. Poor food habits in most children result in not eating whole grains and green vegetables and in the overconsumption of sweets.

Sanjur and Scoma reported (32) a study of the food likes and dislikes of mothers and children and the effect of the mother's food habits on the child, finding that children disliked the same foods their mothers disliked but that the percentage was even greater; for example, 30 percent of the mothers and 59 percent of the children disliked skim milk, and 23 percent of mothers and 43 percent of children disliked raw cabbage.

According to Sanjur and Scoma, the need to individualize teaching applies to members of a family group, in which there may be much variation in food practices. They mention also the need to determine the specific *foods* for attention. In their study they found that adequate amounts of meat and bread were already consumed while amounts of milk and vegetables and fruits needed to be increased. It may be recalled that some of the food groupings, for example, the one used by Roberts in Puerto Rico, were based on the same idea.

There is also evidence that the foods mothers serve do not always correspond to their expressed beliefs. Emmons and Hayes found that "more mothers served foods from the different groups than reported the food groups as being important in their child's diet." They found also that vegetables were served less often than mothers reported thinking them important. (7)

Some writers question whether the mother has as much influence on the child's food habits as has been indicated here; however, it seems probable that the mother has more influence on food habits in early life than anyone else; the father's influence is less direct. Generally the mother prepares what the father and children will eat, while they eat what the mother prepares. When individuals relate to a professional person for advice, they identify the person with father or mother while looking to that person for authoritative scientific advice.

Planning a Nutrition Education Program

The community nutritionist will have many more demands for service than can be filled, so the setting of priorities is very important. Sometimes this is determined by the function of the organization or program, which may be limited to health care for children, education of preschoolers and their parents, or care for men at high risk of heart disease. In some agencies the nutritionist establishes the priorities, using information available about the specific community or information from other sources projected for the community.

In most cases the community nutrition program will cover both prevention and treatment, and time will be divided between nutrition education for individuals and groups and community education through a variety of community and action groups. The nutritionist will need to plan both short-range and long-term programs.

After the priorities have been determined, the steps in planning a nutrition education program are the same for activities with individuals, small groups, or large groups.

Identifying the Audience and Its Needs. Before planning any nutrition education effort, there must be information about the purpose and background of the individual or group concerned. The educator must find out what the learners know, start the learning process there, and provide information that can be put into use immediately. The individual members of a group will probably represent all stages of learning, so there needs to be something offered for all and each helped to move a step or two beyond the current stage.

Setting Goals and Objectives. In any educational program the educator must set one or more general goals to be accomplished. The definition of nutrition education states the general goal as "to influence individuals and groups to eat the kinds and amounts of food that will make a maximum contribution to health and social satisfaction." In a specific nutrition education program, the goal may be to help a mother become more competent and capable of getting the family members to eat the kind of food that is best for them.

The special goal for individual or group should be set by the learners with the educator who then helps them achieve progress toward that goal. The following goals are stated in terms of what individuals can do or should do to promote and support their own nutrition and health. Though these are fairly broad and inclusive, each nutrition educator should state goals that are appropriate to the specific program based on community and individual needs.

1. *Develop the habit of eating a good diet.* A habit is an acquired pattern that has become automatic, so the point of this goal is for the individual to eat food that is appropriate in kind and amount without having to give particular attention to the process. It may include subconscious or premeditated selection by individual foods, food groups, or food combinations. It includes a review during the day that takes note of foods not yet included, or eaten in inadequate amounts, and plans to make up deficiencies or compensate for too high amounts.

2. *Follow good practices in food selection and preparation.* This refers especially to the persons responsible for planning and preparing meals for others, whether at home, in a restaurant, or hospital, or somewhere else. The person who selects the food by menu planning at home or in a group-feeding situation determines the kind and amount that the individual can eat, and the person who prepares it determines how acceptable it will be and the food value of the completed product.

   Individuals are also responsible for selection of their own diets when they choose from an array of foods on a counter, table, or plate. Some knowledge of the relative nutrient content of foods and attention to the selection of those of higher value is needed. A knowledge of preparation methods is also necessary since this is another determinant of the food value of the finished product. Individuals whose food selections are likely to result in foods of lesser nutrient content, or who regularly eat foods high in fat and sugar, or whose caloric intake causes weight gain need more knowledge about nutritional values.

3. *Know effective ways of food purchasing.* The person responsible for purchasing food needs to buy foods that will be nutritious and palatable and suitable for the socioeconomic level. With the proliferation of new foods and food combinations and synthetic and ready-to-eat foods, it is more than ever important that people know how to utilize the new products and how to use new information that is made available on labels. Judicious use of new products will

make it possible for the individual to profit from the good features of technological development and to avoid the products that are of low nutrient content or high in sugar or fat.

4. *Follow good practices about activity and exercise.* Activity is needed by all individuals so that they can eat enough food for their body needs and for personal enjoyment. The values of more activity for the cardiovascular system, the muscles, and general body development, as well as for weight control, have received increased attention since the statement of the Food and Nutrition Board in 1974 that weight control should be accomplished by increased activity along with decreased calories. (26)

5. *Recognize how other health habits affect nutrition.* The individual needs an understanding of the relationship of activity, sleep, appetite, and elimination to the use of food in the body as well as to mental health, dental care, and other health habits.

6. *Be able to recognize reliable information about food and nutrition.* The individual needs to know reliable publications and sources of information, also the signs of quackery and misinformation and how to evaluate what is heard and read. Unless some concept of food and nutrition processes can be gained, the individual is apt to accept any source of information at face value, and to think that all the differing ideas are of equal merit.

Deciding Methods to Be Used. The nutrition educator has a wide choice of methods. The skills used in teaching individuals, counseling small groups, and teaching large groups have already been discussed. Many individuals who cannot be reached directly can be reached by use of the press, television, radio, displays, exhibits, and other mass methods. Some definitions may appear to exclude the press, television, and other mass methods because these media are structured for news rather than being specially structured to produce changes in practices. However, stories reporting the news or social and educational events, and documentaries are attention-getting and provide opportunities for individual learning by making information available, and they are considered as possible methods of nutrition education.

Education for individuals and small groups can be conducted by counseling after the objective has been determined by evaluation of the individual diet. The evaluation can be done by the nutritionist or other diet counselor or aide in the program. Individual instruction is indicated when the diet is complicated, when the needs are unique to the individual, or when timing is such that group instruction is not feasible. Appropriate instructional materials should be used—teaching leaflets, posters, charts, foods or food models, or a visit to a cafeteria. Cassettes or films may be used as supplemental devices to reinforce learning after the counseling session.

In a community nutrition program, it is not possible to educate everyone, perhaps not even possible to educate all who request service. Some nutritionists have many requests for talks to large groups; it is important to select the specific groups that can profit most by this kind of education and to select for each session a limited objective with a few ideas, then to put these ideas across clearly and succinctly.

Two important ideas that should be woven into most nutrition education are (1) having a variety of foods from the Four Food Groups with emphasis on those which have higher amounts of nutrients, and (2) limiting amounts of sugars and fats, which make foods high in calories.

Large-group instruction in the community setting is usually a one-contact activity, so the objectives are to motivate for change in practices by giving knowledge and developing attitudes that will lead to change, but the educator will not usually know what has been accomplished. More than one contact with a large group will occur only when the people are already highly motivated; sometimes the highly motivated have derived their motivation from food faddists. The group will usually consist of persons who have similar interests such as weight control, child nutrition, or food for senior citizens.

The specific method will depend on the available time and facilities and the wishes of the group. In this case, the nutritionist will find it useful to plan these things with a small committee of group members. When the group is from the general public, attracted by an announcement of the program on a specific subject, planning with the group may not be possible.

Group methods may include workshop, symposium, panel discussion, or lecture. The most feasible method for an individual nutritionist to use is the lecture because other methods require additional personnel who may not be available. A possible approach for the nutritionist who finds frequent need for large group instruction is to find or develop resources in adult education or community colleges.

Skill in use of illustrative materials or live demonstrations can make the lecture a vital, exciting presentation. Advance planning for a parent-teacher group could include a survey of food practices among the children, with the results to serve as the basis for the presentation. If poor lunches are the problem, the demonstration could be packing a good lunch; if the deficiency in the diet is in dark-green leafy vegetables, the demonstration could be of ways to use them, with samples of the finished product for tasting.

Involving members of the group such as having a few members of a weight control group prepare low calorie snacks or desserts can provide an effective way to involve the group and change practices. The nutritionist can supply the recipes and distribute copies. A film which illustrates the points to be made can be an effective teaching device. The nutritionist should introduce the film and explain the points it covers that are especially pertinent to the group and after the film conduct discussion of the points to be emphasized. Interviewing teenagers or adults representing the group whose practices are under consideration can be an effective way to illustrate the lecture.

Yee reports the use of a filmstrip with small groups of men in a coronary prevention program. The Blob is the villain, cholesterol, while Corporal Paul of the Royal Polyunsaturated is the hero. Yee tested the men before and after presenting the program and on the basis of an informal evaluation from "attentiveness, enthusiastic participation, and favorable responses in 125 sessions" (statistical results were not complete) considered the education to have been effective. (37)

Group counseling gives opportunity for stimulation from other group members and makes it possible for the nutritionist to work with more people. Dagley reports a group counseling service in an adult education program in Yarmouth, Nova Scotia. She held a series of five 1½-hour classes with 19 persons. Preliminary data at the time of registration indicated interest in all topics, but there were some changes as the classes progressed.

The class reviewed food advertisements, prepared snacks to illustrate the day's topic, and used a bulletin board to disseminate information. A subjective evaluation indicated that the class members had benefitted from attending. The nutritionist is planning a second course in which the content will be planned after the enrollment. (5) In a group of this size, the interchange between teacher and learner is different than in the usual group of three to five for client counseling. Methods used more nearly resemble classroom or workshop techniques than those of counseling.

A nutrition education program that reached 300 people in three months is described by Clamp and Carr. (2) Twenty nutrition aides trained by the community college used a portable demonstration unit to present lecture/demonstrations at various sites in the community (YMCA, homes, churches, city recreation room, and so forth). The classes covered breakfast, meat extenders, whole grains, and other topics. Construction of the light-weight, portable demonstration unit is described. The program was considered to have been very successful as judged from letters of appreciation, requests for additional services, and a program evaluation in one center.

Todhunter reports a joint program of the Tennessee PTA and Tennessee Nutrition Council for a "Nutrition Study Course." The Council planned a study program and made a handbook for the course to be presented to local PTA groups by volunteer instructors. The content of each course was to be based on the food and practical problems of the particular group and on information about the nutritive values of foods. (36)

Mass Nutrition Education

Education of large numbers of people may take place through newspapers, television, and radio and in large events such as food fairs and community campaigns.

Few newspapers have nutrition-trained persons on their staffs, but they are usually interested in nutrition stories that are news. The community nutritionist may foster this channel for education by reacting to the food editor on a news story, for example, to a story on the prevalence of obesity by commenting on why obesity occurs and how it can be avoided. The response to a story on a sudden rise in the cost of eggs could be to discuss the food values of eggs and possible alternates. Being available as a consultant to answer questions and sending the newspaper copies of new educational materials can also provide a story. Offering a leaflet related to the article provides a way to determine reader reaction. Commenting on controversial topics or criticizing specific programs and proposing alternatives are other ways to make the news.

Radio interviews and telephone talk shows provide another means of mass education. The content must be easily understood, however. Sometimes a very short presentation can be used to make a point or to enforce previous teaching.

Television shows need expert direction and production. The nutritionist can participate by providing consultation, or appearing for an interview or other program. Sometimes the interviewer will ask specific questions supplied by the interviewee ahead of time, but often the interviews are unrehearsed. Planned questions and outlines are not always followed. Real food or very simple, eye-catching props can be used. Fruits and vegetables are especially attractive on a color program. As in the case of radio, it is hard to evaluate the impact. Gifft and coauthors believe that television and radio are used mostly for entertainment, especially among the culturally disadvantaged, with education as a frequent by-product. They believe also that reading is used mainly for serious or practical purposes, either for self-education or for intellectual stimulation. (9)

Community Events and Campaigns

The possibilities for large-scale education are limited only by imagination and funding. These possibilities include fairs, displays, campaigns, and expositions. One or more sponsoring agencies, strong leadership, and a large active committee are necessary for smooth operation of large fairs and campaigns, and the event must be carefully planned with meticulous attention to detail. In various programs, funding needs have been met by contributions from food companies or other interested purveyors, by rental of exhibit space, or by charging admission. Attendance is likely to be much higher if the event is free to the public.

Lectures or demonstrations by widely-known popular speakers will help to draw crowds. Exhibits should be educational and should involve action—one popular kind is the board listing questions while pushing a button reveals the correct answer. (Figure 14.1) Exhibits should be carefully screened to avoid controversy and faddism. Individual education can be provided by nutritionists and dietitians who staff booths and talk with visitors. Free educational literature should be provided. There may be an overall theme, with all or many of the speakers and exhibits mak-

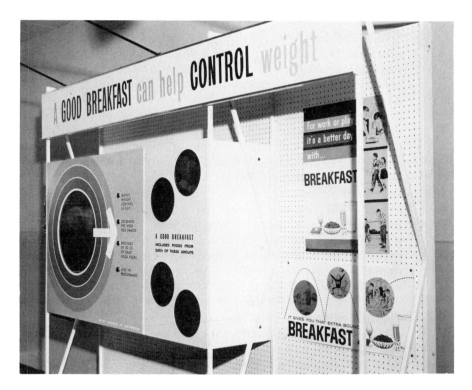

Figure 14.1 Exhibit for Audience Participation—A Light Appears When Correct Answer Is Selected.

ing the same points. A search of the literature will stimulate other ideas for similar programs.

An unusual community program was conducted in Keokuk, Iowa by an action committee of home economists and dietitians. They formed a special sponsoring group to organize the week-long campaign. (19) It was conducted during National Nutrition Week, which provided additional publicity. The program proceeded in two steps.

First, there was a week of nutrition education through schools, civic groups, radio, and newspapers to familiarize people with basic information about nutrition and the need to alter poor food habits.

Second, the week of nutrition education, persons of all ages were invited to sign a pledge card that committed the signer to "adopt a new and good food habit" or to "eliminate an old and bad food habit." After a week and again three months later, a telephone survey was made of a sample of participants to determine how well they had kept their pledges. The surveys showed that during the first week 67 percent of the sample adhered to the pledge most of the time; three months later 59 percent were adhering to their pledges 51 to 100 percent of the time. School children who participated were very enthusiastic about the program. The authors point out that children may present a way to reach their parents.

A booth sponsored and staffed by the Cleveland Dietetic Association during the Greater Cleveland Congress of International Women's Year provided opportunity for nutrition education of many of the 46,000 persons who attended the Congress. Dietitians were available to answer questions or make referrals to appropriate agencies. (18)

Since 1971 the Arizona Nutrition Council, Arizona Dietetic Association and Cooperative Extension, and a local newspaper have co-sponsored an annual Food Fair that has 50 to 60 exhibits and attracts about 5000 persons. Nutrition education is conducted by food demonstrations, talks, and free printed materials. Admission is free with expenses provided by income from exhibitors. Door prizes and a bread-baking contest have helped to attract the public. Further educational value has been provided by radio and television announcements and interviews. (35)

The Los Angeles District of the California Dietetic Association held "Nutrition Expo," a two-day, public exposition, in March 1974, providing nutrition education by prominent speakers and exhibits by food manufacturers and educational agencies. There were also demonstrations on microwave cooking, Chinese cuisine and other food-related topics, and a motion picture about nutrition and activity. Attendance was about 5,000, half professionals and half general public. Income was from rental of exhibit booths and a charge for admission. (15)

Motivation

Methods of motivation in nutrition education must be selected according to the group. Some reasons that may motivate change are:

1. Knowing that good nutrition will help achieve some personal goal of the learner, such as a healthy baby, stronger bones, or weight loss.
2. Trying and liking a new and exciting food, preparation method, or serving method.
3. Emphasizing the pleasures in eating a nutritious diet of basic foods.
4. Helping save money, time, and energy in food purchasing and preparation.
5. Curing or controlling an illness, thereby making the person feel better, for example, an anemic child, a dyspeptic or constipated adult, or a post-coronary patient. This is especially motivating for the adult frightened by an illness as when threatened by hypertension or obesity.
6. Getting approval of family, teacher, or friend for having made good changes.

One factor believed to have little or no motivating effect is characterizing the diet or regimen as "good for health." Apparently the individual needs to have evidence of a tangible reward (healthy baby) or to be scared by some undesirable result (heart attack).

Most community nutritionists work with one or more cultural groups and know that there are differences within each cultural group as well as between groups. Baird and Schultz (1) have provided some useful ideas for understanding and motivating these groups by application of marketing concepts. They studied the responses of Anglo, black, Chinese, and Mexican homemakers to questions about appropriate uses of foods; for example, some foods were characterized as to be eaten by children, or for a snack, or when unhappy. They found that the Chinese attitude was essentially "conservative," the black and Mexican was "enjoyment," and the Anglo was related to the "pleasure-pain principle." The nutritionist could use some of their behavior classifications during interviewing and counseling to find out the attitudes and suggest possible ways of motivating specific individuals.

Evaluation

The direct purpose of nutrition education is change in food practices, but there are other important intermediate and final changes. The kinds of change are:

1. Changes in food practices as in foods consumed and in the way food is selected and prepared.
2. Changes in knowledge about nutrition and food.
3. Changes in attitudes, in what the individual feels and thinks about food and nutrition.
4. Changes in nutritional status as shown by anthropometric and biochemical measures.
5. Changes in how the individual perceives nutritional health, as shown by subjective comments such as "I have lots more energy since I started eating breakfast."

Any of these changes can be evaluated in some way. The nutritionist must use the best available practical methods, modifying them with experience to make them more useful. Since people in nutrition education programs are usually in a free-living situation, a variety of other influences are at work at the same time. These include education by the mass media, especially television advertising and programs such as cooking demonstrations. Though there is no accurate way to assess such effects, the nutritionist should note other programs or activities that have occurred during the same time, or ask the individual about other factors that may have exerted an influence, such as television advertising that stressed a particular food. Because of the problems in determining changes in food practices, changes in knowledge are often used for evaluation.

The best way to determine the effect of a program is to take a food record before nutrition education begins and another afterwards, noting differences in intake of foods and nutrients. Differences in selection of foods (e.g., lean meat rather than fat) or in preparation methods (e.g., using less water in cooking vegetables) can also have beneficial effects on food intake.

Changes in knowledge about nutrition and food are important and should be measured with the recognition that knowledge does not always correlate with practice. Shortridge described a school program in which most learners achieved the learning objectives such as to classify "a variety of foods into the Four Food Groups," measured by practice with food models. (34)

Changes in attitudes are frequently shown by the individual's commenting on a new realization of the importance of nutrition, or a resolution to stop listening to the faddists, or a comment that recognizes the contribution that breads and cereals make to the diet by a person who earlier considered them only as sources of calories.

In a research study, Hunt and coworkers measured differences in knowledge about meal planning and buying, storing and preparing food, and biochemical measurements before and after an educational program with 214 pregnant women. They found significant differences in information in the treatment group and some improvement in the dietary intakes, but little difference in the biochemical measures except a greater increase in red-blood-cell folic acid in the treatment group. It was thought that the ingestion of nutrients as dietary supplements may have obscured improvements due to the improved diets. Differences in the dietary intake of the treatment group and the control group at the end of the study were also in favor of the treatment group, for which intakes had increased. (16)

Whatever kind of change takes place in the individual, it must be satisfying and provide changes that can be seen or felt. Often it is "feeling better," a result frequently heard from a person who takes vitamin supplements, changes diet, loses or gains weight, or starts to exercise. The community nutritionist should evaluate all programs using the best available practical methods, which will be less precise than those used in a research study. Nutrition educators should realize that most efforts will have at least some degree of success but that some individuals are not amenable to change.

SCHOOL NUTRITION PROGRAMS

School would seem to be an ideal time for inculcating good food habits in a child so that they will endure for a lifetime. Unfortunately this does not always take place. The amount and quality of nutrition education are variable, depending on administrators, teachers, parents, school boards, and voters.

Most nutrition educators agree that nutrition should be integrated into subject matter at all grades. Cornely has suggested that there should be requirements for knowledge and state of health as a child progresses through the grades. (3)

The current status of school nutrition education was reported by Johnson and Butler (17) from a 1974 survey that showed that 10 states have legislated policy about nutrition education in schools and many others have a wide range of activities. Requirements for the person responsible for nutrition education have been established in 31 states. The suggested requirements proposed for federal legislation include a bachelor's degree in nutrition or foods and nutrition, a master's degree in nutrition education, public health nutrition, or community nutrition; work experience in applied nutrition; teaching certificate and experience, and knowledge about school food service or experience in the field. The school system in 23 states reported having a nutrition component in the curriculum guide. The schools also reported many nutrition education publications on teaching techniques, units in home economics and health, and nutrition education guides. Administrative placement of nutrition education was most often under school food service, but also under nutrition education specialists, home economists, health educators, registered dietitian, physical education specialist, and school administrator.

The authors suggest that nutrition and education professionals at state and local levels participate in determining placement of nutrition education in the state. They point out that the current interest makes this a good time to develop legislation for school nutrition education. This is especially important because of the impact on the child during years K-12.

When community nutritionists have an official responsibility for the school program, the method of work will be determined by agency policy. When the nutritionist works in a community agency with a broad program, with some time devoted to community activities, various kinds of service may be given to the schools.

It should be remembered that nutritionists are trained to be nutritionists and teachers are trained to teach. Most nutritionists are not specialists in educational methods nor in curriculum planning. The appropriate function for the nutritionist is to act as a subject matter specialist in an advisory capacity, to provide liaison with community agencies, to keep the school informed of pertinent activities and programs, to be informed about school activities and programs, and to give service according to agency policy. Sometimes the nutritionist can encourage the school to participate in a particular program and help them develop the plans.

One public health nutritionist persuaded a school to apply for funds for nutrition education and helped them develop the proposal. Though the funding was not approved, the school was encouraged to find a way to start some nutrition activities. A variety of services have been provided in the schools by nutritionists working in the community.

A health educator asked a nutritionist for help in preparation of a booklet on cultural food practices for the elementary grades. The nutritionist provided resource materials, made a critical review for accuracy of the subject matter, checked recipes, menus, ingredients and methods, and advised on converting the recipes to metric measures.

Two public health nutritionists helped the educational consultant for a religious school system by arranging a workshop to train teachers for followup with children screened under the EPSDT program. The nutritionists planned the program and arranged for three instructors from a nearby university to participate. The workshop included a speaker from the EPSDT program, a physician, and a nurse. There was a demonstration of proper weighing and measuring techniques, followed by a period of practice in weighing and measuring for the teachers and other school personnel who attended the meeting. They were also shown how to use the new growth charts from the Center for Disease Control to monitor growth.

Some nutritionists in one health department have been requested to make a critical review of a school's nutrition curriculum each time changes are to be made. Their review is of subject matter and sequence, rather than of the curriculum itself. Nutritionists have also frequently conducted education in nutrition and related subject matter for teachers and school nurses.

Peck has suggested action to increase nutrition activities in schools by finding out the interest of school administrators and school board members, and investigating the possibility of support for such programs by funding from state or federal governments, voluntary agencies, or local foundations. (29) The community nutritionist could cooperate in these endeavors by assuming leadership for discussing the possibilities with the people mentioned, and organizing other professionals interested in nutrition.

SUMMARY

Community education includes activities designed to educate and inform leaders and citizens how they can solve their community nutrition problems by united action. Professionals concerned about nutrition should utilize the community organization process to identify problems and propose means by which they may be solved. They should then identify community leaders who can organize the community for action.

A function of professional leadership is to collect and organize data about problems so that they can be used by action groups. These groups can educate and inform the public about nutrition problems and help them find their way through the maze of agencies of city, county, state, and federal governments.

Nutrition education teaches individuals and families about personal food and health practices that will lead to good nutrition. Individuals need to know what constitutes food for health and how to select their own food. Mothers and other persons responsible for the family food at home must know the needs of various family members. Persons responsible for the food served in restaurants, cafeterias, schools, and institutions should know the principles of nutrition, meal planning, and food preparation so they can serve attractive, nutritionally adequate food.

Nutrition education must include or be accompanied by information about purchasing, household skills, and home management so the individual can solve these accompanying problems that often interfere with feeding the family. Several ways of teaching nutrition for individuals may be adapted to the food management needs of various groups. The goals in planning a nutrition program have been outlined and some examples of programs have been given.

REFERENCES CITED

1. Baird, Pamela C. and Howard G. Schutz, The Marketing Concept Applied to "Selling" Good Nutrition, *J. Nutr. Educ.,* 8 1–3/76 13.
2. Clamp, Betty A. and Colleen M. Carr, Community College Nutrition Outreach Project, *J. Nutr. Educ.,* 8 7–9/76 130.
3. Cornely, Paul B., Community Concern for Total Health Care, *J. Am. Diet. Assoc.,* 60 2/72 110.
4. Creasy, Donna N., How Will America Eat? *What's New in Home Econ.,* 36 10/74 47.
5. Dagley, Beverly D., Adult Education Minicourse in Nutrition Involves Group, *J. Nutr. Educ.,* 8 4–6/76 79.
6. Editor's note, *J. Nutr. Educ.,* 7 1–3/75 31.
7. Emmons, Lillian, and Marian Hayes, Nutrition Knowledge of Mothers and Children, *J. Nutr. Educ.,* 5 4–6/73 134.
8. Gifft, Helen H., Marjorie Washbon, and Gail G. Harrison, *Nutrition, Behavior and Change,* Prentice-Hall Inc., Englewood Cliffs NJ, 1972, 1.
9. Ibid. 71.
10. Gussow, Joan D., Improving the American Diet, *J. Home Econ.,* 65 11/73 6.
11. Harker, Charlotte S., and Penelope Kupsinel, Nutrition Education for Today, *J. Home Econ.,* 63 1/71 15.
12. Hertzler, Ann A., and Helen L. Anderson, Food Guides in the United States, *J. Am. Diet. Assoc.,* 64 1/74 26.
13. Hill, Mary M., Food Guides—Where Do We Go? *Nutrition Program News,* 3–4/73.
14. Hill, Mary M., ICNE Formulates Some Basic Concepts in Nutrition, *Nutrition Program News,* 9–10/64.
15. Hixson, Sue, Consumer Education: Los Angeles Style, *J. Am. Diet Assoc.,* 66 2/75 167.
16. Hunt, Isabelle F., Mary Jacob, Norma J. Ostergard, Gloria Masri, Virginia A. Clark and Anne H. Coulson, Effect of Nutrition Education on the Nutritional Status of Low-Income Pregnant Women of Mexican Descent, *Am. J. Clin. Nutr.,* 29 6/76 675.
17. Johnson, Mary J., and Jane L. Butler, Where Is Nutrition Education in U.S. Public Schools?, *J. Nutr. Educ.,* 7 1–3/75 20.

18. Keenen, Pamela C., Exhibit of Greater Cleveland Congress of International Women's Year, *J. Am. Diet. Assoc.,* 68 6/76 555.
19. Lambert, Verona E., and Lois O. Schwab, Can We Change Our Food Habits?, *J. Home Econ.,* 67 9/73 33.
20. Leverton, Ruth M., What Is Nutrition Education?, *J. Am. Diet. Assoc.,* 64 1/74 17.
21. Los Angeles County Health Department, unpublished pamphlet.
22. Making Health Education Work, *Am. J. Pub. Health,* 65 10/75 Supplement, 9.
23. Manoff, Richard K., Potential Uses of Mass Media in Nutrition Programs, *J. Nutr. Educ.,* 5 4–5/73 125–29.
24. Medical Auxiliaries Study Nutrition To Teach It, letter from Juno-Ann Clarke, in *J. Nutr. Educ.,* 7 1–3/75 31.
25. Message to Youngsters from ABC: You Are What You Eat, *Los Angeles Times, TV Times,* June 20, 1976, 6.
26. National Research Council, Food and Nutrition Board, *Recommended Dietary Allowances,* 8th ed., National Academy of Sciences, Washington DC, 1974, p. 26.
27. Navarro, Vicente, From Public Health to the Health of the Public, *Am. J. Public Health,* 64 6/74 538.
28. Nutrition Council as a Tool for Change, Report of a Workshop in Effective Action, *J. Nutr. Educ.,* 6 10–12/74, Insert i–iv.
29. Peck, Eileen M., Nutrition Education Specialists: Time for Action, *J. Nutr. Educ.,* 8 1–3/76 11.
30. Position Paper on Nutrition Education for the Public, *J. Am. Diet. Assoc.,* 62 4/73 429.
31. Reed, Leni C., Patients Learn from Recording of Diet Counseling, *J. Am. Diet. Assoc.,* 66 6/75 615.
32. Sanjur, Diva, and Anna D. Scoma, Food Habits of Low-Income Children in Northern New York, *J. Nutr. Ed.,* 2 Winter/1971 85.
33. Ibid., 93.
34. Shortridge, Russell C., Learner Success or Failure, *J. Nutr. Educ.,* 8 1–3/76 18.
35. Smitherman, Alice, Arizona Food Fair, *J. Am. Diet. Assoc.,* 68 6/76 553.
36. Todhunter, E. Neige, PTA and Nutrition Council Cooperate in Study Course, *J. Nutr. Educ.,* 5 7–9/73 208.
37. Yee, Barbara, Firefighters Learn To "Eat Heart-ily," *J. Nutr. Educ.,* 8 1–3/76 31.

ADDITIONAL REFERENCES

Kintzer, Frederick C., Approaches to Teaching Adults, *J. Am. Diet. Assoc.,* 50 6/67 475.

Light, Luise, The "Discipline" of Nutrition Education, *J. Nutr. Educ.,* 6 10–12/74 129.

Martin, Ethel A., *Nutrition in Action,* Holt, Rinehart and Winston, New York, 1971.

Martin, Ethel A., *Nutrition Education in Action: A Guide to Teachers,* Holt, Rinehart and Winston, New York, 1963.

Mayer, Jean, Time for Reappraisal, *J. Nutr. Educ.,* 7 1–3/75 8.

Peck, Eileen B., Nutrition Education Specialists: Time for Action, *J. Nutr. Educ.,* 8 1–3/76 11–12.

Rickie, N. D., Some Guidelines for Conducting a Health Fair, *Pub. Health Reports,* 91 5–6/76 261.

White, Philip L., Why All the Fuss over Nutrition Education?, *J. Nutr. Ed.,* 8 4–6/76 54.

5 THE ACTIVITIES

In conducting a profession, a body of knowledge is applied in services for people who have common problems. In community nutrition the special body of knowledge enables the nutritionist to conduct activities for attack on problems that can be prevented or treated by some nutritional intervention. These activities are based on a mastery of the tools, skills, and techniques discussed in previous chapters. The body of knowledge is applied in health center, clinic, home, and other settings where the nutritionist works with individuals, families, and communities.

The body of knowledge will be used in professional education and public education. Some nutritionists will not conduct all of these activities; for example, many nutritionists will not be working in rural or migrant communities. Other activities, such as working with the poor, advising on food money management, and combatting food misinformation will be used constantly. Knowing about ways to study cultural food practices and ways to use legislation is necessary to recognize when these activities will help to solve problems.

The nutritionist may furnish information on any of these topics to newspapers, or radio or television programs, or to professionals and the public.

CHAPTER 15 SURVEYING FOOD PRICES AND CULTURAL FOOD PRACTICES

The subjects of this chapter are food money management and cultural food practices. The purpose is to describe methods of obtaining information and using it for professional and public education rather than to supply information about prices or food practices. One way to collect food prices and some ways to use the prices in preparing materials will be described. Several ways in which food practices were studied and how the information was used will be reported.

ADVISING FAMILIES ON FOOD MONEY MANAGEMENT

Food money management is the controlled use of food money to provide palatable, attractive meals with sufficient nutrients to cover the needs of the various family members at an appropriate cost. Actually food money is so closely entwined with other needs that the entire family budget must be considered as a unit. In many households the income is too low to provide for the basic needs, which include food, housing, clothing, health care, electricity, fuel, cleaning and household supplies, and either carfare or gasoline for transportation. Other expenses include insurance, recreation, gifts, and, for employed persons, federal and state income taxes, social security taxes, and, often, union dues.

Food is usually the largest item, and the most flexible expenditure, purchased from day to day and often allocated only from what is left after fixed amounts have been spent for other items. Frequently under these circumstances, a family reduces food expenditures below the minimum for health, using the money to provide medical care, school supplies, carfare, or other items, sometimes including alcohol, drugs, and funds for gambling. Reducing food expenditures in this way sets the stage for later malnutrition and illness with their additional expenses.

For many years the USDA has published family food plans at several cost levels. An explanation of the Food Plans was given on page 142.

Nutritionists who teach about food costs must have current food price information. Collecting prices in several markets that cater to various economic and ethnic groups is a great help in understanding food costs. Printed materials that contain low-cost foods should be updated at least once a year, and more frequent pricing at least of some items may be needed when there are unusual changes in the price of basic foods. An unseasonal freeze in a far-off valley or excessive rain in the Midwest may ruin crops of grains or fruits, producing a sudden leap in prices, or non-shipment of hogs or beef cattle to market or a failure of the corn crop due to drought may cause dramatic changes in meat prices. Recent examples of similar changes are increases in the price of dried beans due to a variety of natural causes and in the price of coffee due to unusually cold weather in a major coffee-producing area.

Food Pricing Method

The method and extent of pricing depends on how the prices will be used and how much time is available. An extensive list that includes a variety of food items for the low and moderate cost food plans may have several hundred items. Pricing a list of 350 foods in a supermarket takes an experienced nutritionist a full day or more. Aides or students or volunteers can assist the nutritionist, working under supervision until they acquire enough skill to carry the complete responsibility.

The items priced should be appropriate to the group with which the prices will be used. These include foods used by specific ethnic groups for example, rice for Orientals, coconut for Samoans, and cornmeal for Southerners. It may be advisable to prepare special market baskets for various ethnic groups comprised of appropriate foods. A publication with a week's menus and market order for a family from a local ethnic group makes a useful teaching tool (Figure 15.1, 15.2).

Pricing special limited lists of foods may sometimes be helpful. In one area where day-old bakery goods were available and widely used, the nutritionist regularly priced these foods and prepared a leaflet with prices and information about possible savings through their use.

Good public relations with markets are established by carrying official identification and sometimes a letter from the agency. The market manager is contacted by the nutritionist upon entering the

SUNDAY

Orange Juice	Vegetable Soup	Chicken with Rice
Huevos Rancheros with Tostados	Bologna Sandwich	(Arroz Con Pollo)
Enriched White Toast, Margarine	Celery Sticks	Green Beans Spinach Salad
Milk for children	Canned Peaches	Flour Tortillas Cake
Coffee for adults	Milk for all	Milk for all

MONDAY

Sliced Bananas	Fried Beans (Frijoles Fritos)	Stew (Guisado)
Oatmeal with Milk	Tomato and Lettuce Salad	Macaroni Salad
Enriched White Toast,	Flour Tortillas Cake	Flour Tortillas
Margarine	Milk for all	Milk for all
Coffee for adults		

TUESDAY

Grapefruit Juice	Peanut Butter Sandwich	Picadillo
Cornflakes with Milk	Cabbage, Apple,	Fried Potatoes Sopa de Arroz
Enriched White Toast, Margarine	Raisin Salad	Enriched White Bread, Margarine
Coffee for adults	Milk for all	Canned Apricots
		Milk for all

WEDNESDAY

Sliced Oranges	Bean (Frijoles) Sandwich	Spaghetti with Meat Sauce
Fried Eggs Fried Potatoes	Carrot Sticks	Tossed Green Salad
Enriched White Toast, Margarine	Apple	Flour Tortillas
Milk for children	Milk for all	Milk for all
Coffee for adults		

THURSDAY

Sliced Bananas with Corn-	Deviled Egg Sandwich	Albondigas Soup
flakes and Milk	Carrot Sticks	Beans (Frijoles) Fried Potatoes
Enriched White Toast, Margarine	Orange Cookies	Flour Tortillas Cole Slaw
Coffee for adults	Milk for all	Milk for all

FRIDAY

Orange Juice	Tuna Salad Sandwich	Fried Fish
Oatmeal with Milk	Celery Sticks	Broccoli Mashed Potatoes
Soft Cooked Eggs	Banana Cookies	Enriched White Bread, Margarine
Enriched White Toast, Margarine	Milk for all	Cake
Coffee for adults		Milk for all

SATURDAY

Grapefruit Juice	Potato Salad	Tacos with Meat, Chili,
Pancakes, Syrup	Sliced Bologna	Tomato, Lettuce, Cheese
Bacon	Sliced Tomato	Fried Beans (Frijoles Fritos)
Milk	Hot Biscuits Apple	Milk for all
Coffee for adults	Milk for all	

County of Los Angeles Department of Health Services
Community Health Services
Nutrition Program
2/70

Mexican-American Family: Man, Woman, Boy age 13, Girl age 8

Figure 15.1   Menus for One Week for a Mexican-American Family of Four.

Quantity	Food	Unit Price	Cost
	Milk and Milk Products		
8 quarts	Whole milk	$ .71/½ gal	$2.84
7 quarts (reconstit.)	Nonfat dry milk	3.05/14 qts	1.53
¾ pound	Cheddar cheese, mild	1.49/lb	1.12
			$5.49
	Meat, Fish & Poultry		
1 pound	Beef stew, boneless	1.29/lb	$1.29
1 pound	Chuck steak, blade	.78/lb	.78
1¾ pounds	Ground beef	.83/lb	1.46
½ pound	Bologna, sliced	.99/lb	.50
1-2½ pound	Chicken	.49/lb	1.23
1 pound package	Perch fillets, frozen	1.19/lb	1.19
1-6¼ oz can	Tuna, grated	.45/can	.45
			$6.90
	Eggs		
27	Eggs, medium, grade AA	.55/doz	1.24
			$1.24
	Dried Beans, Peas & Nuts		
4 pounds	Pinto beans	.73/lb	$2.92
½ pound	Peanut butter	.64/lb	.32
			$3.24
	Flour, Cereal & Baked Goods		
5 pounds	Flour, enriched white	.85/5 lbs.	$ .85
6 loaves—1½#	Bread, enriched white	.47/loaf	2.82
1 box—1#, 2 oz	Oatmeal	.48/box	.48
1 box—8 oz.	Cornflakes	.29/box	.29
1 pound	White rice, enriched	.85/2 lbs	.43
½ pound	Macaroni, enriched	.42/lb	.21
½ pound	Spaghetti, enriched	.42/lb	.21
			$5.29
	Citrus Fruit & Tomatoes		
4 pounds	Oranges, fresh	.20/lb	$ .80
2-6 oz cans	Orange juice, Frozen	.20/can	.40
32 oz	Grapefruit juice, Canned	.51/46 oz	.36
2 pounds	Tomatoes, fresh	.49/lb	.98
4-8 oz. cans	Tomato sauce	.11/can	.44
2 pound cans, #303	Tomatoes	.25/can	.50
			$3.48

County of Los Angeles Department of Health Services
Community Health Services
Nutrition Program   Man, Woman, Boy 13, Girl 8
Rev. 7/74
VG:kt

Figure 15.2   Market Order for One Week for a Mexican-American Family of
Four.

Quantity	Food	Unit Price	Cost
	Dark-Green & Deep-Yellow Vegetables		
2 pounds	Carrots, fresh	$ .19/lb	$ .38
1-10 oz package	Broccoli, frozen chopped	.25/pkg	.25
1 bunch, ¾ lb	Spinach, fresh	.33/lb	.25
1	Green pepper	.59/lb	.59
¼ pound	Green chiles	.79/lb	.20
			$ 1.67
	Potatoes		
7 pounds	Potatoes	.14/lb	$ .98
			$ .98
	Other Vegetables & Fruits		
2½ pounds	Onions, dry	.15/lb	$ .38
1-2 pound head	Lettuce	.35/lb	.70
1-2 pound head	Cabbage	.10/lb	.20
1 pound stalk	Celery	.30/lb	.30
1 pound can, #303	Green beans	.26/can	.26
1 pound can, #303	Peaches	.37/can	.37
3 pounds	Bananas	.15/lb	.45
2½ pounds	Apples	.49/lb	1.23
1 pound can, #303	Apricots	.43/can	.43
2 oz	Raisins	.81/15 oz	.11
1-10½ oz can	Vegetable soup	.20/can	.20
2 oz	Red Peppers, dried	.39/1½ oz	.52
			$ 5.15
	Fats, Oil and Bacon		
½ pound	Bacon	.79/lb	$ .40
2 pounds	Margarine	.44/lb	.88
1 pint	Vegetable Oil	.92/24 oz	.62
½ pint	Salad Dressing	.79/qt.	.20
			$ 2.10
	Sweets & Sugar		
2½ pounds	Sugar	1.51/5 lbs	$ .76
1 pound	Brown sugar	.38	.38
			$ 1.14
	Beverages		
½ pound	Coffee, ground	1.05/lb	$ .53
			$ .53
	Accessory Foods		
	One percent of total cost		$ .36
			$37.57

County of Los Angeles Department of Health Services
Community Health Services
Nutrition Program
Rev. 7/74
VG:kt

market and the activity is explained, with assurance that a number of markets are being surveyed and names and prices of individual stores will not be divulged. Usually the manager is interested and gives full cooperation and help. If all stores of the same chain have the same prices, pricing one will suffice. It is important to price in stores in the neighborhoods where the residents shop, to price items used by the residents, and to price standard items including the store brands.

After the prices have been collected, they must be interpreted in ways that will make them useful in professional and public education. They can be used to determine which foods, at current market prices, are the least expensive sources of nutrients, to estimate the minimum and average amounts of money needed for food for a specific family, and to illustrate ways of getting the most for the available money.

Though the average of all prices collected is sometimes used, a more realistic way to tabulate prices so the figures will be applicable to many families, whatever their markets and shopping practices, is to use the price that will cover the cost of an item in three-fourths of the stores studied. For example, prices are collected in eight stores for canned tomatoes: 55¢, 49¢, 47¢, 45¢, 44¢, 44¢, 42¢, and 39¢. The price selected is 47¢, which covers the cost in six of the eight stores. The premise is that most families can purchase the item at or below this price. This method eliminates the very high and very low prices that distort an average.

A market basket composed of foods that might be purchased for a specific period of time or a food order for one week offers a convenient method for comparative pricing, as the foods can be priced at specific intervals, for example, monthly, quarterly, or once a year.

Nutritionists who work with small families or with older persons who live alone or in two-person households should survey the additional costs to the small household caused by purchasing in small quantities. Peterkin reports that one-person households paid 11 percent more and two-person households paid 7 percent more than six-person households. (11) Part of this higher cost is due to the need to purchase in small quantities because of limited refrigeration and other storage facilities.

Community nutritionists who participate in pricing welfare food allowances or in advising about them should recognize the need for frequent pricing and prompt use of the results. These figures can be used by nutritionists in making welfare officials and politicians aware of the health consequences of inadequate money for food.

The Community Council of Greater New York issues an *Annual Price Survey* that gives costs for self-supporting families in New York City. The budget is based on the Bureau of Labor Statistics budget for a moderate level. Another publication, *Family Budget Standard,* is used to evaluate the economic condition of the family before counseling on money management. (5, 6)

Cost of Convenience Foods

Much has been written about the excessive costs of convenience foods. These include frozen, canned, dried, and dehydrated packaged foods that have been partially prepared to reduce work and limit the ingredients to be added in the home. Personnel who work with home-makers, especially those from low income families, will need to keep abreast of their cost and convenience as compared with foods prepared at home.

The increased use of these products has probably been due to the assumption that their use saves time and gives a better, more consistent product. In reporting a survey of use of convenience foods by a selected sample of low income families in New York State, Seoane says ". . . convenience foods are here to stay. Therefore, an effort must be made to assist the homemaker in the selection and use of those foods." (15)

Actually the cost of convenience foods is sometimes less than their counterparts completely prepared in the home. Cromwell and Odlund compared the cost (8) of plate dinners and skillet main dishes, finding that the plate dinners cost more but costs of the skillet main dishes varied, with some costing more and some less than home-prepared counterparts. In all cases, the lower-priced brands of the skillet dishes cost less than the homemade product. Savings in time were considerable for the plate dinners, less for the skillet dishes. The authors suggest that the family evaluate the amount and acceptability of the product before calculating comparative costs. The protein content of a main dish must also be evaluated.

Teaching Food Money Management

The preparation of materials and use of pricing data and other food-cost materials must be planned to meet the needs and interests of the specific clientele with whom it will be used. The nutritionist must be careful before trying to educate a client about food money management to determine whether the real need is for education or money.

Nutritionists and home economists generally believe that planning of menus and shopping lists and careful control of marketing are valuable as the way to obtain better nutrition within the budget. The daily plan should include snacks if they are a part of the individual or family food pattern. In using the Family Food Plans (page 142) as the basis for counseling, the nutritionist or nurse may find it useful to determine the total amount of food for a week from the figures for each person. Showing the homemaker these figures, for example, the number of pounds of green and yellow vegetables recommended per week, may stimulate the homemaker to serve them more often.

Sometimes the homemaker may need help in deciding how much of the family income should be spent for food. Peterkin points out (13) that there are many ways to state the percent of income spent for food and that averages have limitations in their application to any specific family. It has been estimated that 16 percent of disposable personal income in the United States is spent for food. Persons with high incomes spend a low percentage while those with low incomes may spend 35 to 50 percent or more, and large families spend a higher percentage than smaller families.

The federal figures from which these percentages were derived include nonmoney income such as the value of rent for persons living in their own homes and the value of home-produced food and fuel. The expenditures do not include nonfood items such as soap, paper, cigarettes, or alcoholic beverages. Obviously there is no single figure that is applicable to all families. Each family needs to consider its own goals, circumstances, and desires in deciding what proportion of income to spend for food.

Budgeting by food groups is another technique that may be used with some homemakers. USDA food economists showed how some families divided their money among the food groups and compared the results with the costs if they had followed the low-cost plan. (1)

Food Group	Family Practices	Low-Cost Plan
Milk, cheese ice cream	$0.13	$0.18
Meat, poultry, fish, eggs, legumes	.40	.30
Vegetables and fruit	.20	.25
Cereals, bakery products	.13	.16
Other foods	.14	.11
	$1.00	$1.00

Some families may be willing to spend less on one group to allow more for another. "Other foods" include fats, oils, sugar, sweets, coffee, tea and soft drinks.

There are various ways to teach comparison of food costs to both professionals and homemakers. Usually the comparison will be for food portions that supply equivalent amounts of nutrients, but the comparisons may sometimes be between portions with less consideration for food values. A number of food economists have made comparisons by methods and tools that are practical for use in community nutrition programs. The nutritionist can use these methods to develop tools for comparing other foods.

Home economists of the U.S.D.A. have prepared a number of tables to compare foods that can be used as alternates in planning meals. (3) One table compares the cost of calcium provided by one cup of milk with the same amount from cheese, ice cream, and other dairy products. Another table provides information to compare the costs of 3 ounces of cooked lean meat from various kinds of meat, poultry, and fish. Other tables provide methods of comparing the cost of meat from various parts of chicken and turkey, and comparing the costs of a half-cup serving of canned, frozen, and fresh vegetables.

Williams and Justice have developed a worksheet listing 21 protein sources with factors for determining the cost of portions supplying 14 grams of protein. (19) They describe the method for preparing similar tables on other foods. The factor is determined by dividing 14 by the number of grams of protein in 1 pound of the food. This factor is then multiplied by the price per pound to get the cost of the 14-gram portion.

The nutritionist, home economist, public health nurse, or nutrition aide who tries to help a family that appears to lack enough money for food should first analyze the cause for the inadequacy. If the amount of money is actually enough but the homemaker needs help in planning use of the money, the professional or aide can be of assistance in a review of expenses.

The kinds and quantities of food eaten can be compared with a food guide to show that the diet is inadequate. The nutritionist can also estimate which nutrients are low. The amount of money spent for food should be compared with current costs of the foods for the family calculated by using the low cost food plan (page 143) with local prices. When the amount spent appears to be adequate, counseling is in order to change the family expenditure of food money. Often money is expended on vitamins or other food supplements because the mother has been persuaded that these items are necessary to provide good nutrition for the children. Sometimes the family needs to spend less on bacon and more on lean meat, or less on soft drinks and more on milk.

Seoane (15) suggests that many families can benefit from better management of money spent for meat to free part of it for other items using meat alternates, which are often a less expensive source of good-quality protein. She further suggests stressing more nutritious snacks, particularly for low income families.

In other cases, analysis will show that the amount of money is simply not enough. Then the effort should be directed to finding or developing other resources, or to changing legislation to provide more adequate funds. This will fill the need of many families who will purchase an adequate diet when they have enough money. There are some families with inadequate food money whose diet will probably not be improved by simply increasing their income. In such cases there must be a dual attack to increase the family's purchasing power and to improve its practices of meal planning, purchasing, and food use. Purchasing power may sometimes be increased by a change in purchasing practices, for example, patronizing a different market or using different brands. When the family already employs good practices, its nutritious food supply may be increased by finding additional resources such as WIC, or produce at low cost or no cost.

At higher income levels, where there is enough money to meet all family needs, improvement of food practices must be effected by education. Jolly has examined the relationship between income and nutritional levels, finding that there is a strong relationship between the two, and noting that "36 percent of families in the lowest income group had poor diets, but only 9 percent of the high income families." Jolly considers income to be the main determinant of nutritional value, noting also a relationship between income level and inadequate intake of vitamins A and C. (9)

Another question is what motivation can be used to change management practices. Zimmerman and Munro (20) report that mothers in the Missoula Head Start Program responded negatively to discussions on food buying and preparation saying that their families would not accept nutritious food even if they prepared it. It was concluded that their negative feelings were due to their not having the skill, knowledge, and money to prepare the food. Behavior modification techniques were used in a successful program to effect change. One of the key points was not asking for a report of home diets as this produced a negative reaction. Instead, the program was centered on planning the Head Start lunch and the home meals so the two together provided a good diet. Members of the group successfully improved their home meals and continued to support each other by functioning independently as a group.

Taking advantage of current advertising methods and "specials" is one way to extend purchasing power. Recently, both food companies and markets have been using "cents off" coupons for sales promotion. One nutritionist used a bulletin board in the health center waiting room, where coupons supplied by staff and friends were displayed with a sign *Take One*. Some coupons represented a 25-percent saving on the item. Reports in the press have claimed that coupon savings may amount to several hundred dollars a year, but there has been no varification of this statement. Sometimes the stimulus of the cents-off bargain may cause a family to purchase a more expensive item, so there is actually no money saved. Loss-leader and other promotions are also common and may offer worthwhile savings that must, however, be balanced against the time, effort, and transportation costs to take advantage of a special offer.

Perhaps one reason for poor marketing practices, and the unwise expenditure of money, is the amount of time needed for purchasing in today's supermarkets. The variety and extent of foods, the different package sizes, and the number of nonfood items regularly purchased in supermarkets have combined to increase the time required for marketing.

In 1967 Walker studied the time used for homemaking in 1296 husband-wife families of various socioeconomic levels and lifestyles. Two-day records were collected of time used by all family members. Time spent was compared with studies made in 1926–27 and 1952. Time spent on marketing, record-keeping, and management increased between 1927 and 1967, although there was a decrease of 30 minutes per day in time spent on food preparation and after-meal cleanup. (17)

It appears probable that the current practices of reading labels, using coupons, issuing merchandising stamps, and handling government food stamps have increased shopping time even more since Walker's study. The ingenious nutritionist or aide will find ways to help families compensate for these problems. Even for persons on comfortable incomes and eating a good diet, better control of food expenditures can contribute to better family living by making more money available for nonfood expenditures that contribute to the enchment of life.

A more detailed analysis of the complexity of food economics is provided by Burk using systems ideas in consumer education and in evaluation of efforts to improve American diets. (2) Burk says: ". . . a family of four with $106 a month in food stamps will buy a different combination of foods than they did when they had only $50 or $60. They can buy the expensive foods they have seen advertised on TV, or they can buy foods with higher nutrient content per dollar. The latter choices will require more knowledge and skills and probably gradual development of the value sector of the family's human capital."

Myths About Food Prices

There are many myths about food prices, probably arising from surveys that are subjective, limited, or inaccurate. The nutritionist needs first-hand, objective information to use in both professional and public education. Only careful inspection of items and reading of labels will assure that comparable items are being accurately priced in various places.

One example of the kind of myth that may develop occurred in a large city a few years ago, when there were persistent reports that chain markets regularly charged higher prices in the poverty areas of the city than in the more affluent parts of the city and in the suburbs. A survey of markets was conducted to determine the truth of these allegations. Comparison pricing was done on fifty-four selected items that would comprise a nutritionally adequate diet at low cost for a family of four for one week. Prices were collected in supermarkets located in both low income and in more affluent areas.

Some differences in shopping practices were noted; for example, the chain store brands were more easily found or more readily available in the higher income areas than in the lower while the advertised brands were given more emphasis in the lower income areas. Apparently this was due to customer demand. Food expenditure in the low income areas was sporadic because the customers spent most of their food money at the time they received their welfare checks or food stamps.

The cost of the food list priced in low income areas ranged from $24.14 to $26.19, in the other areas from $23.73 to $26.98. The price comparisons between pairs of chain stores were:

	Low Income	Other Area
Chain 1	$25.75	$26.98
Chain 2	26.19	26.19
Chain 3	24.14	23.73
Chain 4	24.78	24.85
Chain 5	24.44	24.81
Chain 6	24.31	24.95

The general conclusion was that there were no significant differences in prices charged by chain stores for the same item in low income and higher income neighborhoods.

The results of the survey confirmed those of the 1966 survey of the Bureau of Labor Statistics, which showed that (1) foods cost the same in low income as in high income neighborhoods if bought in the same type of store and in the same quality and quantity; (2) prices for the same item in stores of a given grocery chain were usually the same in the two kinds of neighborhoods; (3) small independent stores tended to charge higher prices than chain and large independent stores; and (4) relatively few large chain groceries were located in the low income neighborhoods. (16)

It was also noted in the BLS survey that the similarity of costs did not solve the shopping problems of the low income consumer living some distance from a chain store. Some people prefer the neighborhood store despite higher prices because it is friendly or willing to give credit. Often having only a small amount of money at a time makes it necessary to buy food in small quantities even though this makes total food costs higher.

During 1969 the USDA's Economic Research Service surveyed food prices in low income areas of seven (16) cities (Washington, D.C., Jackson, Miss., Boston, Mass., Newark, N.J., Detroit, Mich., Cleveland, Ohio, and Oakland, Calif.) to test allegations that retail food prices were increased after families received their welfare checks. Selected items used frequently by low income families were purchased in stores the week before check issue dates and one week later immediately after checks were issued. Though prices on 14 percent of the items had changed, the net difference for all stores in the seven cities was very small, only 85¢ on a total bill of $1600 for all sample stores in the seven cities. There were marked differences in movement of prices during the week; for example, about 60 percent of the changes in Oakland were decreases but in Detroit 70 percent were increases.

Another allegation heard frequently is that sanitation in stores in low income areas is poorer than in high-income areas. U.S. Food and Drug Administration workers reported a comparison of chemical and microbiological content of five foods (chicken, hamburger, green beans, white grapes, and milk) between a lower-than-average income area (less than $4000 per year) and a higher-than-average income area (more than $8000 per year), and between the days of the week. They found no significant differences between lower and higher income areas. The level of occurrence of disease- and illness-producing organisms was approximately equal in both areas, making both subject to potential hazards. (10)

Resource Materials

Nutritionists will need a continuing source of ideas about helping clients with food money management. These can be obtained from a variety of publications for both professionals and the public. Perhaps the most useful is the USDA publication ARS-NE-36, *Family Economics Review,* issued quarterly for home economists and specialists of the Cooperative Extension Service, but available to other professionals. Many other ideas can be found in magazines for the home, newspaper food columns, and radio and television food programs. Some excellent pamphlets on the subject have been issued by trade organizations, savings and loan companies, banks, supermarkets, and other commercial sources.

STUDYING CULTURAL FOOD PRACTICES

Nutritionists and others who are concerned about changing food practices are well aware that the first step is to find out what a person eats. Several tools for doing this were included on page 150–152. The community nutritionist must have an extensive knowledge of the food practices of the various cultural and other groups in the area served. Before beginning an effort to change food practices, the nutritionist must learn what the existing food practices are.

There is in much of the United States a food pattern that is sometimes called the "Middle-Class American Diet," based on three fairly structured meals a day. It includes a breakfast of fruit juice, bacon and eggs, toast and coffee. Lunch is often composed of salads, sandwiches, soup, or other light foods with dessert of cake, pie or ice cream. Dinner usually includes a large portion of roast meat or steak, potatoes, gravy, salad and, perhaps a vegetable, with rolls or bread, and a dessert. This diet is high in calories, protein and saturated fat, and low in calcium, iron, and some vitamins and trace minerals.

This typical American diet has always been modified by regional practices, but usually in specific foods rather than in structure. For example, in the South grits and biscuits replace potatoes and rolls, and fried fish or chicken replace the roast or steak.

In addition to these regional variations, many immigrant groups brought their own food customs. Some foods are associated with specific groups, such as pasta with Italians, rice with Orientals, dried beans and tortillas with Mexicans, and corned beef with Jews. All of this has resulted in a varied diet, and as Americans have become more mobile, ethnic foods have become known to more people. Perhaps this has reached a peak in big cities where most large markets have sections for International Foods where black beans (Cuban), pinto beans (Mexican), guava paste (Latin-American), rye wafers (Scandinavian), pizza (Italian), pita bread (Arabian), and other ethnic foods are displayed.

The vegetarian diet is an alternative food pattern which, like most other food patterns, provides all necessary nutrients when it is carefully selected, except that the pure vegetarian diet (i.e., one with no animal products) is usually deficient in vitamin B_{12}. The vegetarian diet should not be regarded as extreme or faddish but as one good food pattern among many. The nutritionist must know how to evaluate it by the Four Food Groups, calculate the nutrient content and cost, and suggest modifications to adjust either. There has been an increase in the number of persons who follow the various vegetarian patterns because of concern over the world food supply.

There has also been an increase in the number of persons who follow more unusual eating patterns such as macrobiotic, organic, or additive-free. There are many of these unusual patterns, and new ones constantly appear and old ones recur. The nutritionist would be hard-pressed to be acquainted with all. In addition, the traditional three-meals-a-day pattern is changing and some observers believe that we are in a permanent pattern characterized by many small meals and snacks.

In learning to work under these circumstances, the basic principle in nutrition education is still to start with what the individual eats, identify the missing nutrients, and propose gradual changes that are acceptable to the client. This principle holds true regardless of the method of nutrition education and regardless of the setting for it. To accomplish changes in the food intake of an individual, the nutritionist will need to have an extensive knowledge of the food practices of local cultural groups.

Collecting Information About Cultural Food Practices

When there is a sizeable number of persons in an ethnic or cultural group in the community, the nutritionist will find it helpful to study the food practices of the group. This is best done by a process that involves techniques from various disciplines. The nutritionist will probably find it necessary to plan and conduct the study and adapt the findings with limited help because the need and application are different from those of other disciplines. Often public health nurses or health educators pose the need to the nutritionist, provide much of the data, and help in necessary contacts. The examples that follow show various methods by reporting studies of five different cultural groups.

Thirty Arabic Families. Public health nurses in one health district asked the nutritionist for help in counseling Arabic families. The nutritionist found out from the nurses that there were about 30 families, that they bought most of their food in the one Arabic market near where they lived. The nurses suggested that the nutritionist talk with two English-speaking Arabic women to get information about purchasing, cooking, and eating practices. The nutritionist interviewed the two women to learn the usual food practices, and visited the market to identify the foods and collect prices. This gave her a good picture of the food consumption. The nutrient content was calculated to show what changes were needed in food choices and what foods could be added to provide the Recommended Dietary Allowances.

The nutritionist also calculated food costs and suggested possible alternatives of equivalent nutrient content at lower cost. The information was assembled in a pamphlet and presented to the nurses as inservice education. A glossary of foods was included in the monograph.

Mexican-American Families. At the time this study was made, it was estimated that about 18 percent of the population of Los Angeles County was of Mexican ancestry. In this study there was a language problem as many of the recent immigrants did not speak English. The information was obtained with the help of six members of the nursing staff who provided information and reviewed the pamphlet while it was in progress.

The pamphlet contained a discussion of typical dishes and staple foods, use of protein foods including milk and cheese, and use of fruits and vegetables. The common meal patterns were explained and good practices were listed, followed by suggestions on how to improve the diet. Because of the widespread use of a low salt diet and calorie restriction, a page of suggestions for each was included. Since some of the foods and their uses were new to the nurses, they were classified into the Four Food Groups and suggestions for improving the diet were made. There was a section on chiles, a food much used by Mexican-Americans.

A glossary of common foods was included with a sheet on vitamin content of Mexican foods. There was also a section on evaluating mixed dishes for nutrient content. The nutritionist or knowledgeable nurse identified the foods that are in the mixed dish and considered them separately. For example, in soup there may be 1½ ounces of beef, 1 stalk of celery, ¼ onion, and 2 ounces of zucchini. This would be counted as ½ serving of meat and 1 serving of "other vegetable." To assist in this process, a description of mixed dishes with main ingredients and quantities was given, with instruction on how to count each toward servings of the Four Food Groups. The basic information about the food practices was put into a booklet for use of nurses and nutritionists, and teaching leaflets in both English and Spanish were prepared. The nutritionist orients new nurses to the use of these resource and teaching materials.

Black American Food Practices. A different method was used for this study, because many of the black persons in the area had recently come from the Southeast, and because some information was available from a survey of prenatal patients and other clinic food records. The first step was to obtain information about food practices in the 14 Southeast states from which most of the Black population had come by writing to nutritionists in those states. This information showed that although the foods eaten varied from state to state, there was a common thread of food choices.

After the information from the native states had been compiled, it was used as the basis for collecting information from prenatal patients by means of a questionnaire and one-day food record. A health educator assisted in the preparation of the questionnaire and a community worker obtained some of the food records. From this information it was possible to determine the apparent changes that had been made since the clients had moved to the local area and to identify the good practices and those that needed to be changed. This included points that could be used in counseling. Here are two examples: (1) It was observed that some families made an entire meal from cooked greens and cornbread, a meal which was low in protein. It was recommended that when a family was counseled about meat and meat alternates the counselor suggest adding a protein-rich food to that meal. (2) Many diets were high in calories and saturated fat. It was recommended that in counseling about weight control, emphasis be placed on the use of fewer fried meats and eggs, and the use of very small amounts of salt pork and bacon for seasoning green beans. The latter was a compromise with clients who would not give up fat meat entirely.

A special effort was made in this survey to get information about the use of certain foods associated with Southern eating practices (hog maws, pig's ears and tails, and chitterlings), particularly to find out if these foods were used in the Los Angeles area. It was found that they were used occasionally in special meals but not as a regular part of the diet.

Samoan Food Practices. The information for this ethnic group was hard to obtain because there was a relatively small number in the area, they were quite scattered in the population, and there was a difficult language problem with few interpreters available. Several resources were used. Some information was obtained from health center staff;

then the nutritionist interviewed three homemakers who were community leaders and a minister who was widely known and respected. The nutritionist also visited two markets where Samoans shopped, consulted the professional staff at the health center, and examined the food records of prenatal patients. Many of the foods and names were unfamiliar, so a glossary was placed at the beginning of the resource pamphlet.

Much checking was necessary because of a problem of identifying several banana-like foods that were used frequently in a number of ways. Although adults commonly ate only two meals a day about eight hours apart, with nothing but beverages between the two, it was revealed in the study that large amounts of food were eaten, for example, an adult might have three pork chops and three or four bananas for breakfast.

It was also learned that although the adults continued to eat according to the native patterns, with two meat-starch meals a day, the children were eating a combination Samoan-American pattern with three meals a day. Another cultural characteristic was the attitude toward obesity in that it was not considered a problem but rather a desirable sign that the individual was well fed.

It was suggested that the nurses counsel toward a change to a three-meal pattern as the goal because of the great problem of getting all of the recommended foods into two meals. The counseling was directed toward increasing the consumption of milk, increasing foods with good iron content, and using a greater variety of vegetables. One source of much saturated fat and many calories was the coconut cream pressed from grated coconut and used in many cooked foods. Reducing the amount and encouraging cooking methods that use less fat was another goal of counseling.

Recently Immigrated Chinese.   A still different method was used to collect the data for this group. The nutritionist made several visits to the stores in Chinatown, trained a Chinese-speaking youth worker to interview patients and collect information by questionnaire, and received consultation and other help from a Chinese-American nurse, nutritionist, and graduate nutrition student.

Comment.   The method used in each study has been described at some length to show the different adjustments necessitated by several specific situations. In each case the nutritionist first reviewed the methods for collecting information about food practices, and the available literature on the cultural group, then assembled as much information as possible from the professional staff members who were acquainted with the families. This was done to give the nutritionist some background before attempting interviews or collecting prices.

Nutrient content and cost were calculated and suggestions were made for counseling in which the good points could be reinforced and the poor ones modified. In each study the method must be developed for the particular circumstances, and often the survey data is only applicable to the specific area surveyed. The studies are well worth the time and effort because the information is necessary for effective nutrition counseling.

Reviews of the food practices of individuals and families of various cultures will be found in the literature. (21, 22, 23, 24, 25)

SUMMARY

The community nutritionist will have frequent need for information about food prices and food practices, thus needs to know sources of information on these topics and methods of surveying to collect data. It is important that food prices be updated at regular intervals and at other times when changes may have occurred because of unusual weather or other reasons. Though price lists are available from the USDA and other sources, the only way they can be made really applicable in a specific area is to use local costs. A method of collecting and processing the prices has been described. Suggestions have been made for teaching families about food money management.

Information about the food practices of specific groups of people is needed as background for teaching those groups about normal or modified diets. There is much variation in food practices, so it is desirable to collect information about the specific group. There is no regular method for such a study, so one must be planned for the occasion. The methods used in studies of five different ethnic groups in one health agency have been described. Examples were given of how the information was used in professional education and in nutrition education.

There are other variations in dietary practices such as the vegetarian diet, which like other diets must be carefully planned to be sure it is adequate in nutrients and meets the calorie needs of individuals.

REFERENCES CITED

Food Money Management

1. Budgeting by Food Group, *Fam. Econ. Rev.,* ARS 62-5, U.S. Dept. of Agriculture, Hyattsville MD, 9/72 21.
2. Burk, Marguerite C., Food Economics Behavior in Systems Terms, *J. Home Econ.,* 62 5/70 319.

3. Chassy, Judy, Cost of Milk and Milk Products as Sources of Calcium, *Fam. Econ. Rev.,* ARS 62-5, U.S. Dept. of Agriculture, Hyattsville MD, 12/72 12.

4. Collier, Linda, and Dianne Odlund, Convenience and Cost of Baked Products, *Fam. Econ. Rev.,* ARS-NE-36, U.S. Dept. of Agriculture, Hyattsville MD, Spr./75 14.

5. Community Council of Greater New York, *Annual Price Survey: Family Budget Costs,* 18th annual ed., 1975.

6. Community Council of Greater New York, *Family Budget Standard, 1970.*

7. Cromwell, Cynthia, Cost of the Lean in Ground Beef, *Fam. Econ. Rev.* ARS 62-5, U.S. Dept. of Agriculture, Hyattsville MD, Win./74 13.

8. Cromwell, Cynthia, and Dianne Odlund, Convenience and Cost of Plate Dinners and Skillet Main Dishes, *Fam. Econ. Rev.,* ARS-NE-36, U.S. Dept. of Agriculture, Hyattsville MD, Sum./74 10.

9. Jolly, Desmond, Changing Food Habits, *J. Nutr. Educ.,* 3 Fall/71 51.

10. Messer, James W., James E. Leslie, David F. Brown, James T. Peeler, Marvin T. Green, James E. Gilchrist, and John E. Wimsatt, A Comparative Quality Survey of Five Common Market Foods in Low and High Income Areas., *Am. J. Pub. Health,* 63 12/73 1074.

11. Peterkin, Betty, Food Prices Paid by Large and Small Families, *Fam. Econ. Rev.,* ARS 62-5, U.S. Dept. of Agriculture, Hyattsville MD, 12/72, 18.

12. Peterkin, Betty, USDA Family Food Plans, 1974, *Fam. Econ. Rev.,* ARS-NE-36, U.S. Dept. of Agriculture, Hyattsville MD, Win./75 3.

13. Peterkin, Betty, The Part of Income That Goes for Food, *Fam. Econ. Rev.,* ARS 62-5, U.S. Dept. of Agriculture Hyattsville, MD, Win./74 6.

14. Peterkin, Betty, The Cost of Meats and Meat Alternates, *Fam. Econ. Rev.,* ARS-62-5, U.S. Dept. of Agriculture, Hyattsville MD, Fall/74 11.

15. Seoane, Nicole A., Shopping Practices of Low-Income Groups, for Convenience Foods, *J. Nutr. Educ.,* 3 Sum./71 28.

16. Taylor, Eileen F., Food Prices Before and After Distribution of Welfare Checks, *Fam. Econ. Rev.,* ARS 62-5, U.S. Dept. of Agriculture, Hyattsville MD, 12/70 12.

17. Walker, Kathryn E., Homemaking Still Takes Time, *J. Home Econ.,* 61 10/69 621.

18. Walter, John P., Two Poverties Equal One Hunger, *J. Nutr. Educ.* 5 4–6/73 129.

19. Williams, Flora L., and Catherine L. Justice, A Ready Reckoner of Protein Costs, *J. Home Econ.,* 67 3/75 20.

20. Zimmerman, Robert, and Nancy Munro, Changing Head Start Mothers' Food Attitudes and Practices, *J. Nutr. Educ.,* 4 Spr./72 66.

Studying Cultural Food Practices

21. Cultural Food Patterns in the U.S.A., pamphlet, American Dietetic Association, Chicago, rev. 1976.

22. Raper, Nancy R., and Mary M. Hill, Vegetarian Diets, *Nutr. Rev.* 32 7/74 Spec. Supp., 29.

23. Robinson, Corinne, *Normal and Therapeutic Nutrition,* 14th ed., Macmillan Co., New York, 216.

24. Williams, Sue R., *Nutrition and Diet Therapy,* 2d ed., C. V. Mosby Co., St. Louis, 1973, 250.

25. Wilson, Eva D., Katherine H. Fisher, and Mary E. Fuqua, *Principles of Nutrition,* 3rd ed., John Wiley & Sons, Inc., New York, 1975, 316.

CHAPTER 16
WORKING WITH THE POOR AND WITH RURAL AND MIGRANT COMMUNITIES

All community nutritionists will work with the poor, so they need to have an understanding of their problems and how the problems affect their eating practices and nutrition. Nutritionists who work in rural areas or with migrant workers need to understand the problems of these particular groups and how the mobility or isolation affects the individual and family.

WORKING WITH POVERTY FAMILIES

Community nutrition programs may be concerned with people at any income level, but many nutrition problems are related to hunger and lack of food due to poverty, so it is important for the community nutritionist to be informed about its origin, its characteristics, and how to work with poor people.

Definitions of Poverty

Poverty is sometimes defined simply as the lack of money, but some persons, such as those in religious orders, may choose a life of poverty, while others, such as students, may choose to live temporarily on a small income and do not see themselves as disadvantaged.

Christakis (5) has defined poverty as "a situation in which the level of living of an individual, family or group is below the standard of living of the community either in terms of subsistence or in contrast to normal standards of income required for at least modest participation in community life."

The federal government has defined poverty (16) in terms of specific dollar amounts, which are updated at intervals. These income levels were developed in 1964 by the Social Security Administration for use in estimating the extent of poverty in the United States. These levels, called *poverty lines,* show the incomes below which families of a specified composition are defined as being in a state of poverty.

Originally the economy food plan of the U.S. Department of Agriculture formed the basis of the poverty line. The cost of food in the economy plan was multiplied by three to compute the poverty line for most types and sizes of families. This method was based on the Household Food Consumption Survey of 1955, which showed that the average food expenditure by U.S. families was one-third of their total expenditure. Smaller proportions were assigned to food for single persons and two-person families.

The income for determining the poverty line for farm families was set lower than for nonfarm families, first at 60 percent of nonfarm, later raised to 70 percent and then to 85 percent. These changes acknowledged the decreasing dependence of farm families on both money and nonmoney farm income. In 1969 the poverty line was modified and based on the Consumer Price Index rather than on food cost alone. (16) The 1976 poverty guidelines are shown in Figure 16.1.

Lewis distinguishes between internal poverty and external poverty, which he considers to represent two distinct categories. (12) *Internal poverty* is the culture of poverty into which one is born, characterized by living only in the present, having little feeling of self-worth, lack of ability to provide for the future, and lack of interest in doing so. *External poverty* is outside the culture of poverty and has different causes, for example, a family that has just enough income for basic necessities is deprived temporarily of part of it, as when the wage-earner is laid off. The family adjusts to the reduced income, but when the wage-earner returns to work the family resumes its former lifestyle.

Walter reports (21) a study of deprived young people in Colombia that showed that social and cultural factors had more influence on the food eaten than did the amount of money. Variety was important; the more kinds of food liked, the greater was the probability of having a good diet. Girls were more likely to have better diets than boys. Having a job did not correlate with eating a good diet, but improvement in diet went along with even a small increase in amount of education.

Walter saw no correlation between income and diet with internal poverty, but he believes that in external poverty diet may deteriorate

Family Size	Secretary's Guidelines	Guideline Levels When Increased By	
		25 percent	95 percent

48 STATES, DISTRICT OF COLUMBIA, TERRITORIES EXCLUDING GUAM			
1	$2,940	$3,680	$5,730
2	3,860	4,830	7,530
3	4,780	5,980	9.320
4	5,700	7,130	11,110
5	6,550	8,190	12,770
6	7,390	9,240	14,410
7	8,160	10,200	15,910
8	8,920	11,150	17,390
9	9,610	12,010	18,740
10	10,300	12,870	20,090
11	10,990	13,730	21,430
12	11,680	14,590	22,770
Each additional family member	690	860	1,340

Source: Child Nutrition Guidelines, *Federal Register,* June 14, 1976 (41 F.R. 23988).
[1] Author's note: Different Guidelines were published for Alaska and Hawaii (used also for Guam).

Figure 16.1 Income Poverty Guidelines July 1, 1976–June 30, 1977 for 48 States, District of Columbia and Territories Excluding Guam.[1]

during a period of reduced income. However, when the external factor is removed (i.e., when the wage-earner returns to work), the family resumes its previous eating habits. Here there is a connection between income and diet, at least when the homemaker is skilled in food money management.

Walter believes that some of the problems with the Food Stamp Program are due to the inability of poor people to plan ahead as they must do if they participate in the program. He recommends that nutrition education be a part of all income maintenance or income supplement programs.

Welfare Programs To Relieve Poverty

Efforts of the federal government to deal with poverty started in the depression of the early 1930's and continued through the New Deal, the New Frontier, the Great Society, and later poverty programs. Descriptions of poverty problems in the U.S. in the early 1960's can be acquired by reading *Hunger U.S.A.* (8) and various portions of the Hearings of the Senate Select Committee on Nutrition and Human Needs. (19) These reports were emotional and subjective, but they caught the imagination of Americans with resulting pressure for action to alleviate the problems of the poor.

Until the 1960's, the poor were, for the most part, unrepresented and voiceless. Since the Hearings of the Senate Select Committee on Nutrition and Human Needs, their voice and representation have been growing and large appropriations have been made for various poverty programs. Some, such as Head Start (p. 101) and the Food Stamp Program (p. 97) have improved the quality of life supplemented the income of many poor people. The poverty programs have resulted in a vocal group of the poor who are now able to make themselves heard.

Thus far poverty programs and social action have made little progress in increasing the inadequate income and reducing the high unemployment that constitute the basic problems of the poverty groups, although the Congress has made some earnest attempts at their solution. There is considerable agreement that reform of our welfare system is needed, but there is little agreement on how this can best be accomplished. Politicians waver between the need for solution with its vast cost, and reductions in the cost of government; and between measures to obtain the support and votes of the poor, or those of the taxpayers who must pay the bill. For 1974 it was estimated that the poor in the U.S. population numbered over 24 million persons, almost 12 percent of the total population. The cost of public social welfare programs in the U.S. has increased steadily since 1950. (17)

An extensive review of welfare and its problems has been made by Ferguson, who traced the history from the Elizabethan poor law to the contemporary movements. (7) Berger gives (1) a brief review of current welfare problems and the major components of the present public assistance programs. Three have been reported in this book, namely, Aid to Families with Dependent Children (p. 81), Food Stamp Program (p. 97), and Medicaid (p. 80). Berger comments that welfare assistance headed the list of unsolved domestic problems until the crisis in energy and the increase in unemployment that occurred in 1974–75.

Vatter has proposed three criteria for a family assistance program: (1) the poor should be better off or at least no worse off with it than without it, (2) incentives to work should be increased, and (3) the cost of assistance to states and taxpayers should not be increased. (20)

Perhaps the most promising approach to solving the problems of social welfare and poverty is through *income maintenance,* which is based on the premise that everyone has a right to a guaranteed annual income with need as the only criterion of eligibility. It encourages a family to work and earn, but supplements income when the basic amount is not reached.

The supplementation may be by cash payments or by providing food, medical care, or housing. Questions raised about the guaranteed income center on whether it would reduce the incentive to work, or result in less work on the part of low-income persons. A three-year study (1968–71) in New Jersey and Pennsylvania was designed to obtain information on these questions. (1).

Eight different support plans were tested with 725 welfare families in the experimental group, while 632 families, serving as controls, continued under the regular welfare program. The head of each family was an "able-bodied, nonelderly male."

Only small differences were found between the experimental families and the control families. Although some men in the experimental group worked fewer hours, and some earned less money than those in the control group, it was concluded that changes under the conditions of the study would have little effect on the labor supply.

There are many stereotypes and exaggerations about people on welfare. One of the frequently heard statements is that once a family gets on welfare it remains there. Actually only a small percentage of families have been on welfare for ten years or more and many of those are disabled persons. Another stereotype statement is that being black or of Hispanic origin is, of itself, conducive to poverty. The relationship of ethnic group and poverty really stems from accompanying factors such as amount of education, kind of work, and size of family. Some problems of the Hispanics and blacks as poverty groups can be seen by a look at these characteristics. The figures are from March 1971. (3, 4)

Spanish in U.S.—4.4 percent of the U.S. population, or 9 million persons, were of Hispanic origin; of these, 5 million were of Mexican origin and 1½ million of Puerto Rican origin.

Families with children under 18—72 percent of Spanish, 61 percent of Black, and 9 percent of all families had children under 18.

Families with four or more children—20 percent of Spanish, 17 percent of Black, and 9 percent of all families had four or more children.

Incomes below poverty level—in entire U.S. population one in eight families was below the poverty level; in Hispanic-origin families the figure was one in four, while in black families it was one in three.

Kind of employment—58 percent of persons of Hispanic origin were in blue-collar jobs, 23 percent were in white-collar occupations and 5 percent were farm workers.

Education—48 percent of the persons of Hispanic origin were high school graduates, compared with 58 percent of the blacks and 77 percent of the entire U.S. population.

Still another stereotype is that persons on welfare do not want to work. Actually in recent times there were few able-bodied males on welfare until there was widespread unemployment in 1974–75. There are numerous one-parent families, many headed by working women whose wages are too small to support the family. Others are headed by women with small children who could take employment if low-cost child care were available. The number of one-parent families has been increasing. Kline (10) wrote in 1974 that the proportion of families headed by a man or a woman without a spouse present was 15 percent in 1973 compared with 13 percent in 1962, with the increase entirely for families headed by a female. Some of the problems in management in a one-parent family are limited money resources, limited time and energy for household tasks with a consequent change in patterns of meal preparation, greater need for convenience foods, increase in meals eaten out, and need for more household help.

Most poverty is the result of social and economic conditions over which the individual has no control. These include disease, unemployment, death of family head, loss of savings, poor housing, lack of education, and exploitation. The earlier point of view that poverty is the result of personal failure and that hard work and self-denial can overcome it has long been abandoned by most health professionals.

One of the blocks to a permanent solution to poverty is that succeeding generations do not learn how to break out of this culture. The child, raised in the culture group of the family, learns the existing survival techniques used in that culture rather than the techniques that are necessary for survival in the dominant culture. An example is the attempt to provide a Spanish-language environment for the Spanish-speaking person rather than to help that person learn English. Then the Spanish speaker can survive in the Spanish-speaking community but still cannot cope with the dominant English-speaking one, so finds no way of escape from that particular ghetto.

Poverty tends to make people brutal, harsh, and indifferent, and the results are seen in the proliferation of youth gangs, substance abuse, and violence. Thus the worst characteristics of society are repeated and continued because the child who grows up in this environment will probably follow the same pattern.

Activities for the Poverty Community

A major difficulty to solving the problems of the poor is that middle and upper class Americans do not know how to motivate the poor for change because they do not comprehend the value systems of the poor or their perceptions of what is important. This includes even health professionals with extensive background about social welfare programs and ways that have been tried to solve the problems of poverty.

In the past, few community nutritionists had experienced poverty because most came from middle or upper class homes. Now this is changing; more community nutritionists have had first-hand experience, either coming from poor families or spending time in work with them. This helps the nutritionists understand the effect of poverty on personality, family relationships, home life, attitudes, and values.

As the members of the nutrition staff get to know families and become better informed about community resources that are available for meeting needs, they can show the poverty group that society cares about their basic problems of food, clothing, and shelter. Then the poor will be more likely to accept the help they need in home management, money management, and child rearing. Program planning must involve the clients and other persons who influence their behavior as well as the staff of the agency concerned.

Nutrition programs should bring to the poor not only services but also direction about living and opportunities for personal enrichment. The nutritionist must find out what people perceive as valuable to them to get suggestions on how to proceed. For example, one group of low-income homemakers requested help with weight control as well as education for food selection and preparation. (9)

As already noted, it is difficult for the poor to purchase the necessary food so they can participate in a plan to change their food practices. Inadequate diet is often accompanied by other family problems based on poor management and housekeeping, which must be solved before the family can progress. Often there are community resources that might help, but the family does not know about them and needs a referral. (2)

The community nutritionist must be aware of the limited resources of the poor to purchase an adequate diet and must recognize that changing food practices usually means finding more money as well as changing cherished habits. Often, solving a nutrition problem must be preceded by solving problems of handling money, getting to market, controlling children, obtaining equipment, or learning new skills. (6)

Meyers discusses some extra costs of being poor (14) and suggests some ways to work for change. The poor consumer has less money to spend, less choice of when and where to spend it, and little opportunity to learn from mistakes in spending. There are also psychological, educational, and physical costs of being poor. In discussing possible leverage for change, Meyers suggests that help be given by education for its benefits through family interaction, economic help for its ability to reduce the costs of being poor, and motivational help to cause the poor to seek their own ways out of poverty.

There are many layers and segments among the poor and in each ethnic group, in the middle class. The community nutritionist needs to look at each person, each family, and each subgroup as an entity recognizing its specific characteristics, adapting approach and teaching techniques in ways that will be appropriate and effective. Cason and Wagner have compared the lower class family with other families in the community noting that it is generally less stable and less goal-oriented, and that the families are larger and health poorer. (2)

Another study reports that health is important in the value systems of some poor mothers and may provide motivation for them to modify food practices when they learn that these practices may cause retarded growth, obesity, anemia, or other health problems. (9)

In working with low income groups, the approach must be suited to the specific group and the methods adapted to their interests. The material must be presented in small units in an informal permissive situation. The low income people are often insecure and dependent, with a low opinion of themselves, and many times they have little control over their resources. In many families the husband is dominant and must give permission or approval before the wife will participate in education or attempt changes.

Moffit (15) has reported an innovative institute for training teachers of occupational home economics in ways to teach disadvantaged children, that combined work experience with classroom demonstrations and lectures. The teachers actually worked one day in a local industry in a job appropriate for one of the students. Nutritionists could plan similar inservice education for nutritionists and dietitians who work with the poor.

Larson and Massoth report (11) use of bilingual Mexican-American aides to work with poor migrants in the lower Rio Grande Valley of Texas. They found that cooking and eating practices were limited by equipment problems, such as ovens that did not work and lack of enough dishes, tableware, and chairs for the family to eat a meal together. The aides worked with the homemakers in their own homes, teaching new dishes, helping to obtain food stamps, and encouraging the purchase of nutritious foods.

In working with poverty groups, the nutritionist should first look at how they cope with their problems. Many families have a great deal of fortitude, astuteness, endurance, and skill in handling their problems. Second, they should be encouraged to identify what they perceive to be their biggest problems. Third, they can be helped to identify existing resources they might use directly or adapt, or to find new resources. The nutritionist must be a helping person rather than a missionary and should help the client focus on the goal or the task. The only way the health professional can change behavior is through personal involvement.

Poverty is not a thing set apart, but must be dealt with in every program as it exists, and an understanding of its causes and characteristics, and an ability to analyze how it affects the people and community, will enable the nutritionist to help individuals and families change their nutrition practices for better health.

A current problem is the apparent lull in progress toward solving the health and nutrition problems of the poor. "The excitement and frenzied bandwagon activity of the '60's to develop health services and programs for the underserved, poor and disenfranchised slowed to the pace of survival tactics in the early '70's. Now the focus has shifted to evaluating what can be done within the limited financial and manpower sources which most health education programs have available." (13)

WORKING WITH RURAL AND MIGRANT COMMUNITIES

A recent notice of a position for a nutritionist-food services supervisor described the position as a combination of administrative and field work in nine child care centers with much "people work" on a one-to-one basis with cooks and other staff. The program was seasonally funded from March to November. Other duties were to provide inservice education to staff in infant care and preschool programs and to help public health nurses handle nutrition-related problems.

That is the kind of challenge that faces nutritionists who work in programs for migrants and cope with seasonal work and the movement with the seasons.

Most of the migrant and seasonal workers are concentrated in ten states: Texas, California, Florida, Michigan, Arizona, Oregon, Ohio, Washington, New Mexico, and New York. Their problems are shown by much higher mortality rates among infants, and among victims of tuberculosis and other infectious diseases. (26)

It was estimated in 1965 that there were about 2 million seasonal agricultural workers in the United States, that perhaps 20 percent of the school age children did not attend school, and that these families were among the most deprived persons in the nation, with a low standard of living and health care. (28) There has been some improvement, largely due to the increase in the minimum wage and the legislation on housing, but there is still a great need to improve the nutrition of this group. About 390,000 migrant and seasonal farmworkers were cared for in 1975 through special health projects funded by the USDHEW. Migrant workers are not classed as categorically needy so many are not eligible for Medicaid benefits. (26)

Kaufman and coworkers described an 18-month program designed to diagnose the nutritional status of migrant workers and to intervene for correction of the food and nutrition problems identified. They observed that the families seemed to live from day to day without planning for the future. The nutritional survey revealed that iron deficiency anemia was the most serious problem, there was some folacin deficiency, and some retarded growth; obesity was common, and there were many dental problems. (24)

Intervention in the project took several forms including nutrition education, provision of food, and counseling on other problems related to nutrition. Recommendations for future work with this group were regular nutritional surveillance, expanded nutrition education, and dietary counseling as a part of health and other programs, consistency between schools and community with school and parent nutrition education programs, and improved school feeding programs.

Rural areas also have unique health problems. The traditional view of rural areas in the United States has sometimes resulted in favored legislation that worked more to the benefit of the higher income groups than to that of the poor. Resources in rural areas are limited and in many states the large metropolitan areas overwhelm the smaller rural areas. Standards and methods for health programs are often designed for urban areas. Frequently both migrant and permanent farmworkers lack money and resources to obtain health care or nutritious food.

The changing climate for rural people and the interest of clients in the preventive aspects of health care are shown when a farmworkers' union makes preventive health measures a part of a health benefit package. (25) How families learn was stated by Solis, an instructor in community medicine, who commented that the rural family structure often has great strength and that family members learn from each other. (22)

Wilber suggests two basic strategies to help solve the problems of persons who live in rural areas. First, a "catchup strategy" is needed to bring nonmetropolitan residents to higher levels, and second, a "go-ahead tactic" should be developed to anticipate demands for new services. (27) The DHEW has a program to demonstrate that small rural health systems can meet the need for health services in many rural areas. Grants are made to various types of organizations that can provide comprehensive health care. One hundred and five projects in rural areas are for migrant farm workers without previous access to health care. (26)

The "Services for Living" section of the *1971 Yearbook of Agriculture* contains several chapters on problems of rural areas. (27) Wilber discusses the great need for social services due to the greater severity of poverty and fewer services in rural as compared with metropolitan areas; for example, one in five in the rural area was poor compared with one in ten in the metropolitan area. Medical, clinical, and family planning services are comparatively lacking in rural areas along with library services, legal aid, welfare counseling, and others. There are more widowed and aged in rural areas.

The preference of professional persons to live and work in cities, the lack of transportation, and the isolation all add to the problems of rural dwellers. According to Wilber, the poor whites are even more disadvantaged than other groups, who are "organized, vocal, and relatively effective in presenting their case."

Nutritionists who work in rural communities must develop innovative programs to meet their special needs. More programs are needed. They must be implemented by national action, perhaps by providing health services in mobile units, and opening additional clinics and hospitals.

SUMMARY

The individual or family without enough money for all the necessities of life often finds that food is the only flexible budget item, so spends less than is necessary to buy an adequate diet. The federal government issues yearly guidelines for the definition of poverty in terms of dollar income.

Persons in the culture of poverty are characterized by little thought for the future and, unless the cycle is interrupted, will pass the same mode of living to their children. Some persons on minimum or inadequate incomes still manage to eat a good diet, but many lack milk, meat, or other foods. Some investigators have found that the amount of education of the planner most nearly correlates with the quality of the diet.

Welfare programs have become complex and unwieldy, and many economists believe that the system should be replaced by a guaranteed annual wage. There are many stereotypes about people on welfare that have little basis in fact.

Most migrant workers are concentrated in ten states. The health problems are greater than among other groups, characterized by more deaths among infants, and more infectious diseases.

Rural areas also have special problems due to their isolation and lack of health facilities. The federal government has funded a number of projects designed to provide comprehensive health services for rural areas.

REFERENCES CITED

Poverty

1. Berger, Peggy S., Guaranteed Income: Does It Work? *J. Home Econ.,* 67 7/75 18.
2. Cason, David, and Muriel G. Wagner, The Changing Role of the Service Professional Within the Ghetto, *J. Am. Diet. Assoc.,* 60 1/72 21.
3. Characteristics of the Low-Income Population: 1972, *Fam. Econ. Rev.,* ARS-NE-36, U.S. Dept. of Agriculture, Hyattsville MD, Sum./74 23.
4. Characteristics of Persons of Spanish Origin, *Fam. Econ. Rev.,* ARS 62–5, U.S. Dept. of Agriculture, Hyattsville MD, 6/72 9.
5. Christakis, George, The Community Nutrition Team, *Annals N.Y. Acad. Sciences,* 196 4/7/72 78.
6. Family Survival in Today's Urban Crisis, *J. Home Econ.* 62 10/70 584.
7. Ferguson, Elizabeth A., *Social Work: An Introduction,* J. B. Lippincott, Philadelphia, 1975, 61.
8. *Hunger, U.S.A.: A Report by the Citizens' Board of Inquiry into Hunger and Malnutrition in the United States,* New Community Press, Washington D.C, 1968.
9. Ikeda, Jeanne P., Expressed Nutrition Needs of Low-Income Home-makers, *J. Nutr. Educ.,* 7 7–9/75 104.
10. Kline, Kristin L., Other Families: Families Without Spouses, *Fam. Econ. Rev.,* ARS-NE-36, U.S. Dept. of Agriculture, Hyattsville MD, Sum./74, 18.
11. Larson, Lora B., and Donna Y. Massoth, A Nutrition Education Program for Texas Migrant Families, *J. Home Econ.,* 65 11/73 36.
12. Lewis, O., The Culture of Poverty, *Scientific American,* 215 10/66 19.
13. Making Health Education Work, *Am. J. Pub. Health,* 65 10/75, Supplement, 1.
14. Meyers, Trienah, The Extra Cost of Being Poor, *J. Home Econ.,* 62 6/70 379.
15. Moffitt, Marie D., How to Teach the Teachers of the Disadvantaged, *J. Home Econ.,* 65 11/73 23.
16. Poverty Statistics Revised, *Fam. Econ. Rev.,* ARS 62–5, U.S. Dept. of Agriculture, Hyattsville MD, 12/69 16.
17. Social Welfare Expenditures Under Public Programs: 1950 to 1974, *Information Please Almanac 1977,* Dan Golenpaul Associates, New York, 91.
18. Suter, Carol B., and Helen F. Barbour, Identifying Food-Related Values of Low-Income Mothers, *Home Econ. Res. J.,* 3 3/75 198.

19. U.S. Congress, Senate, Select Committee on Nutrition and Human Needs, *Part I—Problems and Prospects,* 90th Congress, 2nd Session, Dec. 17, 18, 19, 1968, 5.

20. Vatter, Ethel L., Income Maintenance in the 1970's, *J. Home Econ.,* 63 1/71 19.

21. Walter, John P., Two Poverties Equal One Hunger, *J. Nutr. Educ.,* 5 4–6/73 129.

Rural and Migrant Workers

22. A Conversation with Faustina Solis, *Healthnews,* Calif. Dept. of Health, Sacramento, 2 5/75 3.

23. Hassinger, Edward W., Health Services for Rural Areas, in *A Good Life for More People,* USDA 1971 Yearbook of Agriculture, 92nd Congress, 1st Session, House Document, No. 29, 181.

24. Kaufman, Mildred, Eugene Lewis, Albert V. Hardy, and Joanne Proulx, Florida Seasonal Farm Workers: Follow-up and Intervention Following a Nutrition Survey, *J. Am. Diet. Assoc.,* 66 6/75 605.

25. Plumb, Bill, Health Services—for the Workers, By the Workers, *Healthnews,* Calif. Dept. of Health, Sacramento, 2 5/75 6.

26. U.S. Dept. of Health, Education, and Welfare, *Promoting Community Health,* USDHEW Pub. No. (HSA) 75-5016, 1975 12.

27. Wilber, George L., Social Services—the Great Lag, in *A Good Life for More People,* USDA 1971 Yearbook of Agriculture, 92nd Congress, 1st Session, House Document No. 29 149.

28. *Working with Low Income Families,* Am. Home Econ. Assoc., 1965, 113.

CHAPTER 17

CONSULTING ON ENRICHMENT, FOOD-RELATED HAZARDS, AND FOOD MISINFORMATION

These three topics are the subject of much notice in the media and nutritionists should be prepared to answer many questions about them. They may need to conduct specific programs to promote enrichment or explain or allay fears of the public about food-related hazards. Correcting misinformation of public and professionals is a part of many programs, since misinformation must often be corrected before correct information can be taught.

PROMOTING ENRICHMENT AND FORTIFICATION

Instituting programs for enrichment and fortification of foods provides a mass method of attack on nutrition problems of inadequate intake of nutrients, or deficiency of a specific nutrient as shown by biochemical evidence. When such problems have been identified in the diet of a large number of people, nutritionists should consider the possibility of intervention through improvement of a food that will make a significant improvement needed in the diet. The effect of such an addition on individuals whose intake is already adequate must also be considered to avoid the possibility of a harmful excess.

The term *enrichment* is usually used to mean increasing the amount of nutrients in a food to a higher level than they naturally occur. *Fortification* means adding nutrients that do not naturally occur in a food or that occur in extremely small quantities. The community nutritionist will need to develop a philosophy about these programs and to decide which should be promoted in the area included in a specific program.

The NRC Food and Nutrition Board issued a policy statement in which it endorsed "the enrichment of flour, bread, degerminated corn meal, corn grits, whole grain corn meal, white rice, and certain other cereal grain products with thiamin, riboflavin, niacin and iron; the addition of vitamin D to milk, fluid skim milk and nonfat dry milk; the addition of vitamin A to margarine, fluid skim milk, and nonfat dry milk; and the addition of iodine to table salt. The protective action of fluoride against dental caries is recognized and the standardized addition of fluoride to water in areas in which the water supply has a low fluoride content is endorsed." (1)

The purpose of the enrichment and fortification of foods is to supply nutrients that are apt to be lacking in the diets of many persons. Guidelines for enrichment and fortification state that the food to be used as the vehicle should be one that is eaten in quantities that will supply a significant amount of the nutrient, while the amount supplied is not likely to be excessive. (3)

Though enrichment was first inaugurated by the federal government during World War II, such programs are now under state control. The laws vary, but the general policy is to enrich white bread and flour, cornmeal, corn grits, farina, macaroni and other pastes, and rice. It appears that this group of foods is most suited for enrichment because there is high consumption of these foods by those most likely to be deficient in these nutrients. State laws for compulsory enrichment of white flour and all products in which it is a predominant ingredient, along with cereals, paste products, and rice, can make a considerable improvement in the nutrient intake for persons who consume these foods as an important part of their diets.

One unsolved problem is that many persons who follow Oriental food patterns based on large amounts of rice prefer the unenriched product. Thus the present enrichment methods for rice do not contribute to the nutrition of the groups to whom this food is most important. Nutritionists in communities where unenriched cereal products are an important part of the diet may find it worthwhile to advocate enrichment programs and use of the enriched products.

The NRC also endorses the addition of nutrients to new and formulated foods to make them at least equal in food value to the foods for which they are alternates; for example, a meat analog should have the nutritional value of the meat replaced. (1)

There has been a trend to fortify snack items, mainly products that are high in sugars and fats but almost devoid of protein, vitamins, and minerals. The fortification of such foods to provide the daily allowances of the nutrients for which the RDA have been set does not conform to the endorsement of the Food and Nutrition Board and should not be supported. The reason given for such fortification is that these foods are consumed instead of basic foods, but the community nutritionist should continue to promote a good diet of a wide variety of basic foods as the best way to get the recommended amounts of nutrients.

The nutritionist should keep informed about trends and action on enrichment and fortification and organize efforts for support or opposition when they are indicated.

ADVISING ON FOOD-RELATED HAZARDS

A primary role of the community nutritionist is to encourage consumption of an adequate diet of a variety of foods. Except when the nutritionist is responsible for institution food production and service, the position includes few official responsibilities for the safety of food although safety in food handling should be a part of all nutrition education. In education about problems of additives and pollution, the nutritionist must try to see that these problems do not keep the public from eating a good diet. This occurs because people are concerned about the safety of the food supply and its effect on health, so omit many foods from the diet.

Probably it is the fear of cancer that has caused the attitudes of the concerned general public; however, the existing Food and Drug Law requires that any substance found to induce cancer in animals must be removed from the market immediately even though the amount used with animals is proportionately far more than any human could consume. (5) The current evidence that saturated fat may be more significant than chemicals in the etiology of some types of cancer is mentioned on page 27.

The nutritionist's responsibility is to identify potential problems, to inform the public, and to encourage the community to take appropriate action for an adequate supply of safe foods.

There are several ways in which food-related hazards may affect nutrition. In the present context, *a food-related hazard* is defined as any substance or action that makes food harmful. Hazards include addition of chemicals during production or processing, accidental contamination during production or processing, and contamination in the home.

Use of Additives and Chemicals

An *additive* is a substance that is added to a food to produce a specific desired result, such as increasing nutritional value, or improving the quality of the finished product. *Chemical* is often used as an alternative term. (7)

There is a continuing controversy centered on additives, questioning their safety and demanding that their use be discontinued. Many persons who have an undue concern about the harm from chemicals overlook much more serious and prevalent sources of harm such as overeating, inactivity, excess saturated fat, use of alcoholic beverages, and cigarette smoking. The nutritionist needs to help clients put all of these factors into their proper perspective in the total health regimen.

People need to understand that the human body and all foods are composed of chemicals, that there are hazards in natural foods, some of which contain allergens or other substances harmful to some persons, and that an excess of any substance is harmful.

Many additives are used for varied effects and specific purposes. Additives are constantly in the news, often with prominent persons decrying their use or testifying to their safety. A pronouncement in favor of or against additives or chemicals in food can almost always make the public media, in news columns, feature stories, editorials, or even comic strips.

The scientific point of view about additives holds that they make it possible to provide the qualities that consumers want in their food, such as good taste, ease of preparation, long shelf life, and good nutrient content. Some consumers fear that a cumulative effect may cause cancer, hyperkinesis, or vague feelings of non-well-being. Often the same persons who decry the use of additives and chemicals take vitamin pills or other food supplements every day to compensate for the poor values of the food they consume, seeing nothing inconsistent in supplementing with products that are themselves composed of chemicals.

Probably no one would deny that food should be safe and that any substance convincingly demonstrated to be harmful or dangerous should be removed from the food supply. Actually it is hardly realistic to say that a food additive is safe or unsafe because for most products it is the *level* that is safe or unsafe and only a toxicologist or a chemist is qualified to determine the safe level. Safety must be evaluated according to the proposed use of a substance in foods with consideration of the highest amount that might be consumed under any conditions of use.

The Food and Drug Administration is responsible for the safety of food additives. The manufacturer must prove the safety of each food additive before using it. The GRAS (Generally Recognized As Safe) list includes all additives in general use in 1959, when the Additive Amendment was passed. (3) Miles of the FDA says that today consumers and the public question both people and institutions and that they want answers to their questions. (5)

Concern about additives may be a luxury afforded only by better-educated citizens with adequate incomes and enough leisure time to consider the subject. Learning about chemicals and additives was of little concern to low income homemakers in one survey. However, these homemakers were interested in food safety and wholesomeness, a broader topic, which in some cases requires the use of additives to achieve. Perhaps the topic of food additives may be approached in nutrition education from the standpoint of food safety. (4) The American Dietetic Association booklet *Food Facts Talk Back* has a brief explanation of additives that will help the nutritionist explain the subject to the public. (3)

Contamination During Food Production and Processing

Contamination during production may occur from substances used to protect the plant during the growing period, and also from substances used during the processing, or added to the finished product. A basic problem is the need for measures to protect and fertilize crops during growth so that enough food can be produced to feed the population. The alternative to the use of pesticides and chemical fertilizers is reduced production with resulting lower food supplies. Action and education should be directed at proper use, which will keep foods safe for consumption. (8)

Processing refers to the procedures used during commercial preparation of foods for consumption. It includes cooking, freezing, canning, dehydrating, removing or adding substances, changing the physical characteristics, and washing and chopping raw foods. Though there is the possibility of contamination at every step manufacturers attempt to control processing in order to avoid such problems.

Food poisoning from microbiological contamination during processing is an important problem. It occurs because of unsafe handling or use of improper production and storage practices. Contamination may also occur from mycotoxins produced by molds that develop during growing, storage, or processing. Harmful chemicals may also get into food during handling or storage from substances that are used in equipment or packaging.

The federal government is responsible for the safety of food supplies that move over state lines, while state and local governments are responsible for local products. The community nutritionist needs to know the sources of control over food supplies in the area served and be able to advise the public how to identify unsafe or impure products. Individuals should be encouraged to report problems to the appropriate local, state, or federal agency. The actual number of problems is very low in relation to the total amounts of foods used.

Contamination in the Home

Food poisoning from microbiological agents is probably the most prevalent form of contamination in the home. (8) This occurs because of poor practices in food storage and preparation. Proper food handling should be incorporated into all teaching about food and diet. Unwashed fruits and vegetables are one source of contamination. Some people are unaware of the importance of washing fruits and vegetables before use. Washing in running water or scrubbing with a brush when practical will remove contaminating substances. The public is mainly concerned about pesticides, but there are probably greater hazards from contamination from the natural fertilizers used in organic gardening. Another problem is contamination from unclean hands of fruit and vegetable pickers, store personnel, and. customers. Washing will also remove the wax used to preserve some fruits and vegetables.

Another potential source of contamination in the home is uncooked poultry and meat. Many homemakers do not understand the importance of clean hands and kitchen equipment, such as knives, cutting boards, and other kitchen work surfaces. Knives and cutting boards can transmit organisms that cause food poisoning. Though it is fashionable to eat raw meat, this is a dangerous practice because of the possibility of contamination. Eggs are another source of contamination; careful storage of eggs in both uncooked and cooked products is necessary.

Public Education About Safety of the Food Supply

The biggest problem is that the information and understanding of the public is based on information from the public media. Many problems occur because of misleading information that is continually directed at the public, some politically motivated. Many science writers, editors, and television and radio personnel are well informed, but some are misinformed or irresponsible, and report unsubstantiated studies that receive the same credence as other stories that report sound scientific information because all news stories are of generally equal credibility at the time they are published. The community nutritionist should become acquainted with the persons responsible for scientific stories in the press, radio, and television. Sometimes they are interested in consulta tion or training. Most are eager to see that their copy is scientifically correct.

Many organizations arrange for speakers on the food supply. They are concerned with making a responsible contribution to their members or to the community and may need help in planning their activities. They may be referred to local resources such as the public health department, Cooperative Extension, local Dietetic Association, nutrition committee, or a college or university. Many times the problem is that they do not know the reliable sources for information.

The nutritionist and other professionals can interpret to the public the various kinds of risks from chemicals with possible results and the alternatives. The alternative to use of chemicals in food processing may be stale, moldy, or rancid foods, and higher food costs because of spoilage. Discontinuing use of chemicals in food production and processing would reduce the variety and quantity of food products available. Though a reduction in the number of fatty, salty, sugared, and high calorie products would be desirable, it is likely that the keeping qualities of these products would hold them on the market while the number of basic foods in various forms would decrease. Perhaps the interest and zeal of groups about safety of the food supply could be redirected to concern about overconsumption of saturated fats and sugars.

A few scientists, physicians, and other professional persons have joined consumer groups and other organizations in causing public apprehension about the food supply. Consumers have been alarmed by reports in the media of controversy on food safety among scientists. Many scientists believe that such debates should be kept within the scientific community for evaluation by qualified boards of review. Often these reports have been based on preliminary findings that need further investigation to confirm or deny. (2) It has been suggested that there is a need for regional clearing houses that could publish pamphlets and bulletins for the public, and that nutritionists and other scientists should give the public better explanations of their work and clearer interpretation of new developments.

Food safety must be a joint responsibility of government and the individual. Government should assure protection when the individual cannot provide self-protection, for example, inspection of food manu- facturing operations. However, the individual should be well enough informed to make decisions when a nonexpert depth of information can be sufficient, for example, to reject food that shows evidence of spoilage or improper handling.

Points for Public Education

There are risks in use of additives, but there are also risks in not using them.

Food manufacturers must solve problems of manufacture and distribution that produce unsafe foods.

Fat in present diets is a greater hazard than additives or pollutants.

The public must support programs to identify toxic substances and establish safe levels.

In the case of some pollutants, the hazard may be in the interaction of a substance with a food rather than in the substance itself.

One of the best safeguards is to eat a varied diet to avoid concentration of harmful substances that may be in a particular food.

COMBATTING MISINFORMATION AND QUACKERY

Many problems occur because of misinformation on food and nutrition on the part of some professional persons—physicians, nurses, home economists, dentists, and teachers—as well as the general public. An extensive review of the sources of the problem with answers to the commonly asked questions was published in 1974. (14)

Misinformation and quackery exist in other professional fields such as medicine, psychology, engineering, and architecture. However, there are reasons for the particular proliferation in nutrition because food is intimately entwined in living, so all people know something about food because they eat it every day. Some think that this eating qualifies them as authorities, while others deliberately mislead for personal gain. (12)

The concern here is mainly with the nutritionist's own point of view and method of handling this problem. Recently there has been a rejection of established views, with criticism of some government agencies. There is also a tendency for many persons to yield with implicit faith to the irresistible, mystic teaching of the amateur. In a field as broad and deep as nutrition, it is not possible to make an exhaustive literature search on every question, so the nutritionist needs to develop a system for keeping the answers to the questions most often asked, and for handling misinformation.

Perhaps hardest to accept, or endure, are the professionals in other fields who are aware of the nutritionist's extensive study in the field, but who nonetheless adopt misinformation sources as their authorities.

Much misinformation is passed along by professional perons who are not well informed on nutrition, but who are expected by many individuals to be authorities on the subject. Nutritionists need to work for better background for these professionals through basic training, personal contacts, and the provision of resource materials. They should also promote the use by other professionals of dietitians and nutritionists as sources of expertise.

Both professionals and public need to be able to identify misinformation. The informed person recognizes statements about the miracle qualities of specific foods, the complete omission from diets of basic foods such as white bread, the cure of disease by foods, and the superiority of natural and organic foods as signs of a misinformed person. Professionals and public also need to know reliable sources of information on food and nutrition such as nutritionists in public health agencies, The American Dietetic Association and local affiliate, Cooperative Extension, nutrition departments of state colleges and universities, Food and Drug Administration, and The American Medical Association.

The nutritionist must also be concerned with the correction of food misinformation in professionals and in the public. Henderson points out that some people are so emotionally involved in their search for a health-promoting miracle that they are unable to change, but that there is another group whose misinformation can be corrected by appropriate methods. The nutritionist must learn from experience how to recognize the strategic time to challenge the individual about misinformation, and present the correct facts as convincingly as possible. (11)

Sources for help for the nutritionist on problems of misinformation are professional colleagues, university teachers, the FDA, and related agencies at state or local levels.

As in all community programs, handling the overall problem of misinformation should include analysis of the specific and most influential sources of the problem, program planning for the most effective attack, community organization to mobilize resources, professional education to strengthen this source of help, and public education to help the health consumer use wisely the available resources for good nutrition. Each nutritionist must decide whether the program approach will be militant or low-key, to many or to few, through mass approaches or a one-to-one basis.

SUMMARY

In states where there are no enrichment laws or where the laws are not inclusive enough, the community nutritionist may find it desirable to promote enrichment. Nutritionists should follow the policies on enrichment and fortification issued by the NRC Food and Nutrition Board. A current problem is the tendency for manufacturers to fortify many items besides the basic foods covered under the NRC policies.

Fears of the public about the possible carcinogenic properties of all chemicals added to foods cause some persons to omit foods or groups of foods that are needed in a good diet. The nutritionist should interpret the significance of various substances and explain the present belief that excesses and deficiencies of nutrients are more hazardous than additives and chemicals. The public also needs to be informed that the greatest hazard is food poisoning from contamination during manufacture or in the home, usually due to poor sanitation practices.

Food misinformation in both professionals and the public is ever present; both must be taught to recognize and deal with misinformation.

REFERENCES CITED

Enrichment and Fortification

1. National Research Council, Food and Nutrition Board, General Policies in Regard to Improvement of Nutritive Quality of Foods, pamphlet, National Academy of Sciences, Washington DC, 1973.

Food-Related Hazards

2. Benarde, Melvin A., and Norge Jerome, Food Quality and the Consumer: A Decalog, *Am. J. Pub. Health,* 62 9/72 1199.
3. *Food Facts Talk Back,* pamphlet, American Dietetic Association, Chicago, n.d., 21.
4. Ikeda, Jeanne P., Expressed Nutrition Needs of Low-Income Homemakers, *J. Nutr. Educ.,* 7 7–9/75 104.
5. Miles, Corbin I., Food Additives and Fortification, *Fam. Econ. Rev.,* ARS-NE-36, U.S. Dept. of Agriculture, Hyattsville MD, Spr./74 9.
6. National Research Council, Food and Nutrition Board, *The Use of Chemicals in Food Processing, Storage, and Distribution,* National Academy of Sciences, Washington DC, 1973.
7. Robinson, Corinne, *Normal and Therapeutic Nutrition,* 14 ed., Macmillan Co., New York, 1972, 272.
8. U.S. Department of Health, Education, and Welfare, *Forward Plan for Health, 1977–81,* Aug. 1975, 112.

Misinformation and Quackery

9. Enloe, Cortez F., Leslie and Betty and the Hobgoblins, *Nutr. Today,* 11 1–2/76 16.
10. *Food Facts Talk Back,* pamphlet, American Dietetic Association, Chicago, n.d.

11. Henderson, LaVell M., Programs to Combat Nutrition Quackery, *J. Am. Diet. Assoc.*, 64 4/74 372.
12. Huenemann, Ruth, Combating Food Misinformation and Quackery, *J. Am. Diet. Assoc.* 32 7/56 623.
13. Mayer, Jean, *A Diet for Living,* David McKay Co., Inc., New York, 1975, 1–61.
14. White, Philip L, ed., Nutrition Misinformation and Food Faddism, *Nutr. Rev.,* 32 7/74 Spec. Supp. 1–73.

CHAPTER **18** USING
LEGISLATION
TO ACHIEVE
NUTRITION
GOALS

Legislation is the process of establishing rules of conduct which are called laws. Since the structure for health programs including nutrition requires authority and money, it involves a complex legislative process which is influenced by political interests, government health agencies, business, and many other forces. The legislative process in the U.S. Congress will be discussed. States have similar processes; the community nutritionist will need to become familiar with the process in the specific state.

LEGISLATION IN THE U.S. CONGRESS

Legislation of importance to nutrition may originate in the Federal Congress, the executive branch, or in the interested department. Frequently the first proposal for legislation on a particular subject is prepared by the personal staff of a legislator, sometimes with the assistance of outside agencies and organizations. Often several similar bills are under consideration at the same time.

Most of the work on legislation is done by committees of the Senate or House. A bill or resolution is introduced by a Senator or Representative in the legislative body, then referred to the appropriate committee. The committee considers the proposed legislation and returns it to the originating body with a favorable or unfavorable report, or with recommended amendments, or takes no action, which allows the bill to die in the committee. (9)

A bill usually includes authorization of the money necessary to carry out the specified programs. After the bill becomes law, the Congress must *appropriate* money to carry out its provisions though the amount may have already been *authorized* in the bill. Sometimes the appropriation is less than the amount authorized.

After a bill is reported by the Committee and returned to House or Senate, the vote is taken. If the bill passes, it is sent to the other body of Congress, where it goes through a similar process. If amendments are added by the other body before it is passed, it must then be returned to the original body for reconsideration and another vote.

When the bill has finally been passed by both houses, it goes to the President who may sign it, veto it, or take no action in which case the bill becomes law in ten days. (9) Laws are usually known by numbers, for example a bill may be called Public Law 90-248, 90 being the number of the Congress in which it was passed.

Miller, a freshman Congressman, reports his action for an appropriation to extend WIC financing by unanimous consent. (3) He points out that the need for the legislation had been identified earlier by a lobby of physicians, nutritionists, and welfare organizations, which had persuaded legislators that this was an important program deserving of support. He contrasts this with the attitudes of members of Congress toward the school lunch program. Miller points out that nutritionists and he himself had failed to persuade the Congress of the importance of that program. He suggested that Congress must be persuaded that additional money spent for education in the school lunch program would increase the cost benefit of the food service.

How The Nutritionist Influences Legislation

The nutritionist may enter the legislative process at either federal or state level by promoting legislation to solve a specific problem or by providing leadership to develop activity for passage of a bill. The nutritionist needs to be familiar with the procedures of the Congress or state legislature where the bill is introduced.

The nutritionist's role may be as enabler to help the community state the need for legislation, planner to develop the components of a law, or advocate to promote activity that brings about change. In some public agencies and other organizations, activities for legislation or advocacy are against agency policy. However, the role of the community nutritionist includes community action, so participation in activities related to legislation should be accepted.

The first step when the nutritionist contemplates the use of the legislative process is to find out the kind and extent of action that are consistent with the policies of the employing agency. This point may have been established by the job specifications, during the interview before employment, or in general policies of the agency. Sometimes changes in laws are necessary to change policies and procedures that determine how medical care is delivered, how food is processed, or merchandised, or how or whether grain products are enriched.

The nutritionist may promote legislation directly by letters and calls to legislators, by serving as a consultant on food and nutrition matters, by giving testimony at hearings, or by advising an action group. The latter is a good approach because much time and effort are needed to influence legislation and it is better to relinquish the actual process to someone who can devote a great deal of time and effort to the activity.

Giving testimony at public hearings may or may not be in accord with agency policy. When a hearing is on a controversial subject such as fluoridation of water or banning an additive, the audience often consists mostly of persons who are against the measure. The questioning in such a case may be very abrasive. The nutritionist might follow a practice of politicians by having a group of advisors who supply information at critical moments. Usually the person presenting testimony is asked to submit it in written form ahead of time and it is distributed to the committee and audience. Often the testimony is simply read, but it may be possible to speak extemporaneously and give additional facts or state the facts in a different way.

If the nutritionist wants to engage in the actual process of legislation or suggest bills, it may be expedient to do so through the employing agency if it has a means for such action. In some agencies the nutritionist is regularly asked to review bills with a nutrition component and prepare recommendations as to whether the agency should or should not support the bill.

In order to participate in influencing legislation, the nutritionist must know how laws are developed and passed. Since the passage of most bills takes considerable time, the nutritionist must find a way to keep informed of the status and progress of a particular bill. This may be done by reading various publications or by checking with the office of a legislator for the area. Letters and calls to legislators can bring copies of bills and laws, information on current status of bills, newsletters, and helpful brochures such as one showing the legislative process and advising the voter how to enter the process. When writing a legislator about a particular bill, a constituent may ask for a statement of the legislator's official position on the bill.

A letter to the legislator can explain the need for legislation, suggest specific changes that should be made in the bill, and affirm support. The nutritionist can also urge other professionals who are concerned with the same kind of legislation to support the bill. Persuading interested community leaders to write their legislators that they favor passage will provide additional support.

Lobbying for Passage of a Bill.   *Lobbying* is a persuasive activity that tries to influence the passage of a bill. Though it is often used to refer to persons working in contact with legislators, the nutritionist or other person who tries to promote passage of a bill is also lobbying. The nutritionist may lobby to start legislation for a particular problem by getting support from the legislators. Several kinds of action may be taken. The nutritionist may prepare a concise statement of the issues and the needs, or develop a statement about the legislation desired and submit it to a legislator as from a constituent, or send information to legislators that confirms the existence and extent of the nutritional problem addressed by the bill. Another kind of action that may be helpful and therefore influential with a legislator is a description of how a program could work to solve the problem, defining the types of staff and resources needed.

After legislation has been introduced, the nutritionist may participate in the politics of supporting the legislation by persuading a number of voters to urge their legislators to vote for the bill.

In the U.S. Congress, all bills die at the end of a session regardless of their position in line, and they must be introduced again in the next Congress as if they were new, going through the whole process of hearings, reports, and passage by one house and then the other. When a bill fails to pass in a Congress, there is often less interest the next year, although occasionally there is a determined effort to force action. Lobbyists should build up strength in advance for the action desired, either to pass the bill or to develop enough opposition to defeat it. A congressional election is usually a good time to lay the groundwork since a voter can find out then what position a legislator takes on an issue. Before voting for a public official, the nutritionist should know how the candidate stands on health needs, especially in the area of nutrition. If such activity is permissible, the nutritionist may inform other voters who are concerned about the same matters.

The nutritionist may also work for legislation through the legislative committee of an organization such as the state or local Dietetic Association, Home Economics Association, Public Health Association, or other group interested in the same problems or organized for the purpose. The American Dietetic Association maintains a Washington representative and is very active in testifying, suggesting bills for members to support, and reporting Washington action. ADA can also provide state associations with guidance on legislative action. Current action of ADA is summarized in the Legislative Highlights section in the *Journal of the American Dietetic Association.*

Examples of Legislative Action.   Here is an example of legislative action at state level by one committee, planned to solve a specific problem in California. Nutritionists in one county encountered problems when teaching about the bread group because corn tortillas were not enriched. The committee decided to try to get legislation enacted to require this enrichment. They discussed the problem with a number of professional persons, manufacturers, and legislators to get necessary information about the action needed. They received considerable support for the project from university students and from a company that made packaged tortilla mix. After some communication with one legislator, they learned that the legislation for this enrichment was already in effect but that it could not be applied to corn tortillas because specifications as to enriching ingredients had never been filed. The committee was asked to write the specifications on which to base the standard of identity that must be added to the State Code. These were prepared by the committee and submitted. The standard of identity is now being prepared. (6)

A similar effort in New York State resulted in the enrichment of rice, paste products, wheat flour, bread, rolls, and related products. (4) The effort started with evidence from over 30,000 diet histories of Negro and Puerto Rican patients that showed that white rice was their staple carbohydrate food. The nutritionists taught the use of enriched rice but found that it was difficult to identify and that large packages were difficult to obtain. They obtained the support of state legislators, physicians, nutrition and other health personnel, and the state commissioners and governor. It was expected that the legislation would especially benefit the poor and the vulnerable sex-age groups.

Helps for the Nutritionist

There are a number of publications of the federal government that explain legislation and provide reports of action. The proceedings of the Congress and action before each committee and subcommittee are published in the *Congressional Record,* which is issued daily when Congress is in session. The *Federal Register,* published daily, makes available to the public, federal agency regulations and other legal documents of the executive branch. The Government Manual (9) explains the structure of the federal government and how the Congress functions, including the preparation and passage of legislation. Soon after the President signs a bill into law, it is printed in an annotated pamphlet (called a slip-law print). At the same time the law is published in the *U.S. Statutes at Large.* (8)

The *Catalog of Federal Domestic Assistance* (10) reports the ways in which grants are made available for various programs. It gives the name and number of the federal laws that authorize each program, explains who is eligible for help under it and how to apply for a grant. These publications are available in public and academic libraries. Each nutritionist will need to locate the sources of similar information about legislative processes within the state.

Public opinion polls in early 1976 indicated a high interest in health for priority in spending when federal money is available. Congress has responded to this interest by overriding presidential vetoes of several health bills including the child nutrition amendments. (2)

Action at Local Level

Policies are also determined and funds appropriated by many local groups such as city and county governing bodies, school boards, and university regents. Nutritionists need to be active, influential advocates for local changes that will improve health and nutrition, especially for the poor and the minority groups. Groups that can have an influence include voters, consumer organizations, health agencies, labor unions, industrial corporations, women's organizations, and civic clubs.

The Nutritionist as an Advocate

Advocate means one who speaks out in favor of, or promotes. Sometimes it has a connotation of aggressive action that may be against the policies of the employing agency; then nutritionists who conduct such activities may risk dismissal. They should consider the objective and decide whether the risk is more likely to produce the desired result than a more conservative mode of action. Even if dismissal does not result, the nutritionist who has defied agency policy may experience reprisals such as lack of support for future nutrition programs.

Nutritionists should be vocal in their agencies and attempt to change policies for better nutrition programs, but a slow change in a nonaggressive atmosphere often works better, generating support among colleagues over a period of time. Sometimes other staff members are also concerned about policies and procedures that are adversely affecting clients. Then advocacy may be in order to change such restrictions.

Using the concept of advocate as aggressive action through confrontation of the health system on behalf of patient care, Springer and Segal studied the attitudes of dietitians toward such activity. (7) They reported the results of a questionnaire study of 64 dietitians, finding that most had never acted as advocates but that 90 percent had positive attitudes toward such action, that 38 percent had often tried to change policies, 33 percent had sometimes done so, while 23 percent had never done so.

Most who had assumed this role felt no repercussions although a few were discouraged, reprimanded, or threatened with dismissal. Perhaps some had not made a careful enough appraisal of a situation before making demands for what appeared to administrators or co-workers as extensive and radical change.

NATIONAL HEALTH INSURANCE (NHI)

Important legislation that is currently before Congress is *national health insurance,* a system of health care financing that would reimburse policy holders for all or part of the cost of medical care. It is usually assumed that the federal government should establish a compulsory NHI system that will cover each individual with a specific group of basic benefits and provide payment for catastrophic illness.

NHI has been under discussion in the Congress for many years, and several bills are always under consideration. The various bills must be evaluated on the basis of who is covered, what benefits are provided, how the quality of care will be regulated, and what the plan costs the individual directly for insurance, and indirectly through taxes and other ways. Some plans propose universal voluntary participation while others propose universal compulsory coverage, the latter of which has the advantage of leaving no doubt about eligibility.

It seems to be generally agreed by politicians, the medical community, labor, and the public that NHI will come. However, some way to control costs must first be established, perhaps by education and motivation of the public for individual preventive efforts that will reduce the need for health services, and the cost. (12, 14)

Need for National Health Insurance

NHI is especially needed by persons who have no resources for meeting the costs of health care. These include the poor who are ineligible for Medicaid, the unemployed, employed persons on marginal incomes, which make them medically indigent, and persons with high health risks. (18) Moreover, persons who currently have health insurance have inadequate benefits that usually lack preventive services, dental care, ambulatory care, nonprescription drugs, and medical devices. (16, 18)

Medicare, the present national insurance for persons over 65 who receive Social Security, provides only partial benefits after the individual has paid a deductible amount (page 81).

Other problems with present insurance programs are excessive costs for persons who have insurance, lack of coverage for many who need it, lack of provisions for controlling costs, and inadequate controls over the quality of service. (11)

Evaluation of Proposed Bills

The possible effects of a bill should be evaluated by consideration of the benefits it provides, the persons covered, and the costs. The basic benefits should include services of physicians, dentists and other health professionals (including dietary counseling), drugs and supplies, laboratory procedures, hospital care, nursing facility care, and home health services.

It has been suggested that a bill that will receive the support of the Congress will be fiscally conservative and will provide for catastrophic insurance for medical bills above $2000 or hospital care exceeding 60 days. It will also provide noncatastrophic insurance to replace Medicaid for low income individuals. The insurance package may be provided by the insurance industry or by the federal government. (15) Some mechanism is also needed to increase the bargaining strength of the insured against hospital, physician, and other providers.

Furthermore a health insurance plan should provide an efficient means for protection at a controlled cost, should be adequate in quality and quantity, should be efficient in terms of production, and allocation of funds and facilities should provide equal care for all in the place where it is needed. Use should be determined by need, but the amount of payment should correspond to the means of the individual.

Some plans give the insured health consumer the opportunity to choose between contract care provided by a health maintenance organization, and care under the conventional fee-for-service system. Competition among HMO's and other systems of health delivery is expected to help in cost control.

Meeting the Cost

There has been much discussion as to who will pay for NHI. It is sometimes forgotten that regardless of the system the cost of medical care is paid by individuals and families. When government pays, the public pays through more taxes. When business pays, the public pays through higher prices or lower wages. Insurance is simply a method of sharing the risk. The most frequently mentioned method of payment is a payroll tax of 1 or 2 percent paid by the employer. Currently the cost of health insurance is often shared by employer and employee. Many persons like having health care insurance paid by payroll deduction, regarding it as an easy, systematic way of paying for their medical care.

Use of health insurance poses a problem because it encourages use of service, thus contributing to a rise in prices. The increase in use is greater by the poor than by the affluent, whose needs are already being met. Insurance must cover all services; otherwise the covered services will be used regardless of cost. An example is the current use of hospital care (a covered item) when ambulatory care (a service not covered) could provide equally good care. This proliferation of use of services encourages unrestricted use of services and uncontrolled costs. Medicare is considered an "uncontrollable" item in the Federal budget. (11, 17)

Decision on what health services should be provided by health insurance has been compared to the decision about how much education should be provided at public expense. This requires a political decision that sets a limit on the amount of money for this purpose, then allocates it for the greatest benefit of all citizens. (11)

Two points of view have been advanced about the purpose of NHI. One assumes that the present medical care system is sound and will adjust to provide care in a satisfactory manner, with the major role of health insurance being to provide protection against unpredictable costs. The second asserts that the present medical system is inefficient in providing health services and in distributing them equitably, and that a major objective of NHI should be to reform the medical care system.

Nutritionists need to be informed about the needs, the problems, and the various plans under consideration. They must also support efforts of professional associations and other groups that are working for adequate nutritional care within the system.

Kerr (1) points out the need for advocacy by health personnel, using their personal knowledge of health conditions, to provide leadership in informing the community about the need for better provisions for the health care of minorities and the poor.

SUMMARY

The community nutritionist needs to use legislation as a way to accomplish long-range goals by the removal of legal barriers to their accomplishment.

Legislation in the U.S. Congress and at state level is a complex process that the nutritionist must understand to be able to use it to achieve goals. A bill may originate in either House or Senate, must be passed by both House and Sensate, and signed into law by the President.

The nutritionist can influence legislation at federal or state level by promoting a specific bill, working for passage of a bill, or giving testimony. The nutritionist may lobby for passage of a bill by preparing statements of need, preparing specifications for the law desired, or providing information about need for the bill. One of the best ways for the nutritionist to work is as a member of a legislative committee of a professional or community organization. The nutritionist can get information about legislation from a number of federal or state publications.

Nutritionists may use advocacy to bring about changes in their own agencies or in other institutions that affect health care of their clients.

A number of bills for National Health Insurance are currently before the Congress. It is generally agreed that the federal government should establish such a program, since present health insurance programs have narrow coverage, are available to relatively few persons, and are expensive.

Bills for NHI should be evaluated on the basis of benefits provided, persons covered, and costs. Some way must be found to control costs that escalate because health insurance encourages use of service. Some bills are designed to provide care within the present health system while others are designed to reform the system. Nutritionists need to be informed about NHI and work for an adequate plan. It must be remembered that, whatever the system, the cost of NHI will be paid by the public.

REFERENCES CITED

Legislation

1. Kerr, Lorin E., The Poverty of Affluence, *Am. J. Pub. Health,* 65 1/75 19.
2. Legislative Highlights, *J. Am. Diet. Assoc.,* 68 5/76 471.
3. Miller, George, Legislation for Nutrition: It Depends on You, *J. Nutr. Educ.,* 8 1–3/76 8.
4. Page, Stella, Dietary Histories Inspire Legislative Action, *J. Am. Diet. Assoc.,* 62 1/73 15.
5. Schlossberg, Kenneth, What It Takes To Pass Nutrition Legislation, *J. Nutr. Educ.,* 5 10–12/73 228.
6. Personal Communication from Virginia Gladney, 2/77.

7. Springer, Ninfa, and Robert M. Segal, Dietitians' Attitudes Toward Advocacy, *J. Am. Diet. Assoc.*, 67 11/75 445.
8. U.S. General Services Administration, Office of the Federal Register, *United States Government Manual 1975–76*, Government Printing Office, Washington DC, 1975, xii.
9. Ibid., 28.
10. U.S. Office of Management and Budget, *1976 Catalog of Federal Domestic Assistance*, Government Printing Office, Washington DC.

National Health Insurance

11. Donabedian, Avedis, Issues in National Health Insurance, *Am. J. Pub. Health*, 66 4/75 345.
12. Fuchs, Victor R., *Who Shall Live? Health, Economics, and Social Choice*, Basic Books, New York, 1974.
13. Kline, Kristin L., National Health Insurance: Issues for Consumers To Consider, *Family Economics Review*, ARS-NE-36, U.S. Department of Agriculture, Washington DC, Fall 1974 14.
14. Legislative Highlights, *J. Am. Diet. Assoc.*, 64 6/74 668.
15. Legislative Highlights, *J. Am. Diet. Assoc.*, 68 1/76 61.
16. U.S. Department of Health, Education, and Welfare, *Forward Plan for Health, 1977–81*, Washington DC, Aug. 1975, 112.
17. U.S. Department of Health, Education, and Welfare, *Forward Plan for Health, 1978–82*, Washington DC, Aug. 1976, 37.
18. Who Lacks Health Insurance Coverage? *Family Economics Review*, ARS-NE-36, U.S. Department of Agriculture, Washington DC, Fall 1974, 3.

CHAPTER 19 MAKING COMPREHENSIVE PLANS FOR HEALTH AND NUTRITION

The purpose of this chapter is to provide a background in overall health planning to help nutritionists plan for nutrition and integrate it into overall health plans.

There is considerable present emphasis on nutrition at the federal level. Much progress has also been made toward developing nutrition policies and plans at federal, state, and local levels. Nutritionists are participating in development of HSAs and in planning for the health service area. This is necessary so they can present nutrition data and standards to the health planners who may be unaware of the value of and indifferent to the need for nutrition in the health plan. Nutritionists must see that nutrition representation comes from qualified persons rather than from self-styled nutrition experts who present a narrow or faddish or at least unrealistic thrust toward nutrition programs. Such distortion may lead to concentration on elimination of additives and white bread, and on the promotion of health foods, rather than on broader, basic problems such as ignorance and indifference about nutritional needs, inadequate income to purchase a good diet, and quality and safety of the food supply.

COMPREHENSIVE HEALTH PLANNING, 1966–1974

National planning for health started with PL 89-749, the Comprehensive Health Planning Act of 1966. (24) At first it appeared that this would bring a new era in public health, but the structure provided by the Act was unequal to the task and health care had more attention for its political values than for its health values. The Act was designed to bring about reform in the health system, but it lacked provisions to make the necessary changes in the usual practices of health practitioners, so did not accomplish this purpose. (14, 19)

The two major parts, Comprehensive Health Planning and Regional Medical Programs (PL 89-239), which constituted the system, made impressive progress in some areas, accomplishing overall planning at state and local level, conducting programs to improve education of professionals and the public, developing new facilities for health care, and collecting data about needs and how to meet them.

NATIONAL HEALTH PLANNING SINCE 1975

Congress developed a new Act that was enacted on January 4, 1975 as PL 93-641, the National Health Planning and Resources Development Act of 1974. The structure provided by this Act was described on page 78. The Act includes Title XV, which covers health planning, and Title XVI, which provides for development of health resources. (25)

National Health Planning

Under Title XV a new system of health planning was established at national, state, and local levels. In the Preface to this new Act, the Congress describes its findings as to health needs. These are equal access to quality care for all citizens as a priority, effective ways to deliver health care with equal distribution of facilities and personnel, provider-participation in developing plans, and public education about individual responsibility for personal health care and use of services.

Congress states the purpose of the Act as "to facilitate the development of recommendations for a national health planning policy, to augment areawide and State planning for health services, manpower, and facilities, and to authorize financial assistance for the development of resources to further that policy." (Section 2)

The Act specifies that planning is to proceed from a data base that states the health conditions in the health service area, the status of health resources and services, and their utilization. (Section 1513) Certain provisions of the Act are of particular significance to community nutrition. The Secretary of Health, Education, and Welfare is responsible for developing and revising guidelines with recommendations and comments from health agencies, associations, and specialty societies. (Section 1501) The American Dietetic Association is one of the specialty societies.

One of the priorities is "promotion of activities for the prevention of disease, including studies of nutritional and environmental factors affecting health and the provision of preventive health care services." (Section 1502) Other priorities include provision of primary care services for the medically underserved, development of health maintenance organizations, training and utilization of physician assistants, especially nurse clinicians, development of various levels of care (intensive, acute, general, and extended), activities designed to bring about needed improvements in quality of care, and development of effective methods of educating the public about personal health care.

Health Resources Development

Title XVI, the second part of the Act, provides for financial and technical help for improvement of health facilities by modernizing medical facilities, constructing new outpatient and inpatient facilities, and converting existing medical facilities to provide new health services.

Discussion

It remains to be seen whether the health planning structure established by PL 93-641 will produce significant improvement in the current health care system. It will be several years before the effectiveness of the new law can be evaluated, but some health planners believe that there will be few innovations and that changes in the health care system will be small and slow. (6, 14, 15, 19, 36, 37)

Community nutritionists will have to work within the new system for the nutritional benefit of the public. Vladeck (36) believes that each individual on an HSA governing body will represent a different constituency and that action will be through "logrolling" that is, supporting each other's interests. Nutritionists will need to develop channels through which to accomplish nutritional goals. They should try to put on the governing body a person who places nutrition interests first; otherwise they will have to rely on another person by supporting the primary interest of that individual and being supported in turn.

As the Act is implemented at the local level, it is important that nutritionists and dietitians participate in leadership. Health planning and subsequent action must be directed into channels that will provide the best service and health care rather than allowed to become political issues or sources of large revenue for individuals or organizations. This can best be done through the influence of the persons to be served using the process of community organization. Nutritionists and dietitians can help in monitoring at the local level to assure that the provisions of the act are followed.

Ginzberg considers it doubtful that there will be an early resolution of the problems that prevent the poor from achieving the goal of quality health care. (6) He points out that the problems are in local production and distribution of health services and that neither national health planning, nor national health insurance, nor PSRO can solve these problems. He considers the real need to be for "improvements in the quality of life, not in the health delivery system," and says that removal of the various barriers that are preventing changes in the system will disappear slowly, and that even a more extensive health delivery system cannot produce the necessary improvements in the quality of life.

Nutritionists should recognize the potential of their work, not only to bring health services to the poor but also to influence healthful family living and increase opportunities for personal enrichment that contribute to the quality of life.

Nutritionists who participate in comprehensive health planning will need to be well versed in the science and art of planning. Waters believes that health planners must first of all be *planners* but need also a knowledge of community organization, agency administration, and health and service problems. (37)

Nutritionists and other health professionals who wish to obtain further insights into the complex subject of national health planning will find Canada's *Working Document* of interest. It is a policy plan document, organized under two broad objectives, five main strategies, and 74 specific proposals. (18) Like the U.S. plan, it emphasizes that the underlying causes of sickness and death must be attacked by improving the environment and reducing the risks in the lifestyle of individuals.

Guidelines from DHEW

PL 93-641 provides that the Secretary of DHEW must issue periodic guidelines for national health planning policy. They are to cover standards for health resources and national health planning goals, with the goals prepared with suggestions from state and area planning groups, professional associations, and other organizations that represent health care providers.

Three sets of guidelines for health planning have been issued under the title *Forward Plan for Health*, the latest for 1978–82. (29, 30) The plans are intended as guidelines for examining major health issues, rather than as plans in the usual sense. They are designed to present issues and facts on which decisions can be made at the Federal level on budget and legislation. The public is invited to express itself on health matters by reaction to the documents.

Forward Plan for Health 1978–82

One of the major points in the 1978–82 Plan is the need for an aggressive program of prevention. The goal of the Plan is to "help improve the health of the American people." The objectives are "to assure access to quality health care at reasonable cost" and "to prevent illness, disease, and accidents."

In the Plan the Secretary points out the impact of the cost of health care that in 1975 was $118.5 billion, more than three times the cost in 1965. The annual per capita cost rose an average of 10.7 percent, from $198 to $547. In 1975 the federal share of health financing was double that in 1966. Three fourths of the DHEW budget was used for medical care under the Medicare and Medicaid programs.

The problem of reducing costs is further illustrated by the report of a proposed consolidation of 15 health programs and Medicaid under a single block grant. (10) It has been estimated that this would result in the elimination of funds for the other 15 programs because in 1975 Medicaid used $7 billion of the $8.2-billion expenditure for all 16 programs. As pointed out in Chapter 18, the structure of Medicare makes its cost an uncontrollable expense.

The major problem that must be solved is the current uncontrolled and excessive costs of health care. The cause is the traditional structure of the health care system in the United States, which has resulted in the use of hospitals for a high amount of illness that, with current techniques, could be treated elsewhere if appropriate alternatives were available. This uneconomical tendency has been increased by the structure of present health insurance plans, which provide higher benefits for hospital care than for ambulatory care in local centers. Two methods of control have been proposed. One is the Professional Standards Review Organization (PSRO), a plan for evaluation and monitoring of the use and quality of services provided. The second control would be accomplished through the local Health Systems Agencies as they are expected to balance the need for various kinds of health care and see that appropriate facilities are available. These facilities would include ambulatory care centers and home health care as well as hospitals and extended care facilities.

Such economic considerations will limit federal health action until ways can be found to control the cost. The solution to health care appears to be through a total systems approach such as comprehensive national health insurance, discussed in Chapter 18.

The methods proposed for controlling cost are developing a nationwide allocation of resources on a need basis, modifying the delivery and use of health services, educating both providers and consumers on proper use of the services, equalizing the cost of malpractice problems and the cost of health services, utilizing current and new technologies to help contain cost and prevent disease and illness, increasing the quality of health care, and strengthening the necessary resources such as health data systems, research, medical institutions, and manpower. (32) Fuchs believes that the financial system of new health plans must be used to modify the behavior of physicians and hospitals before the cost of medical care can be controlled. (5)

These and other proposals made in the DHEW Forward Plan for Health cannot be implemented unless the Congress passes enabling legislation, establishes regulations, and makes the necessary appropriations.

A new law, PL 94-317, the Health Promotion and Disease Prevention Act of 1976, established an office for coordination of all health education and health promotion activities. It is suggested in the document that one of the tenets of the federal position should be to remove the present emphasis through advertising on "indiscriminate consumption of liquor, food, drugs, or tobacco smoke with little regard for the consequences." The relationship of medicine and individual responsibility is also discussed, the point being made that a medical advisor cannot offset the results of a long-continued unhealthful lifestyle. (26)

The theme of the Forward Plan for 1978–82 is prevention based on the premise that the greatest benefits will accrue from improvements in health habits and environment. It names four areas of major importance, which are health education, nutrition, child health, and environmental health. It points out that each individual must assume responsibility for personal health, and society for the safety of the environment. Two kinds of programs are needed, those directed at the general public and those directed toward specific high risk groups.

The priorities proposed in the Plan include the following: (1) Children, women, minorities, and the aged, (2) Environmental and occupational health, (3) Nutrition, (4) Health education and promotion, (5) Dental health, and (6) International health.

COMPREHENSIVE PLANNING FOR NUTRITION

Comprehensive planning for nutrition needs and programs should be established. It should outline a course of action on nutrition by government, organizations, and individuals, provide a way to unify the nutrition programs in the federal government, and to coordinate all nutrition programs in the country.

National Nutrition Policy

In 1974 the National Nutrition Consortium proposed guidelines for a National Nutrition Policy. (17) Five goals were listed: (1) to assure an adequate wholesome food supply at reasonable cost, (2) to maintain food resources for emergency needs, (3) to develop public knowledge and responsible understanding of nutrition and foods, (4) to maintain a system for control of food quality and safety, and (5) to support research and education in foods and nutrition.

Seven major programs were suggested to implement the goals. These included (1) monitoring and reporting on nutritional status, (2) nutrition services as part of the health care system, (3) nutrition education in schools and for the general public through many media, (4) federal support of basic and applied research, (5) national planning for food production and distribution, (6) study and assessment of food values, quality and safety, and (7) assistance to other countries with their nutrition problems.

Schlossberg suggests (21) that national policy and planning for nutrition are needed to coordinate and monitor all nutrition-related programs of the federal government, which are currently constituted in limited programs influenced by special interests of many groups including food producers, processors, consumers, the medical community, and the poor. Current programs such as WIC, Food Stamps, Child Nutrition, and School Lunch were designed as part of a system of income maintenance rather than as ways to solve the underlying problems.

Schlossberg has stated that the first priority of the Select Committee on Nutrition and Human Needs was the development of an annual comprehensive National Nutrition Plan to be presented to Congress at the beginning of each year. This Plan should include a "formal assessment of the nutritional state of the union" with specific goals. Goals should be health, adequate food, satisfactory food quality, and freedom of choice in distribution and allocation of food. The Plan should represent what *is* rather than what *should be,* and provide a basis for identifying necessary changes.

The Committee also proposed establishing a Federal Nutrition Office at Cabinet level to provide guidance on nutrition policy, to speak for nutrition, and to provide a focus for activities.

Community nutritionists should keep informed about the National Nutrition Policy and Plan. Action is reported in various professional journals as well as in special reports from the Congress. Nutritionists will also need to see that nutrition professionals are appropriately represented in local plans for implementation of related programs.

Nutrition in the Forward Plan For Health, 1978–82

The Plan recognizes that the food consumption of many Americans is unsatisfactory, resulting in undernutrition or obesity, and that there are problems with the quality and safety of the food supply.

Prevention this year will be focussed on:

1. Fostering more healthful food consumption practices.
2. Integrating nutrition concerns into the planning, organization, and implementation of health care systems, including the training of all health-related personnel in nutrition.
3. Determining the nutritional status of the nation.

Improvement in food consumption practices will be attempted by work with school authorities for better school nutrition education. Public education will be promoted by having nutritionists establish the content, and health education and media experts work with nutritionists to determine the best communication methods. Research will be considered to develop more effective methods of making long-term changes in food consumption.

Another phase of nutrition programs is the integration of a nutrition component into local and state health planning. This component should include the training of all health-related personnel. It was also pointed out that studies are needed to determine the extent and content of patient nutrition education carried out by health personnel.

Nutritional surveillance was stated to be a necessary part of a program to improve the health status of Americans. It was suggested that there should be surveys to determine nutrition problems according to region, income, sex, race, food availability, and cultural habits. Results of the surveys will provide data for evaluating local nutrition efforts and for planning programs. Another action of interest to nutritionists is the FDA plan to develop methods for surveying problems connected with excessive intake of vitamins and minerals.

Action Needed at State and Local Level

Community nutritionists, even those working in programs of limited scope at the local level, can influence the development of local nutrition policies and plans. There must be able leadership at the local level if improved nutrition is to be achieved, for nutrition can only be strong at the local level when it is strongly represented in the local government.

Miller (14) points out that in many communities the public (the health consumer) has little opportunity to influence health planning by participation in determining policies and priorities for allocation of funds. This holds in even greater measure for nutrition; careful guidance of health consumers by nutritionists is needed to develop the consumers' ability to plan wisely for a comprehensive approach to achieving better nutrition for the community through community organization.

Nutritionists can work at the local level to provide program information and the data base for the state and local health service agencies. State and local Dietetic Associations and nutrition councils are working on these programs.

One way in which nutritionists can wield influence is by providing expert technical advice either through a technical committee or by consultation. The governing body will settle technical and professional questions about health planning by voting on them.

Oregon dietitians provided the chief planner for the state with information on services needed. They assessed available services and estimated the number of dietitians and nutritionists necessary to provide the recommended level of services. They pointed out the need to provide for assessment of the food practices, nutritional status, and education of the public. The "public" was described as persons not directly reached through formal education, including persons with cardiovascular diseases, and diabetes, pregnant women and infants, persons interested in weight control and weight reduction, the physically handicapped, Food Stamp recipients, persons who need help with food money management, migrant workers, and foreign-speaking persons. (4)

Dietitians and nutritionists in Arizona were able to have nutrition services included in the state plan for health services that became the state's health care delivery system. Nutrition was included among the recommendations of the Comprehensive Health Planning Authority in the following statement: "Standards for nutritional care services should be included in all appropriate state guidelines and regulations for health care." (22)

Community nutritionists must marshall support for the nutrition plan from the nutrition and dietetic community, from other professionals, and from community leaders. If this is not done, rival plans presented by other groups with more vocal leadership may receive more favorable attention and may be selected as the official position.

Coordination of Nutrition Programs

An important part of community planning is coordination of health programs. The community nutritionist should participate in coordination of food and nutrition activities. Sometimes many programs are taking place in a community, duplicating services and dispensing conflicting information that confuses the public and does not promote the cause of good nutrition. A united position of nutrition and medical communities on dietary fat, meat analogs, minimum number of calories for weight control diets, and other controversial matters will give the public a basis for action without the confusion that often accompanies nutrition advice. It will also lessen the possibility that the public will see a specific nutrition program as just one alternative competing with other programs that come from faddists or extremists.

Coordination may be needed for services within an agency, between a number of agencies, or for all programs in the community. The community nutritionist should know the nutrition services of agency and community and plan to avoid duplication and conflict. The nutritionist in the official health agency is the logical person to provide leadership for coordination. It may also be accomplished by a small nutrition coordinating committee with representatives of various agencies that have nutrition programs. The committee could be organized under the auspices of a local nutrition council or as an adjunct advisory group to the public health agency. If neither of these is possible, a community nutritionist or other nutrition-trained person could assume the leadership for coordination.

THE HEALTH MAINTENANCE ORGANIZATION (HMO)

The name reflects the present emphasis on preventing illness rather than on treating it. The *health maintenance organization* was conceived to fill an important role in the national health system. It is defined as an organization that contracts to deliver comprehensive health care, emphasizing preventive services, primary care, and efficient operation, through specific services to an enrolled group upon the prepayment of a set fee for each individual or family. An HMO may be sponsored by a group of consumers, an insurance company, a group of physicians, a hospital, an independent corporation, or various other organizations. (16)

The prepaid group care concept has existed for some years in the Kaiser Health Plans of California, the Group Health Cooperative of Washington State, the Health Insurance Plan of New York City, the Group Health Association of Washington, D.C., and others. Federal support for expansion of this method of providing health care has been increased since 1970.

The various names that were applied to these organizations during the Congressional discussions help define their functions. They were called "comprehensive health services organizations," "health care corporations," and "health services and health education corporations." (16) They were conceived in the early days of comprehensive health planning as an important part of the health delivery system. Their purpose was to provide prepaid, organized, comprehensive health care systems as an alternative to the fee-for-service private practice system. They were designed to produce a more efficient system with quality control, to provide a mechanism and incentive for cost control, and to place emphasis on health care rather than on disease care. It was also believed that as part of the national health insurance system they would bring incentives for innovative methods of care. Research has shown that HMOs lower total health care costs while covering a greater percentage of costs. (33, 34)

In the early 1970s Congress made appropriations for feasibility studies of the HMO concept. During 1971 and 1972 the DHEW funded some programs and established the Health Maintenance Organization Services within the Department. Legislation with an appropriation of $325 million to assist in development of HMO's was enacted as PL 93-222 on December 29, 1973. (27, 34) The purpose was to stimulate development of experimental health care delivery systems. The DHEW planned to assist in establishing 150 HMO's during a five-year period. By February 1975 it had made 95 grants to study feasibility, initiate plans, or help meet the operating costs of each HMO for the first three years, after which an organization is expected to be self-sustaining. At that time there were 142 HMO's in the U.S. serving over 5 million people. Priority was given to organizations serving medically underserved populations since a major purpose of the legislation is to provide facilities and health personnel for underserved areas.

The requirements for HMOs imposed by the legislation led to higher costs for members compared with other health insurance. Evidence of the slow development of these organizations is shown by the demand for only $18 million for 1977 compared to the $85 million that was originally authorized for the year. (11)

The success of the early HMO's will point the way to further development of this concept of health care delivery. Mass development will be delayed until the results are known. Further legislation will be needed to regulate the types of prepayment and quality of care, but the extent of government control needed is still in question. Present regulations require employers of 25 or more persons to include HMO membership as one of the available health care plans. In some states care to Medicaid recipients has been provided by contracts with HMO's that provide quality care at lower cost than the usual fee-for-service arrangement.

Nutrition Services in the HMO

Functions of the dietitian or nutritionist in the HMO include planning with other team members for overall care, establishing criteria for members who need special attention to nutritional care, assessing needs for nutrition services, and determining priorities for food and nutrition services. (20)

Kunis has reported on the counseling services in a large private corporation that provides a comprehensive medical care program. Nutrition counseling is available for all stages of health care—crisis, remedial, maintenance, and preventive. They have developed a model they believe can be adapted to any health center or medical practice in public, private, or prepaid systems. (8)

Treacy (23) reports her experience as nutritionist on the primary care team in a health maintenance organization. The nutritionist gives nutritional care to members referred from other primary care providers. In addition to the usual individual and group counseling, the nutritionist measures blood pressure and orders diagnostic studies to facilitate monitoring of patients. The nutrition services are covered by insurance whether care is given in office, home, extended care facility, or hospital.

SUMMARY

National health planning has been under way since 1966, but since January 1975 it has gained new direction from PL 93-641, the National Health Planning Act. Title XV of the Act explains that the purpose of the Congress was to develop national health planning and authorize financial assistance. Title XVI provides financial help for HSA's to update health facilities. Planning must start from a data base for which community nutritionists should supply the data on nutrition needs and resources. One of the priorities for action is nutrition and other aspects of prevention. Nutritionists will need to develop ways of working with the HSA governing body to assure that nutrition is given the greatest possible impact to improve the quality of life of the poor, and the health of all Americans.

DHEW presents issues and facts about health in annual guidelines that are intended to give information rather than to offer a blueprint for action. The 1978–82 Plan includes many suggestions about nutrition activities.

A way must be found to control the cost of health care before there can be much federal action. Prevention of disease especially by health and nutrition education, utilizing new technologies, and developing new health delivery methods such as the health maintenance organization are some of the ways that will be used for cost control.

Proposals have been presented to the Congress for a National Nutrition Policy, a Federal Office of Nutrition at Cabinet level, and a National Nutrition Center in the DHEW.

REFERENCES CITED

1. A.D.A. Comments on DHEW's Five-Year Health Plan, *J. Am. Diet. Assoc.,* 68 4/76 352.
2. Concepts of Comprehensive Health Planning, editorial, *Am. J. Pub. Health,* 58 6/68 1011.
3. Dwyer, Johanna T., and Jean Mayer, Beyond Economics and Nutrition: The Complex Basis of Food Policy, *Science,* 188 5/9/75 566.
4. East, Dorothy, and Virginia F. Harger, Oregon Dietitians Respond to Call for Health Care Planning Data, *J. Am. Diet. Assoc.,* 69 10/76 400.
5. Fuchs, Victor R., *Who Shall Live?, Health, Economics and Social Choice,* Basic Books, New York, 1974.
6. Ginzberg, Eli, What Next in Health Policy?, *Science,* 188 6/75 1184.
7. Kerr, Lorin E., The Poverty of Affluence, *Am. J. Pub. Health,* 65 1/75 19.
8. Kunis, Beila S., Family Nutritionist on the Primary Health Care Team, *J. Nutr. Educ.,* 8 4–6/76 77.
9. Legislative Highlights, *J. Am. Diet. Assoc.,* 68 2/76 163.
10. Legislative Highlights, *J. Am. Diet. Assoc.,* 68 4/76 326.
11. Legislative Highlights, *J. Am. Diet. Assoc.,* 69 12/76 661.
12. Lum, Doman, The Health Maintenance Organization Delivery System, *Am. J. Pub. Health,* 65 11/75 1192.
13. Mayer, Jean, ed., *Nutrition Policies in the Seventies,* W. H. Freeman and Co., San Francisco, 1973.
14. Miller, C. Arden, Issues of Health Policy: Local Government and the Public's Health, *Am. J. Pub. Health,* 65 12/75 1330.
15. Mott, Peter D., Anthony T. Mott, Jonathon M. Rudolph, Edward R. Lane, and Robert L. Berg, Difficult Issues in Health Planning, Development, and Review, *Am. J. Pub. Health,* 66 8/76 743.
16. Myers, Beverlee, Health Maintenance Organizations: Objectives and Issues, *HSMHA Health Reports.* 86 7/71 585.
17. National Nutrition Consortium, Inc., Guidelines for a National Nutrition Policy, *Nutr. Rev.,* 32 5/74 153.
18. *New Perspective on the Health of Canadians: A Working Document,* Ministry of Health, Ottawa, Canada, 1974.
19. Pickett, George, Toward a National Health Policy—Values in Conflict, *Am. J. Pub. Health,* 65 12/75 1335.
20. Position Paper on Nutrition Services in Health Maintenance Organizations, *J. Am. Diet. Assoc.,* 60 4/72 317.
21. Schlossberg, Kenneth, Progress Toward a National Food Policy—Its Implications, *J. Am. Diet. Assoc.* 68, 4/76 326.
22. State Legislation in Arizona Recognizes Nutrition. *J. Am. Diet. Assoc.,* 62 1/73 26.
23. Treacy, Lois H., The Nutritionist in a Comprehensive Health Care Plan,

No. V in series: Dietary Counseling in Ambulatory Care, *J. Am. Diet. Assoc.,* 68 3/76 246.

24. U.S. Congress, The Comprehensive Health Planning and Public Health Services Amendments of 1966, PL 89-749, Nov. 3, 1966.
25. U.S. Congress, The National Health Planning and Resources Development Act of 1974, PL 93-641, Jan. 4, 1975.
26. U.S. Congress, Health Promotion and Disease Prevention Act of 1976, PL 94-317, June 23, 1976.
27. U.S. Congress, Public Health Service Act to Amend and to Extend Health Maintenance Organizations and to Establish a Commission on Quality Health Care, PL 93-222, Dec. 29, 1973.
28. U.S. Congress, Senate, Select Committee on Nutrition and Human Needs, Toward a National Nutrition Policy, May, 1975, Government Printing Office, Washington DC, 1.
29. U.S. Dept. of Health, Education, and Welfare, *Forward Plan for Health, FY 1977–81,* Washington DC, Aug. 1975.
30. U.S. Dept. of Health, Education, and Welfare, *Forward Plan for Health, 1978–1982,* Washington DC, Aug. 1976.
31. Ibid., 8.
32. Ibid., 19.
33. Ibid., 50.
34. U.S. Dept. of Health, Education, and Welfare, *Promoting Community Health,* USDHEW, Pub. No. (HSA) 75-5016, 1975, 9.
35. U.S. General Services Administration, Office of the Federal Register, *United States Government Manual 1975–76,* Government Printing Office, Washington DC, 1975.
36. Vladeck, Bruce C., Interest-Group Representation and the HSAs: Health Planning and Political Theory, *Am. J. Pub. Health,* 67 1/77 26.
37. Waters, William J., State Level Comprehensive Health Planning: A Retrospect, *Am. J. Pub. Health,* 66 2/76 142.

6

THE PRACTICE

The primary focus of a community nutrition program is maintenance of health through good nutrition and prevention of conditions and diseases caused by inadequate or improper nutrition. The goal of malnutrition control is proposed for a more precise approach to the solution of nutrition problems than that of optimal nutrition. The methods are nutrition surveillance and nutritional care. The targets are the conditions and diseases that are the result of nutritional inadequacies, imbalances, or excesses. Many nutrition programs are directed at specific communities based on the sex-age groups when specific programs are needed or when they have the most probability of success.

20 PREVENTION AND CONTROL OF MALNUTRITION
I. METHODS

The purpose of this chapter is to present the problem of malnutrition and the methods by which the nutritionist can plan for prevention and control.

The mission of a nutrition program is usually stated as being to maintain optimal health of the population. The objective is frequently stated as the improvement of nutrition and food habits. These large general goals must be narrowed considerably before they can be attacked. A way of focusing personnel and resources on specific problems is found by setting the realistic mission of *malnutrition control* instead of the more nebulous one of *optimal nutrition*.

Malnutrition is a state of disease caused by deficiency, excess, or imbalance of the supplies of calories, nutrients, or both, that are available for use in the body. It may be due to dietary content, to faulty utilization of food eaten, or to a combination of both. Faulty utilization may be due to poor digestion, impaired absorption, or a malfunction in metabolism. *Undernutrition* is the body condition that results from inadequate amount of calories, or nutrients, or both. *Overnutrition* is the body condition that results from too high an amount of calories or nutrients. Retarded growth, underweight, and anemia are the most common evidences of undernutrition. Obesity is the most common evidence of overnutrition. Problems of digestion, absorption, and metabolism require investigation. (2, 6)

It is generally believed that undernourished people are more susceptible to infectious disease, have a lower level of function, and that they may suffer from apathy, indifference, and lower intelligence. Kallen (3) suggests that apathy and social uninvolvement may be jointly responsible for anomie and that a change in nutrition may be necessary before change will take place in the social conditions. Some effects of improved nutrition are increased production and greater efficiency.

Malnutrition control is the prevention and treatment of malnutrition. The method of approach is identification of nutrition problems by anthropometric, biochemical, clinical, and dietary assessment of individuals. (2, 3, 5) Anthropometric measures identify retarded growth and obesity. Biochemical determinations identify iron deficiency anemia, vitamin deficiency, and other problems.

The clinical examination can identify a variety of physical signs and symptoms of nutritional deficiencies as well as similar signs that are not related to nutritional status.

The dietary assessment gives clues to the reasons for the signs of malnutrition just mentioned and to the dietary changes needed to avoid future malnutrition. Information about individual food consumption may show that intakes of specific nutrients are lower than the RDA; however, if the biochemical data show normal values, the individual is not deficient. The food record can show whether a problem is most apt to be dietary or whether it comes from other causes.

It is important to identify nutrition problems before starting a program and to plan activities to meet the specific needs that are identified. There are a number of conditions and diseases that are especially appropriate for attack by preventive community programs because of their prevalence or the significance of food and nutrition in their development. These include iron-deficiency anemia, retarded growth, obesity, atherosclerosis, hypertension, diabetes, cancer, and dental caries.

Prevention of these conditions and diseases should be a part of any community nutrition program. Persons who have any one of these conditions will constitute a "community" by definition, and prevention (and sometimes treatment) may be approached in community nutrition by incorporating preventive measures into all community nutrition programs, by planning preventive programs for the persons most likely to develop the specific conditions or diseases, or by initiating corrective programs for those who have them. Early symptoms and predisposing conditions include excessive intake of calories, fats, or nutrients, inadequate diet, and too little activity.

Malnutrition control requires nutritional surveillance to identify problems and nutritional care for intervention.

NUTRITIONAL SURVEILLANCE

Nutritional surveillance is a plan for continuous collection of data for evaluating nutritional status similar to the surveillance systems maintained by official health agencies for assessment of communicable diseases. Nutritionists need the data to identify problems, to constitute a baseline, and to use in setting priorities. (2, 5)

The *Forward Plan for Health 1978-82* mentions nutritional surveillance as a necessary part of improving health to receive attention during 1977 (page 341).

Specific objectives (5) of a nutritional surveillance system are:

To obtain information for evaluation of nutrition programs by comparison of data before and after treatment.

To identify existing cases of malnutrition so that treatment can be instituted.

To identify incipient nutrition problems so that preventive programs can be started.

To obtain data as a basis for priorities in allocation of money and personnel.

To improve medical care by identifying and treating nutrition problems.

To identify the nutrition problems that should become the targets for federal, state, and local assistance.

It is desirable to conduct surveillance on an ongoing basis according to some kind of statistical plan; however, maximal results at the least expense using practical methods may be obtained by what Nichaman calls "convenience samples" (5); that is, taking what is available at the time it is available. Thus any pertinent data that can be obtained may be used in nutritional surveillance. Nichaman recommends that the data be analyzed at a central location and compared with the data from samples of similar groups. Dietary data about the kinds and amounts of foods eaten give useful clues to what may be expected in growth and in nutrient levels in the tissues, and provide information for planning a logical intervention program for correction of the identified nutritional deficiencies.

Practical Method for Nutritional Surveillance

The CDC has provided technical assistance to ten states and one large urban area to help them develop surveillance systems using data from ongoing programs such as EPSDT, WIC, and Head Start. (5, 7) The system is based on three measurements made in these programs—height, weight, and hemoglobin or hematocrit—and uses a computer method of analyzing and reporting the data.

Three relationships are used for expressing the height and weight data: height for age, weight for age, and weight for height (the methods and forms were described on page 192). The surveillance system is intended to provide accurate nutrition-related data on children from birth to age 18. The CDC has developed a method for analyzing the data and reporting the results to the submitting agency. Periodic summaries identify the problems when there is need for intervention. Small programs not in one of the states covered might use a similar method with hand-tabulation of data.

NUTRITIONAL CARE

Nutritional care is making provision for the process of getting the proper nutrients by the consumption of a good diet and attention to related health habits. The American Dietetic Association says: "Nutritional care is the application of the science and art of human nutrition in helping people select and obtain food for the primary purpose of nourishing their bodies in health or in disease throughout the life cycle. This participating may be in single or combined functions; in extending knowledge of food and nutrition principles; in teaching these principles for application according to particular situations; and in diet counseling." (1)

A plan for nutritional care may be made for an individual on a normal or modified diet, for a family group, for residents of a group facility, or for a community. The nutritionist should make the plan using information from personal contact, food records and diet histories, and other records such as medical charts, clinical notes, and laboratory reports.

The care plan should include input as appropriate from the individual, family, group or community, the nutritionist, social worker, nurse, physician, and other health personnel. In most cases, the individual or group should participate in the development of the plans or assume this responsibility. This requires commitment from the individual that good nutrition is desirable and that planning for it and achieving it are worth money and time. (1)

A plan is needed when analysis by food record or diet history shows a poor diet, when a medical examination shows signs of malnutrition, when there is evidence of hunger, when diet therapy is part of the medical care, when nutrient needs are increased by body condition, or when there is obesity or underweight as shown by height-weight data or other physical measurements.

The plan for nutritional care should include:

Analysis of regular eating patterns of individual, family, group, or community, which identifies the good points and the problems.

Identification of reasons for the problems.

Proposal of ways to correct problems.

Method for supplementing resources when needed.

Instruction about normal or modified diets for various individuals or groups, and how to provide food for all individuals in one framework.

Counseling on food money management, and instruction for improvement of practices that interfere with a healthful home environment.

Referrals for help with weight control or obesity correction (groups, exercise facilities) or other problems.

Surveillance to monitor nutritional status.

SUMMARY

Malnutrition control has been suggested as a realistic goal for a community nutrition program. Nutrition problems can be identified by anthropometric, biochemical, clinical, and dietary assessment. Dietary assessment that shows inadequate intake of nutrients may explain the problems identified by the other methods and suggest dietary treatment.

A community nutrition program should have a system of nutritional surveillance, which may be established in a practical way by using data available through regular programs such as EPSDT, WIC, and Head Start.

A nutritional care plan should be made when there is an inadequate diet, signs of malnutrition, or other nutrition problems.

REFERENCES CITED

1. American Dietetic Association, Goals of the Lifetime Education of the Dietitian, *J. Am. Diet. Assoc.,* 54 2/69 92.
2. Christakis, George, ed., Nutritional Assessment in Health Programs, *Am. J. Pub. Health,* 63 11/73 Supplement.
3. Kallen, David J. Nutrition and Society, *J. Am. Med. Assoc.,* 215 1/4/71 94.

4. Mauer, Alvin M., Malnutrition—Still a Common Problem for Children in the United States, *Clin. Ped.,* 14 1/75 23.

5. Nichaman, Milton Z., Developing a Nutritional Surveillance System, *J. Am. Diet. Assoc.,* 65 7/74 15.

6. Robinson, Corinne H., *Normal and Therapeutic Nutrition,* 14th ed., Macmillan Co., New York, 1972, 417.

7. U.S. Dept. of Health, Education, and Welfare, Center for Disease Control, *Nutrition Surveillance,* 1/75.

CHAPTER 21

PREVENTION AND CONTROL OF MALNUTRITION

II. HUNGER, RETARDED GROWTH, AND IRON DEFICIENCY

The major manifestations of undernutrition in the United States are hunger, retarded growth, and iron deficiency. Most hunger occurs because of poverty, which may be either a temporary shortage of food money or a continued state of inadequate income to meet family needs. Retarded growth is a complex problem that may have physical causes, but is usually a problem of inadequate food intake. Iron deficiency is usually due to poor food selection with resulting inadequate iron intake. These are preventable conditions and should receive priority in community programs.

HUNGER AND MALNUTRITION

Hunger is discomfort or pain resulting from lack of food. In most cases hunger occurs because the amount of money spent for food is too small to purchase foods for an adequate diet. Hunger may also occur in children because parents punish them by denying food, because they underestimate the amount of food needed by a child, or because they do not recognize the signs of hunger. Health personnel who visit homes or counsel parents elsewhere should be alert to recognize these problems and to report signs of neglect to child welfare authorities, or to counsel the parents about food behavior that indicates hunger.

The basic problem is usually an inadequate wage or a low welfare budget, problems that must be solved by politicians; hence the remedy must come through community action. Sometimes the problem is poor money management, or poor food buying practices. Then the nutritionist, nurse, or home economist may assist by teaching how the available money can be more effectively used (page 189).

The community nutritionist may find it in order to collect data on the extent of hunger, especially when there is extensive unemployment in the area. Information about malnutrition can be collected at the same time.

One nutritionist had received a number of verbal reports of hungry people in the area and requested that nurses, teachers and physicians report persons who came to their attention along with persons diagnosed by the physician as being malnourished. (3) A simple form was used to record information on where the person had been seen, such as child health clinic, youth clinic, home, or school; age and sex; and who identified the problem, as nurse, social worker or physician. For cases of hunger, there was added information about how long it had existed and the probable cause, such as a neglected child, late welfare check, or inadequate income. For malnutrition the record included the signs and probable cause such as inadequate food money, lack of nutrition knowledge, or apathy. Over a period of four months, 109 cases of hunger and 120 cases of malnutrition were reported.

Such factual data on the extent of hunger is difficult to get. Welfare workers, teachers, and nurses are most likely to identify hunger in the course of their regular work, but individuals and families without food may become known to churches, city officials, local politicians, and others. In some areas churches, neighborhood houses, or hospitals keep a supply of food to help families in need. The nutritionist should identify persons and families and assist in referring them to the place where their needs can be met, such as programs in the area that include free or low-cost meals. These include day care centers, school lunch programs, WIC programs, and meal programs for the elderly.

At the same time nutritionists work to solve the immediate nutritional problems of individuals who are hungry or malnourished, they should also begin plans to correct the long-range problem of poverty, which is the reason for most of the hunger and malnutrition in the United States. In the Ten State Nutrition Survey, it was found that the difference between food intakes of well-fed children and those with malnutrition was in the *amount* of food rather than other factors. (11)

All nutrition and health personnel should be alert to recognize the signs of hunger and malnutrition. Christakis states: "One does not have to be a physician to recognize major signs of nutritional deprivation. Auxiliary health workers can be trained in nutritional diagnosis so that they may be alerted to the major signs of clinical deficiencies." (2)

RETARDED GROWTH

Underweight as a sign of malnutrition in the U.S. population at all ages is far less common than obesity, however, there are children in all populations who are underweight or who show retarded growth.

Genetic Potential and Normal Growth

Every human being has a genetic potential determined by factors present from birth that may be different from the potential of all other individuals (8) Growth is dependent on the genetic potential, but whether that potential is achieved is determined by nutrition and other factors. (10, 14)

The National Center for Health Statistics has reported that in the U.S. the end may have come to a 90-year trend for child size to increase and maturation to occur earlier. They believe that this may indicate that the limits of genetic potential have been reached. (13)

The normal growth pattern includes rapid growth in both height and weight during infancy, continued growth at a slower rate until puberty, rapid growth during adolescence, and a gradual decline until growth stops at 15 to 18 years. (13) Growth is also affected by adequacy of the diet, season of the year, climate, illness and disease, and other factors. (18)

Causes of Retarded Growth

Smith points out that although growth is usually normal there may be growth retardation due to any of 59 specific syndromes of either prenatal or postnatal origin. (15) Growth may slow down or stop if for any reason the total nutritional requirements of infant or child are not met. The reason may be illness, lack of food, too small a calorie intake, or other. There may be no clinical or biochemical evidence of deficiency, but short stature or retarded bone development may occur.

Failure-to-thrive is a condition of young infants characterized by retarded growth. The term denotes a rate of physical growth less than expected, as shown by a decreasing rate of growth or a falling weight curve. It may be due simply to insufficient food intake, but there are usually underlying causes. These include physical problems, emotional or physical neglect, mismanagement, or abuse. These cases need individual medical management that either rules out or treats any organic problems and also assists parents in overcoming problems that lead to neglect or mismanagement. Sometimes when there is parental neglect, the child is simply not getting enough food although the parent may think it is adequately fed.

Growth and development retardation are common in city slums and rural poverty areas. They may also retard mental development, learning, and behavior. (7) Failure to grow may be a mechanism by which the child adapts in order to survive unfavorable conditions. Growth retardation is shown by retarded height and weight, inadequate bone development, delayed menarche in females, and other signs. (6) Adult stature is an index of nutritional status depending on how well the individual has achieved genetic potential. The short individual may have lacked the essential nutrients for best development, instead of being short because of genetics. Growth should be monitored and compared with other children from the same racial group of comparable age and size, or preferably with its own growth on a growth chart. (15) Under severe conditions growth in body weight is first affected by a loss of body fat, and later by a loss of muscle tissue. Growth in height continues at this expense of fat and muscle, which changes the contour and composition of the body. Growth in height is most likely to be retarded by malnutrition due to either inadequate diet or disease.

Identification

Growth should be appraised by the best available methods for determining nutritional status. The important sign is that the child should be growing. This can be determined by regular weighing and measuring, and keeping a growth chart (page 195).

When the child does not grow, food intake should be suspected. Growth retarded because of inadequate diet will resume when the diet is improved. The child may then make up all or part of the growth deficit. (9)

Retarded growth in children is usually identified by comparing parameters for a particular child with those in a reference populations. (1, 12, 16) One problem in this practice is the lack of standards for different racial groups. Growth curves are needed for black, Oriental, and Hispanic children. It has been found that black children are smaller at birth than white, but that from age 2 to 14 black children are taller than white. (5) Using a standard for whites may cause some black children who are actually at nutritional risk to appear to be developing normally.

The two most useful measures for evaluating growth are *height for age,* which measures shortness-tallness and *weight for height,* which measures thinness-fatness. Low height for age is defined as being in a range with only 5 percent of the reference population. When weight for height falls in the lowest 5 percent, growth is defined as greatly retarded. When it falls in the top 5 percent, it is indicative of future obesity. (18) *Height for age* is the ratio of height observed to height expected. This is the best measure for use in identifying short stature caused by malnutrition in mother or child. *Weight for height* is the ratio of weight observed to weight expected for the height and sex. This reflects the recent state of undernutrition or overnutrition, while height for age shows the effects of long-term undernutrition that has caused stunting of growth.

In the CDC nutritional surveillance system, it is believed that children whose height for age is in the lowest 5 percent of the reference population have probably had a long-standing undernutrition. Such data on a large number of children in a state or local area indicate the need for intervention to correct undernutrition in the present and to avoid retarded growth in the future. (16)

Prevention

When the graph of the growth record shows that growth is below normal, the cause should be sought, first by appraisal of the intake of nutrients and calories. If dietary inadequacy is found, the diet should be improved. If other factors than diet are involved, there should be a clinical examination to identify the cause, which should then be corrected.

The nutritionist should work to increase the number of children who are monitored and to improve the diet patterns and food intakes of families when needed. This kind of surveillance should be carried on at every family or ambulatory care center and in school, and incorporated into health and nutrition planning.

The nutritionist in one health agency arranged a workshop for teachers, nurses, and school administrators to learn measuring techniques. Each participant practiced the techniques and learned how to record the data on the growth charts and how to interpret the data. Nutritionists can encourage similar training for persons from other schools, can learn the measuring techniques themselves, and teach them to other groups to increase the number of school personnel who can monitor their pupils.

In the past, children in some schools were weighed and measured several times a year, but often the data were not interpreted or used. Under the guidance of a public health nutritionist, the schools in one district started a regular weighing and measuring schedule and set a goal for all children to be of normal weight by the time they finished sixth grade. Following the progress by seeing each child and keeping up its graph was sufficient motivation to get the teachers to participate.

Groups of parents or school personnel can learn to record and evaluate the children's diets and understand the significance of the data in predicting problems and doing something about them.

Treatment

When there is retarded growth, there should be a medical examination and food record with nutritional counseling as indicated to increase the intake of calories and nutrients. Children who attend Children and Youth Clinics or other health programs where direct services are provided will be counseled there for a better diet. Nutritionists who do not provide direct services or who cannot meet all the needs may help solve the problems of children with retarded growth by participating in the teaching of proper techniques of measuring to teachers, nurses, school administrators, and community leaders, or by providing other forms of professional education, or by referring the family to another agency for service.

IRON DEFICIENCY AND IRON-DEFICIENCY ANEMIA

The Ten State Nutrition Survey and the more recent Health and Nutrition Examination Survey both disclosed that iron deficiency is the most prevalent nutrition problem in the United States (page 18). Anemia and iron deficiency are sometimes considered as the same thing; however, iron deficiency as shown by transferrin saturation level occurs before anemia is identified by low levels of hemoglobin or hematocrit. The American Academy of Pediatrics Committee on Nutrition identifies iron deficiency in infants as a transferrin saturation level of under 15 percent. (19) Anemia is the final stage in development of iron deficiency. Its occurrence means that the body's iron stores have been depleted and that serum iron and transferrin saturation are low.

There has been considerable discussion about the levels of hemoglobin and hematocrit that should be used to define anemia, whether it should be 10 or 11 grams hemoglobin and 33 or 35 percent hematocrit for all children or whether there should be a gradation with age. The values used at a particular time should be determined by current practices of the Center for Disease Control. In some cases the state may set the figure, in others it may be done locally. Lower figures will include a few more borderline children.

Anemia in infants is caused by their rapid growth, and anemia in older persons by low iron intake at times of high need, mainly in teenage girls and women. Iron deficiency is believed to cause or be related to a variety of problems in early life, including pallor, irritability, listlessness, sleep problems, abnormal appetite, pica, dislike of eating solid foods, and increased susceptibility to infections. It appears that iron deficiency in some adult women is likewise related to pica, which may disappear soon after iron therapy is started. (25)

Haddy and coworkers report a study of iron status (21) in 109 infants and children from low income families, four months to five years of age. They found that iron deficiency as shown by transferrin saturation levels below 17 percent was not always accompanied by hemoglobin levels of less than 11 grams per 100 milliliters or by hematocrit readings of under 33 percent; ·thus iron deficiency without anemia existed in their infants and, they believe, probably exists in the population at large. They conclude that there is little likelihood of iron overload in this age group and recommend giving an artificial iron supplement. They found also that the results of a single 24-hour dietary record predicted the laboratory findings for each subject. The nutritionist may find that the food record is especially valuable in this situation. Iron deficiency without anemia was found by Haddy and coworkers when protein and calorie intakes met the RDA, but iron intake was at 57 percent, while anemia occurred only when iron intake fell to 40 percent.

Owen (22) found low transferrin saturation levels in 39 percent of upper-middle class children, age one to two years and in 45 percent of lower-middle class children of the same age. He concludes that iron deficiency in preschool children is not related to socioeconomic status.

Theuer (23) has reviewed the literature on iron undernutrition in infancy, concluding that iron deficiency anemia occurs in as many as 60 percent of infants in the United States and that many infants over six months of age have iron deficiency as shown by subnormal transferrin saturation.

These studies suggest that the community nutritionist needs to be concerned with the possibility of iron deficiency in all income levels of infants and preschool children.

Probably a regular diet that provides the RDA of iron will take care of the needs of many girls and women; however, those who need higher amounts should be identified and counseled with emphasis on high iron foods. Anemia must be corrected by an iron supplement since food cannot supply enough iron to meet regular needs and replenish the body stores. The nutritionist must also be alert for low protein intake and for low intakes of other nutrients but the cause of anemia is most likely to be a low iron intake. Special attention should also be given to the iron intake when there is low consumption of lean meat, whole grain products, or dark-green vegetables.

The nutritionist in a health agency where there is central purchasing of pharmaceuticals to be given to patients should check the composition of the iron compounds used to make sure the kind and amount of iron are appropriate. White says (25) that ferrous sulfate USP is the best iron compound for use in oral therapy because it is inexpensive, well absorbed and has few side effects. Supplemental therapy usually involves 30- to 60-milligram doses of ferrous sulfate USP and the tablets should be coated for protection against moisture. According to White, sustained-release preparations should not be used because of the possibility that the iron may be carried past the main sites of absorption in the duodenum and proximal jejunum.

The community nutritionist will probably need to correct in physicians, nurses, and others the belief that hemoglobin and hematocrit levels in the generally accepted range (10 to 11 grams percent for hemoglobin and 33 percent for hematocrit) mean that infants and young children are adequately nourished in respect to iron. As noted above, there is evidence that iron deficiency may exist in the absence of the usual signs of anemia.

Fomon and Egan suggest that efforts for prevention of iron-deficiency anemia in infants and preschool children should be through a nutrition education campaign with parents and professional workers, stressing the need for iron and use of iron-fortified formulas and iron-fortified cereals in preventing anemia. (20)

The high incidence of iron deficiency anemia shown in the recent national surveys has led to a proposal to increase the iron fortification of foods. This has provoked much comment because of possible harmful effects from too-high intakes. The concern expressed is mainly that increased iron fortification of foods might cause excessive iron intake that could result in neutralizing a person's defense against bacteria thus lowering resistance to disease. It appears, however, that possibilities for such side effects are minimal as are those for adverse effects for men who might take in as much as 30 milligrams in a day from iron-enriched foods. The issue of fortification has not been settled.

The USDA has funded a study at Beth Israel Hospital of Boston to evaluate various iron-fortified diets, specifically, to find out whether supplemental iron or iron-fortified foods will prevent the development of iron-deficiency anemia in infants under 15 months. The study will also test the acceptability and safety of various iron-fortified foods. (24)

SUMMARY

Hunger is usually due to poverty or to temporary shortage of food money. Though the community nutritionist may receive many reports of hunger, it is hard to document the reports. The solution may be a matter of finding community resources to provide emergency food or money, but inadequate family income must sometimes be attacked by political means.

Retarded growth occurs in children in all populations in the U.S. This means that the child is not growing at a rate consistent with its potential for growth. This occurs when some nutritional requirement of the child is not met, and is manifested by retarded height and weight or other signs. Prevention of retarded growth must be accomplished by monitoring with regular weighing and measuring.

Iron deficiency is the most prevalent nutrition problem in the United States. Anemia is the final state in development of iron deficiency, caused in infants by rapid growth, and in older persons by inadequate intake of iron. Community nutritionists should be alert for iron deficiency in infants and preschool children in all income groups.

REFERENCES CITED

Hunger, Malnutrition, and Retarded Growth

1. Center for Disease Control, Evaluation of Body Size and Physical Growth of Children, U.S. Dept. of Health, Education, and Welfare, Public Health Service, leaflet, n.d.
2. Christakis, George, ed., Nutritional Assessment in Health Programs, *Am. J. Pub. Health* 63 11/73 Supplement.
3. County of Los Angeles Department of Health Services, *Study of Hunger and Malnutrition,* 1972, unpublished.
4. County of Los Angeles Department of Health Services, *Nutrition of Infants and Young Children,* 1972, unpublished pamphlet.
5. Garn, Stanley M., and Diane C. Clark, Problems in the Nutritional Assessment of Blacks, *Am. J. Pub. Health* 66 3/76 262.
6. Guzman, Miguel A., Impaired Physical Growth and Maturation in Malnourished Populations, in Scrimshaw, Nevin S., and John E. Gordon, eds., *Malnutrition, Learning, and Behavior,* The M.I.T. Press, Cambridge, Mass., Proceedings of an International Conference, March 1 to 3, 1967, 43.
7. Johnson, Howard W., Society, Nutrition, and Research, in Scrimshaw, Nevin S., and John E. Gordon, eds., *Malnutrition, Learning, and Behavior,* The M.I.T. Press, Cambridge MA, Proceedings of an International Conference, March 1 to 3, 1967, 2.
8. Martin, Ethel Austin, *Robert's Nutrition Work with Children,* University of Chicago Press, 1954, 65.
9. Ibid., 130.
10. Ibid., 164.
11. Mauer, Alvin M., Malnutrition—Still a Common Problem for Children in the United States, *Clin. Ped.,* 14 1/75 23.
12. NCHS Growth Charts, 1976, National Center for Health Statistics,

Monthly Vital Statistics Report, (HRA) 76-1120, U.S. Dept. of Health, Education, and Welfare, Rockville MD, 25 6/22/76 Supplement.

13. NCHS Sees End to Trend of Increasing Child Size, *Nation's Health,* 7/76 3.

14. Robson, J. R. K., F. A. Larkin, J. H. Bursick, and K. P. Perri, Growth Standards for Infants and Children, *Pediatrics,* 56 12/75 1014.

15. Smith, David W., Growth Deficiency Including Failure To Thrive, in Smith, David, ed. and Richard E. Marshall, *Introduction to Clinical Pediatrics,* W. B. Saunders Co., Philadelphia, 1972, 148.

16. U.S. Dept. of Health, Education, and Welfare, Center for Disease Control, *Nutrition Surveillance,* 1/75 14.

17. U.S. Dept. of Health, Education, and Welfare, *Preliminary Findings of the First Health and Nutrition Examination Survey, United States, 1971–72,* DHEW Pub. No. (HRA) 74-1219-1, U.S. Dept. of Health, Education, and Welfare, Rockville MD.

18. Watson, Ernest, and George H. Lowrey, *Growth and Development in Children,* 5th ed., 1967, Year Book Medical Publishers, Inc., Chicago.

Iron Deficiency and Iron-Deficiency Anemia

19. American Academy of Pediatrics, Committee on Nutrition, Iron Balance, and Requirements in Infancy, *Pediatrics,* 43 169 134.

20. Fomon, Samuel J., and Mary C. Egan, Infants, Children, and Adolescents, in *U.S. Nutrition Policies in the Seventies,* Jean Mayer, ed., W. H. Freeman and Co, San Francisco, 1973, 29.

21. Haddy, Theresa B., Claire Jurkowski, Howard Brody, David J. Kallen, and Dorice M. Czajka-Narins, Iron Deficiency With and Without Anemia in Infants and Children, *Am. J. Dis. Child.* 128 12/74 787.

22. Owen, George M., A. Harold Lubin, and Philip J. Garry, Preschool Children in the United States: Who Has Iron Deficiency? *J. Pediatrics,* 79 10/71 563.

23. Theuer, Richard C., Iron Undernutrition in Infancy, *Clin. Ped.* 13 6/74 522.

24. U.S. Dept. of Agriculture, *Food and Home Notes,* Washington DC, 12/8/75 4.

25. White, Hilda S., Dietary Iron and Anemia, *Nutrition & the M.D.,* 2 11/75 1.

CHAPTER 22

PREVENTION AND CONTROL OF MALNUTRITION
III. WEIGHT AND OBESITY

Two intertwined problems, those of inactivity and obesity, have a vital relationship to good health and merit attention as an important part of the community nutrition program because there is a higher incidence of heart disease, hypertension, diabetes, arthritis, and other chronic diseases among the obese than among persons of normal weight. Weight control, which includes both prevention and correction of obesity, is an important component of the community nutrition program.

Obesity increases the hazard of coronary heart disease, high blood pressure, diabetes, arthritis, and other diseases. Life expectancy is decreased among the obese in direct proportion to the degree of obesity. (12) In theory, obesity along with most of its ill effects can be reversed, for example, diabetes and high blood pressure frequently disappear when excess weight is lost. In most parts of the United States but not all, overweight is a greater problem than underweight.

In a specific community nutrition program, it is important to identify the existing problems and to program according to the need. This section will consider some aspects of the weight control problem and some suggestions for program planning. Because of the important role of the nutritionist, the subject will be covered in detail. The first emphasis in the community program should be on *prevention,* but many programs will also include clinical care with obesity correction.

IDENTIFYING THE OBESE

The first problem that is encountered is that there are no precise definitions of overweight and underweight. The determining factor is the amount of fat tissue. When there is too much, the individual is obese or overweight; when there is too little, the individual is underweight. An individual may also be overweight from unusual muscle development, which by definition is not obesity.

Mayer uses the term "overweight" saying that people who are too fat will find it easier to use that term in relation to themselves than "obesity" since "they tend to think of obesity as denoting a degree of adiposity far more extreme than their own and, in fact, take it as an insult." (5) This suggests that terminology may be an important factor in the success of those who work with the obese.

Gordon (2) designates any body weight in excess of 20 percent above "normal" as obese, and says that lesser degrees of abnormality should be labeled as "overweight." He states that identification of obesity should be based on total amount of body fat, but often available equipment limits identification to use of the Metropolitan Life Insurance height-weight tables although these provide an inexact measure. Robinson states that the best weight for a specific individual is not known, but it is generally considered that 10 percent above or below the desirable weight for an individual as shown in the Metropolitan Life Insurance Company tables is within the normal range, that 10- to 20-percent deviation marks a danger zone while more than 20 percent below is underweight. (9)

Different nutritionists, physicians, and physiologists use various methods for estimating the amount of fatty tissue, which is the real measure of obesity. Height, weight, and triceps skinfold are used for all ages. Head and chest circumference are used for infants and preschoolers. Arm circumference is used for all ages beginning with preschoolers, while subscapular skinfold is used for adults. *Nutritional Assessment in Health Programs* (1) explains the use of various measures and gives tables for identifying the percent of deviation from a standard for various ages. The new growth tables for children were discussed on page 195.

WEIGHT REDUCTION

The weight control problem exists when food intake provides more calories than are needed for energy expenditure. A review of the literature (10) on weight control programs with exercise components concludes that:

1. Readjustment of energy balance, preferably by increasing activity and decreasing calories at the same time, produces weight loss in most obese persons.

2. Energy expenditure through activity and exercise increases the success of weight control programs.

3. Biochemical differences, psychologically based compulsions, time of eating, and other factors also play a part in weight control.

Treatment of obesity in health center patients is a medical responsibility, but the nutritionist should participate with the physician in developing policies about diet and activity. The diet should be adequate in nutrients and must be one that the patient can follow. Activity should be extensive enough to enable the individual to lose weight on a diet that has enough food to provide all necessary nutrients. Joining weight control groups has proved valuable for some obese persons. One of the valuable functions that a weight control group may perform is to provide emotional support. Attending a group, regular weighing, and exchange of experience with others, or having friendly sympathetic counseling in a salon or gym may provide this emotional support.

Gordon suggests (2) that a weight reduction regime be built around the following principles: a nutritionally adequate diet that provides less food energy per day than is used for metabolic needs; increased energy output through more physical activity; facilitation of excretion of metabolic water as it is produced; resolving of serious emotional problems responsible for compulsive eating; and limited use of drugs since there is little justification for them in the usual case.

There are many reasons for the high rate of failure in weight reduction. Basically, the cause is failure to follow the weight control diet and program of increased activity. Probably the most common reasons for disliking a low calorie diet are that it includes unfamiliar foods such as leafy green vegetables, or it omits foods that are important to the individual such as bacon, ice cream, and butter, or it fails to use familiar methods of preparation such as seasoning foods with large amounts of cream and butter. For success to be achieved, the calorie content must be lowered while the characteristic food pattern is followed so that the individual will eat the diet.

The purpose of increased activity as a weight control measure is to change the body composition by burning fatty tissue while building lean tissue, as well as to use additional energy to prevent its being stored as body fat. This helps to remove flabby fat and build a trim, firm body.

Much time and effort have been spent in attempts to explain the reasons for overeating. It is obvious, however, that there are a variety of reasons for the excess energy intake and that in many cases it is not possible to establish the regime of smaller food intake and greater energy expenditure. One of the most significant reasons is that among both youth and adults obesity is frequently accompanied by emotional problems that must be dealt with before obesity can be attacked. The practice of using food as a panacea for all problems may be started by the mother giving the baby food every time it cries. Coaxing a child to eat more than it wants may later grow into a habit of regular overeating, and using rich, sweet foods as childhood rewards may result in an adult who continues to use such foods in this way.

Young discusses (15) the emotional problems encountered in some patients and the importance of analyzing the real reasons for overeating, avoiding any moral connotation. She believes that weight reduction should not be attempted in persons with deep emotional problems until those problems have been relieved. She recommends a psychiatric screening before the obese patient is referred for counseling to avoid feelings of frustration and failure for both patient and counselor.

The most difficult form of adult obesity to treat and least likely of success is that in the adult who was an obese teenager. When weight reduction is critical from a health point of view, it is a matter for clinical nutrition practice and must be attempted even knowing that the statistics are against success. Reeducation of obese persons must include exercise, design for living, and other interests as well as food.

Prevention of Obesity

The correction of obesity in youths and adults in the United States has generally met with limited success, so prevention is of great importance. A prevention program will be needed throughout the entire life cycle, with an effective weight control regimen of eating and exercise incorporated into all public and professional education.

Prevention must begin in infancy by identifying those who are potentially obese. Obese parents tend to have obese children. If both parents are obese, 80 percent of the offspring will be obese. If only one parent is obese, the figure drops to 40 percent, while if neither parent is obese, there is a further drop to 7 percent. (11) Neumann (7) believes that the incidence of obesity in early life ranges from 3 percent to 15 percent and that intervention is indicated for the obese infant. She recommends breast feeding, postponing solids until four or five months, monitoring weight gain, education of the mother, and allowing free movement of arms and legs for physical activity. She believes that even at this age activity affects food intake.

Infant obesity may be diagnosed from measures of height and weight, history of obesity in the family, emotional relationship between infant and parents, and food intake. When food intake is normal and there is no history of obesity, infant obesity does not present a problem.

Many parents believe that a fat baby is a good baby and that an excess of available food is a sign of good care. They should be helped to learn that normal weight is a better sign and that excessive food for the infant may set the stage for a lifelong weight control problem.

The nutritionist may need to point out to the clinician, nurse, and mother that overfeeding and early introduction of solids may increase the number of fat cells in susceptible infants, laying the foundation for obesity in later life.

Clinicians sometimes prescribe a nonfat or lowfat milk formula to limit the amount of saturated fat, to restrict calories, or for medical reasons. When this is done, the clinician should provide continuing supervision to be sure the infant is growing normally and prescribe a supplement of linoleic acid and vitamins A and D, if necessary. A formula of lowfat milk or half whole milk and half nonfat is preferable to one of all nonfat milk, which may be low in calories, linoleic acid and fat-soluble vitamins. (8)

Winick believes that dietary treatment for obesity should begin in infancy when there is excessive weight gain. (14) He points out that children from poor families are leaner than children from more affluent families, but that some of the differences are due to population group rather than to food intake. For example, black infants are usually fatter than white infants, but the situation is reversed in later childhood. Puerto Ricans are fatter than either black or white.

Stunkard emphasizes that it is important to establish good dietary and exercise patterns in early life and that physical inactivity and a highfat, high caloric diet leads to adult obesity and coronary heart disease. (12)

Agency policies about diet during early life should be developed by physician and nutritionist. Policies should include age for introduction of solids and whether nonfat or lowfat milk may be used instead of whole milk.

The nutritionist should prepare a nutritional care plan when indicated and see that the mother is instructed in fitting the infant's food needs into the family diet.

Preventive measures are needed at other strategic periods such as age 1 to 6, adolescence, early adulthood, and pregnancy. Wilson, Fisher and Fuqua have suggested as an approach to prevention that a gain of three pounds should "be a signal to begin curtailing one's energy intake or increasing one's energy expenditure." (13) At that point a reduction of saturated fats and sugars would probably take care of the excess calorie consumption.

Achieving weight control by prevention will require many changes in the attitudes of individuals and society which can only be accomplished by an all pervasive campaign of public education and information. It will require that people learn that wise eating is knowing when the body's need for food has been met, and that pressing larger amounts of food on anyone, child or adult, is contributing to obesity and ill health. Ikeda (3) has observed that the desire or need to learn about weight control is directly related to the desire or need to change weight. Creating that desire or need may have to be the first effort.

An important influence on everyone is advertising on radio and television and in newspapers and magazines. Some observers believe that this may be the most potent influence for habit change. News and feature stories on radio and television and in the newspapers may also affect practices. Nutritionists may find this a feasible way to spread good information, or may be able to modify poor information by offering suggestions and content for news and feature items. Local colleges or universities may be interested in conducting research or studies on successful weight losers to find out what factors are associated with successful weight loss. The nutritionist may also study the records of successful reducers to learn what regimens are most effective under particular circumstances.

Program Reports.   In one health department, the nutritionist taught normal diet and weight control to representatives of a weight control group who, in turn, taught the same material to the group itself. Volunteer dietitians attended the groups to answer questions. Once it was established that acceptable information was dispensed, the groups provided a resource to which individuals seeking such help could be referred. Thus a weight control group may serve as a community resource provided that the attitudes and information dispensed are acceptable to the nutritionist and the medical community.

The community nutritionist may organize or conduct professional education on the nutritional aspects of weight control, participate with others in planning how to identify needs and how to use available resources, and develop new resources when there are few or none. Health educators, social workers, nurses, and others will be concerned about the same problems and may be interested in cooperating on their solution.

Suggestions for a specific program can be found in reports of similar activities. Even programs with limited success can give valuable ideas. However, there are few reports in the literature on weight reduction programs in a community nutrition setting. Successful weight reduction in a group attending a local health department was informally reported in a letter to the editor by Lovell. (4) The nutritionist counseled low income obese patients, following them for one year, at the end of which period 62 percent of the patients still maintained their weight loss. Lovell concluded that nutrition counseling with physician support can be effective in weight reduction.

The community nutritionist needs to survey the resources for help with weight control. These may be provided by local voluntary agencies such as the Heart Association, Diabetes Association, and hypertension groups, by nonprofit weight control groups such as TOPS (*Take Off Pounds Sensibly*) and Overeaters Anonymous, or by weight control groups or conditioning facilities organized for profit. There are also a host of locally operated spas, medical reducing clinics, camps for overweight children, and similar organizations dedicated to weight reduction.

Yule and coauthors (16) report the results of a reducing program conducted in ten group sessions by the American Red Cross, Rochester (NY) Chapter. Of the 549 women who registered for these classes, 112 attended nine or ten lessons with about one-fifth losing more than 15 pounds. Two years later 25 percent had lost weight since the last lesson and 42 percent had maintained their weight or gained less than 3 pounds. It was concluded that success in weight loss might be expected in participants who completed the program.

The nutritionist who is preparing to lead a group should search the literature for related programs and use them as a source of ideas.

Behavior Modification in Weight Reduction Programs.

Obesity is the result of eating habits that determine calorie intake and of activity patterns that determine calorie expenditure, rather than being mainly a sign of underlying psychologic disorder. Monitoring by outside sources is not a feasible method of control of the amount of food because it is under the individual's control. (25) Jordan points out that obesity is a state of equilibrium acquired over a long period of time, so that it must be accepted that weight loss will also be a long process. (23) Though many persons lose weight using various methods, there has been less success in maintaining the loss. (18) There is some indication that behavior modification and calorie-controlled diet used together for weight loss will be more successful than either alone. (26)

Behavior modification is a method of changing behavior by cultivating the desired behavior through reinforcement with rewards or other methods, and by minimizing undesired behavior through ignoring it or emphasizing the undesirable consequences.

The behavior modification technique is useful for changing food practices. Though it may be used in other programs, its major use in nutrition education has been in weight losing.

Jordan names three related techniques of experimental psychology: behavior modification, behavior therapy, and experimental analysis of behavior, any of which may be applied to changing learned behavior. (23) Operant conditioning therapy and image shaping are related methods.

The theory of behavior modification is that behavior is determined by the environment and is influenced by its immediate consequences rather than by its future results such as weight change, heart disease, diabetes, or shorter life. There must be an immediate reward for changed behavior to reinforce the effort for change or it has no influence. The objective of nutritional behavior modification is to change eating practices by changing lifestyle. The purpose of the method is to help the individual make permanent changes in the practices or habits that result in overeating.

To change eating behavior, the circumstances that surround eating are changed. Blake used techniques of elimination (e.g., no other activity while eating), of suppression (e.g., having another person monitor eating), and strengthening (e.g., making the diet more desirable to the individual). (18) In some programs the behavior was changed without making the individual aware of the change. (34) Behavior modification for weight control includes changes in practice related to both eating and activity. (23)

Program Reports. Behavior modification in treatment of obesity is still in the research stage. Most of the programs reported were research studies with clinic patients. Results in them have been generally better than in individual counseling or other methods of weight loss. (31)

Some behavior modification programs started with analysis and handling of eating behavior followed by extensive nutrition education after changes in practices had been accomplished. Assertiveness training was incorporated into some programs on the theory that individuals who overeat are unable to control their behavior. (21) This corresponds with the long acceptance of the idea that fat people are good-natured and agreeable. A technique used in some programs is to have participants write down what they plan to eat for a meal, but reducing the actual intake by crossing out one food before they eat.

Stern, at the Institute for Behavioral Awareness in New Jersey, conducted a 16-week program with 69 adults in small-group settings. (29) Members identified the consequences of overeating and kept extensive records. The course did not include a diet prescription. The purpose of the course was to help the individuals learn to handle their internal behavior by image building that would enable them to change their own behavior. The women and men in the group lost an average of 16 pounds in 14 weeks and 70 percent retained their losses for a year.

During a course in training nutrition graduate students how to use behavior techniques with patients, the students treated 12 patients using these techniques. All patients made good weight losses. (19)

A nutritionist and a psychologist conducted a weight control group using behavior modification techniques with eight women. They used a group of mixed ethnic and racial composition (four black, four white, and one Puerto Rican) as representative of their regular clinic population. The project was successful for the white and Puerto Rican women who lost from 14 to 40 percent of the intended weight change. There was little change in the weight of the black women. Lack of family support was one reason for this difference. (33) The black women generally received less encouragement at home than did the other women.

Blake, a dietitian, reports (18) that 44 patients who completed a 12-session weight control course using behavior modification lost weight more consistently and in a shorter time (29 percent lost 10 to 20 pounds in three months) than clinic patients on individual counseling (23 percent lost 10 to 20 pounds in five months).

Orkow and Ross used behavior modification, nutrition education, and an exercise program in a Colorado weight control project with six women who were 6 percent to 50 percent above their desirable weights. After the course of eight weekly group sessions, each woman had lost weight. Six months later, five of the six still weighed less than they had at the beginning although only three had continued to lose. (27)

A behavior modification program not related to weight control was used to change the food practices of a group of Head Start mothers with the objective of increasing the use of new and nutritious foods. The mothers later applied the same tactics to change their families' eating behavior. (34)

Orkow and Ross consider behavior modification as "a relatively simple technique which teachers and parents can learn to apply as successfully as specially-trained persons in the field of psychology. It is based on the principle that an individual will continue behavior that is rewarded and discontinue behavior that is not." (27)

The nutritionist or dietitian who wants to use behavior modification must know group techniques and behavior modification techniques. Blake learned these two techniques by studying literature, attending classes, and observing groups. While making specific plans for her own groups, she obtained consultation from a staff psychiatrist. While conducting the groups she was joined by a nurse, psychologist, and a physical therapist. (18)

The possibility of training volunteer leaders to use behavior modification techniques was considered by Jordan and Levitz. They trained a formerly obese business executive in the method, finding that the group with which he worked made a good response in weight-losing. The group members were responsive to the leader's attempts to change their eating behavior. (24)

Discussion. Compared with the results of other methods for weight losing programs, behavior modification appears to offer a way to achieve greater loss in a shorter time. In many cases the weight loss has been sustained for a longer period of time. Used with a group it makes teaching more effective than individual counseling and members are able to support each other. Advance information should include a specific structure for subject matter, an outline of topics, number of classes, and other details about the course. (18)

Behavior modification has proved effective with adults who had an adult-onset obesity, but not with adults with juvenile-onset obesity. Adults whose obesity was the result of continuing their food patterns from adolescence into adulthood profited from nutrition education, but adults whose obesity began in adolescence were unable to do so and some needed psychotherapy. (22)

Levitz has reported the elements of behavior therapy and suggested readings to give the nutritionist a general background in the technique. He emphasizes the need to individualize the method for each client and to have a systematic logical plan for the course. (25)

A problem in using behavior modification is that participants become discouraged when they reach a weight-loss plateau, a common occurrence at various stages of weight loss. Another is that participants tend to drop out when they reach their goals for weight loss. Though the latter disrupts a research study, it appears to be a natural consequence of having reached the desired weight. Various incentives have been used to reward participation for remaining with the group.

Obviously behavior modification is a means to an end, that is, a way to reduce food intake or increase activity, or both; the method does not change the principle that body weight is in balance between energy intake and energy output. Neither is there, as some have believed, a mystic principle at work in behavior modification technique. It would be a good addition to the nutritionist's skills for use also in other areas of nutrition education.

SUMMARY

The hazards of obesity are well known as it is a factor in development of diabetes, high blood pressure, and heart disease. Obesity is usually defined as a body weight of 20 percent or more above normal.

Weight control should begin in early infancy and continue as a part of the everyday lifestyle. It is important because of the hazards of overweight and the difficulty of correcting obesity.

Behavior modification, which concentrates on changing the circumstances that determine eating practices, has been successful in some weight-losing programs, but its long-range effects are not yet known.

REFERENCES CITED

Weight Control and Obesity

1. Christakis, George, ed., *Nutritional Assessment in Health Programs, Am. J. Pub. Health*, 63 11/73 Supplement.
2. Gordon, E. S., The Present Concent of Obesity, *Med. Times*, 97 5/69 148.
3. Ikeda, Joanne P., Expressed Nutrition Needs of Low-Income Homemakers, *J. Nutr. Educ.*, 7 7-9/75 106.
4. Lovell, Helen, Weight Neighborhood Health Program, Letters to the Editor, *J. Am. Med. Assoc.*, 218 11/15/71 1049.
5. Mayer, Jean, Overweight, Causes, Cost and Control, Prentice-Hall, Inc., Englewood Cliffs NJ, 1968, vii.
6. National Research Council, Food and Nutrition Board, *Recommended Dietary Allowances*, 8th ed., National Academy of Sciences, Washington DC, 1974 26.
7. Neumann, Charlotte G., Prevention and Management of Obesity in Infancy, *Nutrition & the M.D.*, 1 7/75 1.
8. *Nutrition of Infants and Young Children*, County of Los Angeles, Department of Health Services, Los Angeles, unpublished pamphlet, 4/72.
9. Robinson, Corinne H., *Normal and Therapeutic Nutrition*, 14th ed., Macmillan Co., New York, 1972, 417.
10. Rodert, Ellen R., and Jessie C. Obert, *Nutritionist's Guide to Activity in Weight Control Programs*, County of Los Angeles, Department of Health Services, Los Angeles, unpublished pamphlet, 10/74.
11. Stare, Frederick J., in *Obesity: Data and Directions for the 70s*, MEDCOM Learning System, Richmond VA, 1974 14.
12. Stunkard, Albert J., The Obese: Background and Programs, in *U.S. Nutrition Policies in the Seventies*, Jean Mayer, ed., W. H. Freeman and Co., San Francisco, 1973, 30.
13. Wilson, Eva D., Katherine H. Fisher, and Mary E. Fuqua, *Principles of Nutrition*, 3rd ed., John Wiley & Sons, Inc., New York, 1975, 447.
14. Winick, Myron, Childhood Obesity. *Nutr. Today*, 9 5-6/74 9.
15. Young, Charlotte M., Norman S. Moore, Kathleen Berresford, Betty McKee Einset, and Betty Greer Waldner, The Problem of the Obese Patient, *J. Am. Diet. Assoc.* 31 11/55 1111.
16. Yule, June B., Ethel L. Marth, and Charlotte M. Young, Weight Control: A Community Program, *J. Am. Diet. Assoc.*, 33 1/57 47.

Behavior Modification

17. Bandura, A., *Principles of Behavior Modification*, Holt, Rinehart and Winston, New York, 1969.
18. Blake, Alma, Group Approach to Weight Control: Behavior Modification, Nutrition, and Health Education, *J. Am. Diet. Assoc.*, 69 12/76 645.

19. Brightwell, Dennis R., and Catherine L. Sloan, Graduate Students and Faculty Learn Behavior Therapy of Obesity, *J. Nutr. Educ.,* 8 4–6/76 71.

20. Dosti, Rose, Behavior Modification a New Way to Diet, *Los Angeles Times,* March 27, 1975.

21. Dosti, Rose, Life-Style Assault on Obesity, *Los Angeles Times,* Jan. 15, 1976.

22. Grinker, Joel, Behavioral and Metabolic Consequences of Weight Reduction, *J. Am. Diet. Assoc.,* 62 1/73 30.

23. Jordan, Henry A., In Defense of Body Weight, *J. Am. Diet. Assoc.,* 62 1/73 17.

24. Jordan, Henry A., and Leonard S. Levitz, Behavior Modification in a Self-Help Group, *J. Am. Diet. Assoc.,* 52 1/73 27.

25. Levitz, Leonard S., Behavior Therapy in Treating Obesity, *J. Am. Diet. Assoc.,* 52 1/73 22.

26. Levitz, Leonard S. and Albert J. Stunkard, A Therapeutic Coalition for Obesity: Behavior Modification and Patient Self-Help, *Am. J. Psychiat.,* 131 1974 423.

27. Orkow, Bonnie M. and Judy L. Ross, Weight Reduction Through Nutrition Education and Personal Counseling, 7 4–6/75 65.

28. Paulsen, B. K., R. N. Lutz, W. T. McReynolds, M. B. Kohrs, Behavior Therapy for Weight Control: Long-Term Results of Two Programs with Nutritionists as Therapists, *Am. J. Clin. Nutr., 29* 8/76 880.

29. Stern, Frances, Weight Control Through Imagery Training, *Nutrition News,* National Dairy Council, 39 12/76 13.

30. Stuart, R. B., and B. Davis, *Slim Chance in a Fat World: Behavioral Control of Obesity,* Research Press, Champaign IL, 1972.

31. Stunkard, Albert J., The Obese: Background and Programs, Ch. 3 in Mayer, Jean ed., *U.S. Nutrition Policies in the Seventies,* W. H. Freeman and Co., San Francisco, 1973.

32. Ullman, L. P., and L. Krasner, *Case Studies in Behavior Modification,* Holt, Rinehart and Winston, New York, 1965.

33. Weisenberg, Matisyohu, and Elizabeth Fray, What's Missing in the Treatment of Obesity by Behavior Modification?, *J. Am. Diet. Assoc.,* 65 10/74 410.

34. Zimmerman, Robert and Nancy Munro, Changing Head Start Mothers' Food Attitudes and Practices. *J. Nutr. Educ.* 4 Spring/72 66.

CHAPTER

23 ACTIVITY AND WEIGHT CONTROL

In the past the role of the nutritionist in weight control programs was concerned mainly with diet for weight losing as planner, motivator, and instructor, a role generally accepted by physicians and other members of the health team. The 1974 recommendation of the National Research Council, Food and Nutrition Board (10) for increased activity for weight control mandated a new responsibility for the nutritionist and dietitian. This was to promote exercise and to plan and instruct for increased expenditure of energy as a regular part of a healthful lifestyle. Weight control, that is, maintenance of normal weight, is recommended as part of a nutritional care plan for all individuals.

This necessitates a new point of view for many nutritionists and other members of the health team. They must correct an impression formerly held by many professionals as well as by the public that increased activity was not significant in weight control because the increase in energy expenditure was small and was accompanied by a greater appetite, which nullified the results of a greater energy expenditure. It is now apparent that the increased activity results in significantly greater energy expenditure and may actually decrease the appetite rather than increase it. For these reasons increased activity should be a part of every weight control program.

Weight control as it is considered here includes a lifelong regimen for achieving and maintaining normal weight as well as correcting weight when it is above the normal range. A moderate degree of underweight is generally considered to be acceptable and perhaps desirable.

The nutritionist's role in weight control indicates that the nutritionist, like the nurse, pharmacist, and other members of the health team, should assume responsibilities previously considered inappropriate. It is just as logical for the nutritionist to counsel on exercise as for the physician, physical therapist, or nurse to counsel on diet. This means that the nutritionist must acquire a background in the principles of physical fitness, the mechanism of calorie expenditure, and the biochemical effects of activity in order to teach patients and clinic staff about the benefits of exercise, and the nutritionist must learn to assess the individual's weight picture by taking anthropometric measurements and planning the exercise program. The nutritionist should look upon increased activity and exercise programs as beneficial for everyone unless prohibited by a medical problem. Exercise is now generally recognized as beneficial to most individuals, including post-coronary patients.

PROGRAMING FOR EXERCISE

Community nutritionists have many opportunities to influence the activity expenditures of both the well public and ambulatory patients. They have also the responsibility and the opportunity to identify existing community resources and to lead the way in developing new resources. Most important, the nutritionist should lead in the development of new attitudes about activity and exercise among both professional persons and the public.

The nutritionist will be in somewhat of a dilemma on reading statements that exercise should be carried out only under medical supervision and only after an exercise or stress test. Following these requirements would prohibit most leisure exercise and recreational sports and would deny most persons their benefits because they do not know a physician who is accustomed to practicing preventive medicine or they cannot afford the cost of the stress test.

Thus the requirements appear to be unrealistic, impractical, and unlikely to be followed. Since weight control is of much importance to good nutrition, the nutritionist is the logical member of the health team to interpret medical recommendations and to assume responsibility for helping individuals and groups develop more effective paths to weight control.

There seems to be little chance of any problem resulting from a gradually initiated, sensibly performed exercise program for the individual who does not have a known cardiac problem, diabetes, or gross obesity. Cummings states it this way: "As long as any exercise program is started gradually and performed sensibly, there is little chance for precipitating any cardiac disaster whether the patient has a known cardiac problem or not." (7)

One physician has suggested that the leader of a weight control group can safely advise a walking program for any member who has not had a myocardial infarction, heart attack, coronary thrombosis, or an abnormal electrocardiogram, and that asking the individual specific questions about these conditions will usually produce sufficient answers. If an individual appears uncertain, it may be advisable to obtain a physician's statement before giving advice about increased activity.

Using another approach Zohman (14) gives a 25-question "Medical Questionnaire" designed to be self-administered and to identify conditions that contraindicate exercise until after a medical checkup and exercise stress test. The questions are designed for "yes" or "no" answers and the individual who answers "yes" to even one question is advised to see a physician before starting an exercise regime.

The nutritionist may be involved in planning and instructing for five types of regimen related to weight control:

1. Individuals and groups, of normal weight or less than 20 percent above normal weight, who are interested in maintaining normal weight or in small weight losses.

2. Parents concerned about the development of obesity in their infants or small children.

3. Individuals for whom weight loss is desirable but not critical, with less serious diagnoses such as moderate hypertension, family history of diabetes or heart disease, or slightly elevated blood cholesterol. Most of these patients will be under medical care and should have had a physician's advice about exercise.

4. Patients for whom weight loss is a critical part of medical care, often grossly or moderately obese with diabetes, infarction, severe hypertension, arthritis or psychological problems. These patients will be under medical care and the nutritionist should cooperate with the physician in determining the weight-losing regimen of diet and exercise.

5. Nonobese patients who want to lose weight for cosmetic reasons. The nutritionist should discourage the desire for excessive leanness by counseling. Consideration of body type, measurement of body fat by skinfold calipers, and comparison with height-weight charts can be used to show the amount of body fat and the effect of further weight loss. The need for an exercise program to modify body composition without weight loss should be emphasized.

The usual concept of exercise fostered by traditional school physical education programs is based on calisthenics and similar exercises. Though these have some value in building muscle and in developing flexibility and joint mobility, the actual increase in energy consumption is small and of little value in weight control. Calisthenics are mainly of value in conjunction with vigorous exercise and may be used as warmup before starting the main exercise.

Considerable attention has also been given to heavy lifting and other isometric-type exercises that derive their benefit from tensing muscles against weights or immovable objects. Though they are of value for strengthening specific muscles and building lean tissue, they should be used with caution in weight control because they present a danger to some individuals by producing a rise in blood pressure, which increases cardiac work.

The most extensive benefit from exercise is from a vigorous type sustained over an hour or more, which achieves two objectives, weight control and stress for the heart and circulatory system. Fast walking, jogging, bicycling, and aerobic dancing can be used. This type of exercise should be vigorous enough to result in puffing and increased body heat, usually evidenced by sweating. Though the greater benefit for the circulatory system comes when the exercise period is of high intensity and lasts at least thirty minutes, if the main reason for exercise is increased calorie expenditure the intensity should be moderated to permit a longer duration, for the longer time results in a greater expenditure of calories than a shorter time even at higher intensity. (13)

Noncompetitive sports are better for energy expenditure than competitive sports such as tennis, basketball, baseball, handball, and badminton because these sports have periods of varying intensity rather than a steady intensity that permits a continuous expenditure of energy.

STARTING A PROGRAM OF INCREASED ACTIVITY

The term "increased activity" rather than "exercise" is used here to point out that the first efforts with many individuals may need to start this way. Except in cases in which individuals or groups are already motivated toward exercise, the nutritionist must be very moderate in the initial suggestions. The first attempts at change may need to be directed at small increases in energy expenditure in daily living, especially when the subjects must depend on individual rather than group programs. Each program should be based on information about the extent of activity obtained along with the food record. This should disclose how much time the individual spends in walking and other exercise, how much in watching television, and in activity on the job or in home chores.

The person who has been extremely inactive may need to start with less lying in bed, less sitting, and more walking. In most cases the nutritionist may encourage individuals and groups to spend calories all the time by taking the stairs instead of the elevator, parking farther from destinations, and doing one's own errands instead of sending a secretary or a child. The increase in activity in the course of regular daily living will be enough to control weight for many individuals. Though vigorous exercise would be beneficial to most individuals and should be promoted, it must be recognized that most persons will not engage in such a program.

Once an individual is motivated to start a planned exercise program by a physician's recommendation or for other reasons, the nutritionist may advise about the value and significance of specific kinds of exercise and about starting the program.

There are several good references for advice about starting and managing an exercise program. Any activity that is familiar to the individual through past or present participation offers a good starting point. The individual who already walks, swims, or plays golf or who has done so in the past should be encouraged to increase the frequency or resume the same activity. (5, 6, 12, 13)

Different procedures are in order in advising individuals about their exercise programs when they are under a physician's care and when they are not. When the patient is under a physician's care, the nutritionist should discuss with the clinician the activity level and the benefit of exercise in the weight control program, then collaborate in making the diet-activity plan. The nutritionist handles or arranges the instruction on diet and exercise and participates in case conferences on patient progress. When an individual in a weight control group is under care of a private physician, the nutritionist may suggest that the patient ask the private physician for approval of an increased activity program.

When there are no apparent reasons for not exercising and the individual is not under immediate medical care, the nutritionist may suggest a walking program starting with 10 minutes a day at a comfortable speed, increasing gradually to 30 minutes. The first 10 minutes should be a warm-up period, the second 10 should be taken as fast as possible without reaching the point of quick, hard breathing, and during the last 10 minutes the speed should be gradually decreased for a cooling down period. The time may later be increased to one hour with 15 minutes warmup, 30 minutes fast walking, and 15 minutes cooling down. There should be at least four exercise periods a week while a daily walk will give even greater benefit. Walking is also the only exercise suitable for a grossly obese person since more vigorous activity will not be possible. (3, 13)

Individuals who are ready for more vigorous exercise can get it by jogging, running, bicycling, swimming, or hiking. Rowing is another good exercise when a rowing machine is available and combined with the stationary bicycle will exercise all the large muscles. The intensity and duration of any of these exercises are easily controlled by the individual. The nutritionist can help the individual learn to evaluate the exercise program by teaching recognition of the level of activity at which stress begins to occur, and can advise about developing capacity for more difficult or prolonged exercise, which is produced by regular training that causes stress. A gradual start on a program with adequate conditioning will avoid muscle soreness, breathing problems, and other difficulties. (13)

Time allowed for warming up in each exercise allows the body to adapt to the stress of going from a resting state to a working one. The cooling off period provided allows for a gradual change from work to rest and specifically avoids accumulation of blood in the feet which may occur when activity is suddenly stopped. This occasionally results in nausea or fainting. Immediate showering or steam baths without a cooling off period may also result in these problems. (13)

Some patients will express concern about their physical safety while engaging in an exercise program. It is true of an exercise period that there is no way activity can be completely safe, but knowing that exercise is prescribed for coronary patients and that they can learn to monitor their own programs by noting symptoms is often encouraging.

EXERCISE RESOURCES

Available resources may be located by a survey of the community. These may include existing exercise groups such as YWCA, YMCA, adult education programs, and health clubs. Many YWCA's and YMCA's now have fitness programs for both sexes and all ages, and some have started aerobic dancing and some clubs for retired persons have exercise classes. The nutritionist should have information about such programs and about those operated as profit-making enterprises. This will make it possible to guide individuals into suitable well operated programs that meet their objectives. When there are no existing resources, it may be possible to mobilize a community to initiate one.

There are a number of factors that the nutritionist can use in evaluating a resource to which individuals may be referred for exercise and instruction. Cost, background and training of the leaders, available facilities and equipment, and nutrition information dispensed are all indicators of the quality of the program. The last-named, nutrition information, is easiest for the nutritionist to evaluate; perhaps no further evaluation need be made when the nutrition information includes the recommendation of a high protein-low carbohydrate diet or a high fat-high protein regime or use of excess vitamin, protein, or other food supplements. However, there are programs that are excellent in every respect *except* for the nutrition information they dispense.

A facility should have some provisions for vigorous exercise, such as a swimming pool, a running track, rowing machines, and stationary bicycles. The usual equipment for flexibility, weight-lifting, stretching, and bending is a good addition, but not necessary for weight control although these exercises help build muscle. Likewise, the presence of other amenities that may add to a facility's appeal—and surely to the cost—such as sauna and steam rooms, a whirlpool, and infrared lamps, do not increase the value for weight control. Showers and hair dryers must be provided.

The function of a facility's staff is instruction, motivation, coaching, and encouragement. Perhaps the most important role of the staff is to teach the necessary skills, encouraging moderation in the beginning, and later encouraging stress and endurance building so that exercise can be continued long enough for real energy expenditure. Often the interest and encouragement of a staff member provide the motivation necessary to make an effective program.

The nutritionist can also evaluate the fees charged and help the individual to a realistic appraisal of a specific program. Often the only facilities needed are available free or at little cost. There is always a place to walk, running tracks are frequently available for the asking, and swimming pools for a small fee. Home gyms are of uncertain value since the equipment is often of limited use and frequently not used after the initial enthusiasm is gone. The small size of many home pools limits their value as a means to consume energy or produce stress. Health clubs with life or other high initial fees should be avoided along with programs of passive exercise, which have little value for weight control.

EXERCISE TESTING

The nutritionist should be familiar with exercise testing even though it will not be available to many individuals. The *exercise or stress test* is a medical test by a physician or exercise physiologist to show how the heart responds to stress on exertion. The equipment may be a treadmill or bicycle with attached sphygmomanometer to monitor changes in blood pressure and an electrocardiograph to monitor heart action, or it may be a stool for the "step test" with the physician keeping watch for signs of overexertion. (4)

PRESCRIBING THE DIET

The calorie level should be decided along with the exercise regime and planned to provide a calorie deficit that will produce a weight loss of about two pounds per week. The frequency and number of meals and the kinds of foods must also be decided. As long as the diet provides 1800 to 2000 kilocalories, nutritional adequacy can be easily achieved. When calorie level is reduced further, as when the physician wishes to produce immediate weight loss as a critical part of treatment, there must be rigid restriction of fat, sugar, and alcohol.

The nutritionist should help the patient plan a diet based on food preferences and patterns that will be acceptable for long-time adherence. The diet can be at a compromise calorie level, low enough to produce a calorie deficit when added to the calorie demands of increased activity while still nutritionally adequate and acceptable for life-long use. When weight loss has been achieved, calorie control for normal weight must become a part of all meal planning, primarily by regulating the amount of fat, sugar, and alcohol. This will necessitate education for normal diet and gourmet cookery that limits fat and sugar, depending for flavor on low- or no-calorie substances. Wines and other alcoholic beverages can be used if the alcohol evaporates in the cooking process.

MOTIVATION FOR INCREASED ACTIVITY

The puritan ethic that suggests that what is good cannot be pleasant accounts for much of the negative attitude against increased activity. Though most individuals who join weight control groups or who seek advice about weight loss are already motivated for weight loss, few will be eager to engage in a program of increased activity or exercise. The best way for the nutritionist to learn what motivates for exercise is observation and experience. One study offers some clues.

Berman reports a motivational survey of 487 participants in Diet Workshop. (2) Most of the findings were based on data collected by questionnaire. The participants were middle class women of the Boston area. About half were below 40, half over 40. About 64 percent had what the investigators call "self-defeating behavior." It was found that 60 percent of the group practiced self-defeating behaviors such as rewarding themselves for weight loss with foods not on their diets or abandoning the diet after the loss of some weight. Older dieters seemed more able to adapt to need for change in eating behavior than younger ones. The author believes that neither diet nor exercise nor therapy alone is enough to help dieters achieve and maintain a permanent weight loss. This is believed to be due to a low self-image and the investigators think that dieters need to utilize community resources to strengthen their self-image. Physical activity including dance and movement to music, working at hobbies and crafts, and enhancement of personal appearance were recommended. This approach might not work with low-income groups because of cost, child care problems, and the need for leisure time for sessions and exercise.

Some persons may be motivated by the excess fat itself. Since carrying the extra weight makes every movement in housework, walking, gardening, and so forth, more difficult and usually produces clumsiness. Some may be motivated by the difficulty of finding well-fitting clothes or by the possibility of relief from foot problems. Older women may be encouraged to start exercise programs by knowing that their capacity for training is similar to that of younger persons. (1) Persons concerned about aging may be motivated by knowing that some authorities believe that exercise helps prevent aging and, especially, the disabilities of aging.

Motivation may also be found in the subject matter of nutrition and exercise physiology. The amount to teach and the level must be carefully geared to the needs of the individual or group. There are only two reasons for teaching this subject matter: (1) for motivation in the immediate situation, and (2) for improved long-range food and exercise practices. Extensive information about nutrition is not necessary to enable a person to eat a good diet nor about body mechanics to have a good exercise program. Some individuals and groups may want a good deal of information about nutrition and may have many questions, others will want only specific information about what they can eat, how to cook it, and how to make it taste good.

The point that weight loss is often accompanied by a drop in serum cholesterol and blood pressure may be strong motivation for persons who have these problems. Exercise may be helpful to the patient who is overeating for emotional reasons although reducing will probably fail until the anger, frustration, or anxiety that is the cause has been resolved. The increased activity may help by releasing physical tension, adding new interest and filling time. However, some of these persons will still need help from a social worker or psychiatrist.

Exercise gives a feeling of being alive and relieves the feeling of just sitting and getting fat. There is also a magnificent sense of satisfaction in having accomplished an exercise objective such as running a mile or swimming ten laps, a feeling of increased physical well-being from the exertion itself and satisfaction from the achievement of self-discipline.

EXERCISE PROBLEMS OF WOMEN

Though many of the old prejudices about women in sports have disappeared, there are a number of problems that interfere with their participation in exercise programs. Many American women and men regard the ability to exercise, the development of muscles, and sweating as unfeminine and undesirable attributes for women. Some women discourage their husbands from engaging in exercise programs and prepare meals that are high in calories and saturated fat resulting in excess weight gain for both. Some men discourage women from participating in exercise by expectations about clothing and grooming such as high heels, tight clothing, and perfection of makeup and coiffure.

There is no easy solution to these problems, but they must be recognized before an attempt can be made to solve them. Misinformation about food and nutrition is also common among women, especially among those involved in weight control and exercise programs.

SUMMARY

The community nutritionist must assume responsibility for promoting activity for weight control as part of a healthful lifestyle for all individuals. One of the hardest tasks will be to get people to set aside time for exercise.

It is often suggested that exercise testing, a physical examination, and an exercise prescription should precede exercise. This means that most persons will never start. Fortunately, more authorities on exercise are suggesting that a program of walking or light exercise may safely be started by any individual who is not a known cardiac.

The nutritionist may include advice about the effect of different kinds of exercise, about exercise resources, and including increased activity as a regular part of nutritional care. The purpose is to motivate the individual to start a program of increased activity or exercise.

Some problems in motivating individuals to start an exercise program have been discussed.

REFERENCES CITED

1. Adams, Gene M., and Herbert A. DeVries, Physiological Effects of an Exercise Training Regimen upon Women Aged 52 to 79, *J. Geront.*, 28 1/73 50.

2. Berman, Edith M., Factors Influencing Motivations in Dieting, *J. Nutr. Educ.,* 7 10–12/75 155.

3. Blankenhorn, David M., Personal Communication.

4. Cooper, K. H., Guideline in the Management of the Exercising Patient, *J. Am. Med. Assoc.,* 211 3/9/70 1663.

5. Cooper, K. H., *The New Aerobics,* Bantam Books, New York, 1970.

6. Cooper, Mildred and Kenneth Cooper, *Aerobics for Women,* Bantam Books, New York, 1972.

7. Cummings, G. R., On Prescribing Exercise, *Manitoba Med. Rev.,* 50 7–8/70 18.

8. DeVries, Herbert, *Physiology of Exercise for Physical Education and Athletics,* W. C. Brown Co., Dubuque IA, 1974, 235.

9. Mayer, Jean, *Overweight: Causes, Cost, and Control,* Prentice-Hall, Inc., Englewood Cliffs N.J., 1968.

10. National Research Council, Food and Nutrition Board, *Recommended Dietary Allowances,* 8th ed., National Academy of Sciences, Washington DC, 1974 26.

11. Rodert, Ellen E., and Jessie C. Obert, *Nutritionist's Guide to Activity in Weight Control Programs,* County of Los Angeles Department of Health Services, Los Angeles, unpublished pamphlet, 10/74.

12. Sharkey, Brian J., *Physiological Fitness and Weight Control,* Mountain Press Publishing Co., Missoula MT, 1974.

13. Skinner, J. S., Exercise Prescription for Middle-Aged Persons, *Del. Med. J.,* 7 1/71 12.

14. Zohman, Lenore R., *Exercise Your Way to Fitness and Heart Health,* American Heart Association and the President's Council on Physical Fitness and Sports, 1974, 12.

24 PROGRAMING FOR DISEASE PREVENTION

This chapter will cover programing for prevention of five nutrition-related diseases, atherosclerosis, hypertension, diabetes, cancer, and dental caries, for which nutrition methods of prevention have been established. It will also report studies and activities in drug and alcohol programs. Though the latter contain limited information on nutrition, they suggest strategies that can be used in nutrition programing.

Policies about prevention of these diseases should be developed by the nutritionist with the appropriate medical staff in the agency. Evidence of a depth of knowledge that shows that the nutritionist is prepared to participate in treatment will facilitate the development of a joint policy.

Some will contend that dietary changes for the prevention of these diseases should be delayed until there is positive proof that such changes will prevent their development. However, reducing the consumption of saturated fats, sugar, and salt is a change toward the levels of these substances that existed before recent high intakes of beef, sugar, and heavily salted foods. Almy recommends that such changes be made in the absence of evidence that a harmful biological action may result. (1)

ATHEROSCLEROSIS

Though there are many references to sudden heart attacks, every episode is based on a slow, progressive disease that probably begins in early life. (3) The cause of atherosclerosis is not known, but it has been shown that the danger of heart attack and stroke increases with the presence of certain risk factors. Basic prevention in the population involves changes in four risk factors which can be modified by the individual or family: diet, exercise, cigarette smoking, and stress. The nutritionist can integrate prevention by diet and exercise into nutrition education for both individuals and groups.

The community nutritionist is in a strategic position to promote among the general public the design for living that is currently recommended by the American Heart Association for prevention of heart disease and stroke. (5) This life pattern includes eating a diet with the RDA of protein, vitamins, and minerals, with an energy intake to keep weight at optimal level while being low in saturated fat and cholesterol. The diet is recommended for prudent action by the general population.

Fat control is accomplished by using fish, chicken, turkey, and veal often, with moderate portions of beef, pork, lamb, and ham less frequently; avoiding deep-fat frying; using margarine made with liquid vegetable oils instead of butter; and replacing regular milk and cheese with skimmed milk and skimmed milk cheeses. Cholesterol control is accomplished by limiting egg yolks to three a week and restricting use of fatty meats, shellfish, and organ meats.

This diet recommendation was formulated by the American Heart Association's Nutrition Committee on the basis that there is "substantial evidence" that these modifications will help to reduce the number of heart attacks. (5) The earlier in life such a pattern is established, the better.

While the AHA recommendation is for the general public, each community nutritionist will need to decide with medical personnel how and whether to implement the recommendation in the agency. At least some control of the amount of saturated fat is necessary for calorie control when diet modification is needed for weight control or weight loss.

Information, materials, and help with professional and public education may be obtained from the state or local affiliates of the American Heart Association. The nutritionist may also cooperate with the local Heart Association in its programs, serve on committees and boards, or provide consultation on nutrition.

There are other risk factors of nutritional significance—high serum cholesterol, high blood pressure, electrocardiogram abnormalities, and diabetes, which can be changed under medical supervision. The other risk factors—sex, age, race and heredity—cannot be changed.

Terris has proposed (16) the establishment of "environmental barriers" between the person (host) and the problem (agent) by regulatory measures. One of these would require that unsaturated fats be used in commercial baking and that details about type of fat be stated on the labels of other foods. He further suggests awarding financial benefits to farmers for production of beef low in saturated fats and subsidies to reduce prices for foods rich in unsaturated fats. Such drastic measures would require changes in the nation's political orientation before they could be accomplished. Further stimulus for changes in fats will follow current emphasis on the prudent diet for the prevention of cancer. This will be reported in the section on cancer. If changes in practices of individuals about saturated fat, alcohol, and tobacco are to be accomplished, it may also be necessary to ban counter-education in advertising and to provide a large government budget for education.

Many studies and programs are under way to gather new information about heart disease. The educational program outlined above conforms to current knowledge. The nutritionist should be prepared to modify teaching and programs when new information suggests that changes are in order.

HYPERTENSION

Hypertension, or high blood pressure, is a major cause of morbidity and mortality in this country. (4) Part of the problem is that hypertension may exist for years without sympsions. Haughton (8) cites a Chicago study that showed that more than 50 percent of persons with hypertension were not aware of their condition. The American Heart Association estimates that only 10 percent of those afflicted receive the treatment which is necessary to arrest and control the disease. While there are effective methods of control, it is difficult to persuade persons who feel well and have no symptoms that they have a serious condition and should be under regular medical supervision. There are effective treatments, but they must be continued over long periods of time.

There is currently emphasis in some areas on making the measurement of blood pressure a part of every medical care contact. Screening programs are another method of identifying the disease. In screening programs, blood pressure is frequently measured by aides and other personnel. Nutritionists can learn to take blood pressure and screen some persons who would otherwise not be reached. Screening is easy as it requires only learning to measure with a mercury or aneroid sphygmomanometer.

Nutritionists can participate in community hypertension screening and control programs in a number of ways, most often by promoting and helping plan programs and by incorporating into their regular teaching and promotion these points about blood pressure:

1. High blood pressure is a dangerous condition as it may lead to stroke and failure of heart and kidneys.
2. "Essential" hypertension means that there is no recognizable cause.
3. High blood pressure may exist without symptoms, but it can be detected by a simple test.
4. A person with hypertension requires medical supervision to control blood pressure.
5. Moderation in salt intake is desirable since excessive salt intake over a long period of time may be one of the causes of hypertension, although the evidence is not widely accepted. Either reduction in excessive salt intake or reduction in weight will reduce high blood pressure.
6. Regular moderately vigorous exercise of considerable duration, for example, an hour of jogging daily, has been noted to help in reducing blood pressure and may be advised by a physician.

In some programs it may be appropriate for the nutritionist to serve as monitor for a diet-exercise regimen designed to reduce both weight and blood pressure.

Salt

The fact that sodium restriction will reduce high blood pressure has led to suggestions that a reduction in table salt be made to reduce the risk of developing hypertension.

The Committee on Nutrition of the American Academy of Pediatrics said in 1974 that evidence did not indicate recommending a change in dietary salt intake for the entire population. The Committee did suggest that on the basis of incomplete evidence there might be benefit from a low salt diet for children in a family with history of hypertension. (14)

The NRC Committee on Dietary Allowances reported in 1974 that there was little evidence that the usual salt intake would produce hypertension in persons with normal blood pressure. (12)

Nevertheless there are frequent suggestions for reduction or moderation in salt intake as a preventive measure against the development of hypertension. It is in order to pause here and attempt to define what *moderation* is.

The importance of salt as a seasoning and its use as a carrier of iodine makes it desirable to consider carefully the implications of reducing the amount of salt. The purpose of salt in cooking is to accentuate the flavor of foods by adding a small amount. Salt is also used in larger amounts to give a salty flavor, to preserve foods, and to control the fermentation of yeast in baked products. Many individuals have become so habituated to salt flavor that they enjoy food only when it is heavily salted. From this have come several *misuses* of salt which should be the target of a salt education campaign toward a rational use of salt for its original purpose. These suggestions are for persons for whom therapeutic salt restriction is not necessary.

The first of these misuses is *cooking all food without salt,* a common practice in institutions, restaurants, and homes. Though many persons in the United States would be well advised to reduce the amount of salt they use, this is not the best method. There has been an attempt to sell this practice to the public under the premise of "enjoying the natural flavor of foods," but this results in many persons salting heavily at the table so that it defeats its own purpose, resulting in little reduction of salt intakes for those whose intake is heavy.

The second misuse is *heavy salting at table*. This practice of salting food at table, usually before tasting, results in addition of much more salt than if food were properly salted during the cooking process. Individuals should be taught to taste before salting, to salt only foods not salted before cooking, and to use salt only to accentuate the natural food flavor. The cook also needs to learn what foods have been salted in processing, as occurs with frozen vegetables.

The third misuse is *consumption of high salt foods*. This needs a two-pronged approach, one for the individual to limit consumption of heavily salted foods by using alternative foods such as unsalted nuts instead of salted ones, crackers with unsalted tops instead of salted tops, fresh cabbage rather than sauerkraut, raw vegetables rather than pickles, unsalted popcorn instead of salted, and fresh meats instead of lunch meats. The second prong of this attack should be the development by food processors of ways to prepare foods with lower salt content.

Regular teaching by the community nutritionist should attempt to replace the three misuses with practices that will result in better food and lower salt intakes. Intakes of salt in the United States have been estimated at 10 to 14 gram, about 2 or 3 teaspoons, per day. (6) Realistic goals for family food practices for a moderate salt intake might be to season with no more than 1 teaspoon of salt per person per day, use no salt at table, and use no highly salted foods. In the home setting it is easy to identify and control these practices. This would allow ⅛ teaspoon for each of six servings of meat and vegetables, and ¼ teaspoon for all other foods, such as sauces, and home baked products. These changes in practices would result in a lower salt intake for individuals who currently consume high amounts. Other strategies would need to be used for families which purchase many foods that are already seasoned.

If investigation shows serious effects from a high salt intake, an environmental barrier against heavily salted foods may be needed, similar to that proposed by Terris for saturated fat (page 393).

CANCER

While it appears that the public is mainly concerned about the carcinogenic properties of food chemicals, especially additives, scientific opinion is more concerned with the nutritional effects of food consumption (page 27). Wynder says (18) that present epidemiological evidence indicates more danger from deficiencies and excesses of calories and specific nutrients than from food additives or other known carcinogens. He points out that the quantities of food additives are stated in parts per million while excessive nutrients occur as grams or kilograms over a year's time.

Nutrient deficiencies of most importance are iron, iodine, riboflavin, vitamin A, and pyridoxine. Deficiencies of the B vitamins may be implicated in the relationship between alcohol, smoking, and the risk of cancer of the mouth, larynx, and esophagus, while correlation has been observed between vitamin A deficiency and cancer of the cervix. The greatest danger of excess appears to be from a high consumption of combined animal fat and protein which may be implicated in cancer of the colon and rectum, and high fat consumption may also be associated with breast cancer. Despite some confident statements about fiber, many cancer researchers believe that its relationship to development of cancer is yet to be demonstrated. One of the problems in epidemiological studies of cancer is that of getting histories of dietary intakes from many years before.

The Diet, Nutrition, and Cancer Program of the Cancer Institute of the NIH has established goals for the Program. They are to assess the role of nutrition in cause and care of cancer, to define requirements for nutrition and diet, to study the use of diet and nutrition in cancer, and to educate health professionals and the public in preventive diet. (7, 10)

Diet for Prevention

It has been suggested that the prudent diet currently prescribed by many physicians for prevention of cardiovascular disease should be prescribed also as a prudent diet for cancer. (9, 18)

DIABETES

The cause of diabetes is unknown so there are no specific methods for prevention. However, there is believed to be a genetic predisposition to diabetes, and obesity is considered to be a predisposing factor. Public Law 93-354, the National Diabetes Research and Education Act, was passed by the Congress in July 1974. This was the first step taken by the federal government in an extensive attack on diabetes. The National Institutes of Health will be responsible for the program. (2, 17)

Help with programs for professional education and public education is available from the American Diabetes Association and its branches. The Association stresses public awareness that diabetes is a major public health program, that early detection is important, that it can be controlled by diet and medication, and that complications can be avoided.

Many nutritionists have frequent opportunities to participate in screening programs for detection, and they can encourage people to participate in the screening process and counsel on normal family diet.

Prevention of diabetes must be attacked in two ways, first, to keep it from developing and second, to prevent complications in the person who has the disease. Weight control throughout life by proper food and suitable activity appears to offer the best possibility for prevention. There is some evidence that sucrose may trigger the disease in genetically susceptible individuals. McGandy and Mayer (11) suggest that establishment of better patterns of eating and activity in infancy, childhood, and adolescence is very important.

The community nutritionist will find a number of ways to conduct public education for the prevention of diabetes, such as (1) teaching good diet patterns with controlled amounts of sucrose and saturated fats as a means of good nutrition and weight control, (2) education in the values of activity and exercise, (3) consumer education in label reading so that sources of sugars and saturated fats are identified, (4) promotion of screening programs that include measures for diabetes detection, (5) motivation of persons identified in screening programs to have further tests and to obtain appropriate medical care. The nutritionist can also participate in seeing that continuity of dietary care is provided for ambulatory patients by patient education, professional education, and interpretation of problems to patient, family, physician, nurse, or others who give care. Many times the patient and family need reinterpretation of previous instruction, help in fitting the diet into the family pattern, or in finding community resources to meet specific needs.

Prater reported (13) a five-day live-in course for small groups of diabetic patients, family members, and allied health professionals. Participants ranged in age from 3 years to 65 years. She described the daily schedule and the special activities such as field trips, sports and walks. Though this was a live-in project, some of the techniques and ideas could be adapted for use in community programs.

DENTAL CARIES

Diet has two relationships to caries, first, in the effect of nutrition on tooth formation during the prenatal period and in early life, and second, in the effect of some kinds of food that provide a favorable climate for tooth decay. Thus programing for prevention must include two approaches, proper diet for the pregnant woman, infant and small child, and control of fermentable carbohydrates throughout life.

Di Orio and Madsen state: "Most people are unaware that all dental decay and most gum disease is preventable. The dental profession has reiterated that good oral hygiene, control of food habits, use of fluorides and regular visits to the dentist provide the means for controlling dental disease." (19) The nutritionist can include these facts in a nutrition counseling session, emphasize the need for regular visits to the dentist, and help find or create resources for care when such action is appropriate.

Programing for Prevention

Nutritionists can contribute to dental health by promoting fluoridation of public water supplies, or use of fluoridated water from other sources, and by developing education in diets that include minimal amounts of sugar and de-emphasize sweet snacks in favor of those that provide vitamins, minerals, and protein. Encouragement of good dental hygiene (brushing after meals and brushing or rinsing after sweets) and use of detersive foods can often be a part of nutrition counseling.

Fluoridation should be regarded as comparable to the provision of a nutrient that is not supplied by food or water. It has become an emotional issue and a political one.

Scism reports the events in a small city on the fluoridation issue during consideration and balloting in the city council. (23)

The episode took place in a small city where fluoridation of the water supply was promoted by health professionals with virtually no opposition from the health community. A fundamentalist Baptist preacher led the opposition, characterizing fluoridation "as part of a Communist plot to take over America." The council did not act on the proposal.

The Jaycees conducted an educational campaign in favor of fluoridation and petititioned the council to vote or to hold a referendum. Again the effort failed because of no action by the council. The author's conclusion from a study of the motivations of the council is that pressure groups had little or no influence on its decisions since members of the council relied on other advisors for their information.

Scism comments that physicians and dentists must recognize the political nature of the issue, and must play politics and be able to make the government body feel "politically safe to vote for it."

The community nutritionist needs to be aware of the kind of nutrition teaching done by dental hygienists and dentists, to try to reconcile varying instruction, and to work for teaching of authentic nutrition subject matter in schools of dentistry and dental hygiene. The nutritionist should be alert for conflicting instructions by different professionals; for example, in one health program the dentist advocated popcorn or nuts for dental health, but the pediatrician disapproved these foods because of the danger of aspiration by small children.

Shaw (24) suggests the daily consumption of a good diet from the Four Food Groups for both oral health and general health, discouraging between-meal eating and taking fruit and vegetable snacks rather than sweets.

Madsen emphasizes use of snack foods that provide essential nutrients without excessive dental hazards. He recommended snacks of milk and cheese, meats, nuts, hard cooked eggs, peanut butter, fruits and vegetables, and their juices without added sugar. (20)

Nizel recommends (21) the use of nonplaque firm foods at each meal, such as toast or steak or salad or raw fruit. Fresh fruits such as apples, oranges, and peaches are noncariogenic while the sucrose of dried fruits sticks to the teeth and is cariogenic. His general principles for preventing caries are to have only three eating periods a day, avoid snacks, increase meat, fish, and milk, eliminate sticky sweets, pastry and dried fruits. Carbohydrate should be maintained at the RDA, but by using starches rather than sugars.

Nizel and Shulman (22) describe the nutritional guidance techniques used in a program at Tufts University and the steps in the dietary counseling process. These were (1) to explain the process of dental decay, (2) identify the sweet foods and the foundation foods in the reported intake, (3) assess the adequacy of the diet, (4) analyze the intake of sweets, and (5) diagnose the reason for the problem and prescribe a personalized diet. The authors state: "It is incumbent upon nutritionists to assist the dentist in caries control, just as they do the physician in the management of diabetes and obesity."

SUBSTANCE ABUSE

The community nutritionist may be called on to work with patients seen in the substance-abuse programs, either alcoholics or drug addicts. While there is much pessimism about whether or not these persons can be cured or even helped, there have been enough successes to warrant trying. Leading an alcoholic or an addict back to consumption of proper food is of material help in correcting the conditions of malnutrition that often occur.

Carroll points out that coffee, beer, aspirin, tranquilizers, marihuana, and heroin are all drugs and that alcohol, marihuana, and opium have been used for thousands of years. "Throughout recorded history man has used pleasure-giving and pain-killing substances for comfort and protection against the hardships of life and its strains." (27) The new phase of drug use is experimentation by young people and consequent addiction that accompanies a lack of interest in traditional patterns about education and work. Use of drugs and alcohol by all age groups is a problem and adults who follow the practice of casual use of pills or excess alcohol are setting the pace for similar practices by the younger generation.

Drug use has spread to younger age groups, with the 8- to 14-year-olds now believed to be the fastest growing group of drug users. Marihuana has become a "drug of mass consumption" comparable to alcohol and nicotine; a recent "survey of 16,000 high school seniors revealed that 6.2 percent smoked "pot" daily and 6 percent drank alcoholic beverages every day." (32) Programs of the federal government on alcohol and drugs are many and fragmented, with its efforts said to be divided among seven cabinet departments and 17 agencies.

Most of the need and opportunities for nutrition services in alcohol and drug programs are in treatment. However, the community nutritionist has opportunity for preventive teaching in family and youth clinics, and nutrition counseling can play an important role in helping both youth and adults find satisfactory alternative life styles. The nutritionist needs to be informed about both national and local agencies that deal with these problems.

Drugs

The community nutritionist may encounter drug users among many groups and in many places and should have some background in the subject. Heroin use is generally regarded as the greatest problem because its use is illegal, it has degrading effects, and users commit many crimes in their efforts to get money to meet their need for the drug. Marihuana is the most widely used drug, but it is not addictive and does not seem to produce serious physical problems. However, it has been estimated that 20 percent of people over 11 have tried marihuana.

The nationwide heroin problem had its start about 1965. Government treatment programs were started in 1969. At one point it was believed that stopping the influx of heroin from Turkey had alleviated the problem, so the programs were stopped in mid 1975. Meantime, however, dope smuggling from Mexico increased and reached an all-time high and seems to be increasing, especially in the Southwest. Also, many youths are now turning to "polydrug abuse," which means drug abuse other than alcoholism or heroin addiction. (32)

There is some optimism about the progress that has been made in alleviating the problem of drug abuse, which has been characterized as endemic. It has been suggested that concentrated drug usage is now shifting from the larger Eastern cities to middle-size cities in other parts of the United States. (30)

Einstein (29) reviews the definitions used in drug abuse education and gives a framework for developing a drug education program with ten content areas. He suggests also a technique for selecting the focus of intervention, proposes several drug training programs, and provides a model for program development. Nutritionists who will work with drug abusers will find this a valuable resource. Einstein points out that drugs have usually been defined in terms of the legal-criminal system, in which drug laws and rituals are abused, sometimes as self-abuse, sometimes as abuse of others. He gives also a scientific definition of a *drug* as ". . . a substance which through its chemical activity alters the structure and/or functioning of a living organism." He characterizes the definition as meaningless because the U.S. has decided not to be concerned about coffee, tea, tobacco, food, or other substances that also meet that definition. Perhaps drugs are no more harmful than the other substances named.

Though there are many community drug programs, few have nutritionists. Three situations will provide most of the occasions for the community nutritionist to work with drug users. These are the family setting, the youth clinic, and the therapeutic residential community sometimes known as a "halfway house." The nutritionist's role in the first two cases is usually to work as a member of the team, which may be as a diet counselor, but which may sometimes be expanded also to include treatment of the community of users. Ideas for the nutritionist in both situations will be found in the reports of specific programs. One of the common elements in these programs is the importance of giving these young people the feeling that someone cares how they eat and what they do. The halfway house more nearly resembles a home than an institution. Usually the residents do part or all of the cooking. The nutritionist can advise the person in charge about meal planning, food purchasing and getting the addicts to eat.

Frankle and Christakis report a New York City program by a community nutrition team that included a nutritionist. (30) The nutritionist was the first person to interview a client on the first visit to the storefront clinic, since previous experience had indicated that the client could more readily discuss nutritional patterns than other matters. Food intake data before, during, and after the drug addiction were recorded along with data about drug usage and lifestyle. The diet was evaluated by a food group pattern, and diet recommendations were made as indicated. The diet histories showed that almost half of the clients had in early life eaten inadequate diets even when adequate food was available. Diets were usually low in vegetables, citrus fruits, and milk products. The diet records also revealed that addicts craved candy, cake, cookies, potato chips, sodas, and other high-carbohydrate, low-nutrient foods. These were preferred for their low cost, ready availability and a belief that they enhanced the effects of the drugs.

The authors believe that the nutritional deficiencies of these clients were due to the poor diets caused by use of money for drugs rather than for foods, to disinterest in food, and to the pharmacologic and toxic effects of the drugs that affect metabolism in a number of ways.

Washburn reported (38) her experiences in counseling the residents of a drug rehabilitation center in Atlanta, and helping them plan and prepare their meals. The program included continuous nutritional therapy as a positive health measure and as a supplement to other attempts to interrupt the addiction. Many of the youths entering the program were malnourished due to poor food intake or to liver disease, which resulted in failure to use ingested nutrients. Others were malnourished possibly due to increased nutrient requirements caused by the drugs.

Frankle and coworkers report some experiences with youth drug addicts at "The Door," a free clinic with extended services in New York's Greenwich Village. (31) The nutritionists counseled the clients about general diet, modified diets, weight control, food money management, meal preparation with limited facilities, and prenatal nutrition. Many of these young people were or had been on drugs. The nutritionists helped them develop an acceptable new lifestyle, based on living in harmony with a healthy body, with which they were able to replace a drug-centered existence. The authors give case studies of four persons who were counseled.

The nutritionist should be aware of the signs by which drug abuse may be recognized. Wollman and Steindler (40) give several signs: increased appetite, impaired judgment and memory, inability to concentrate for long periods of time, and loss of interest in recreation. The increased appetite is said to be due to food deprivation during drug intoxication; however, other observers point to signs of craving for sweets and loss of appetite. (30) If the nutritionist is working in a situation where there are likely to be drug users, there should be inservice education on how to deal with them.

Alcohol

Public Law 91-616, the Comprehensive Alcohol Abuse and Alcoholism Prevention, Treatment, and Rehabilitation Act of 1970, became effective in 1971. Responsibility for prevention of alcoholism is divided among a number of federal agencies. The Act provides for grants to states to help them establish more effective programs for prevention, treatment and rehabilitation. Chafetz says "... the problem of alcoholism is ... a microcosm of every social-health issue facing our society today. It cuts across all economic and social classes, and includes highly complex social, environmental, psychological, and physical phenomena." (28)

In a study of 2200 tenth-grade boys with later resurvey, Johnston (34) found that 81 percent reported using alcohol during high school, with 33 percent using it weekly. The year after high school the figures increased to 89 percent and 44 percent. The author comments on the higher use of "the traditionally acceptable drugs, alcohol and cigarettes" as compared with any of the illicit drugs, naming this as one of the most important findings.

Iber (33) reviews the physiology of alcohol, "the metabolic chain of events that puts the alcoholic on the slide downhill to severe malnutrition" and suggests medical treatment for rehabilitation. He points out that alcohol has some of the characteristics of both food and drugs and characterizes alcoholism as "the most prevalent *drug* addiction in the Western world." He mentions three fallacies, that vitamin deficiencies are the cause, that beer drinking does not cause alcoholism, and that most alcoholics eat adequately. The poor diet is due to lack of appetite and inadequate food money because it is used for alcoholic beverages.

Brenner reports (26) a national survey of drinking practices during 1964-65 that disclosed relationships between income and drinking. There was a higher proportion of heavy drinkers at lower socioeconomic levels and fewer heavy drinkers among middle and upper income groups. Excessive drinking and alcoholism were low among Italians who grew up in Italy and also among first-generation Italians in the United States because their drinking habits and values were established according to different cultural patterns, in which drinking was acceptable but drunkenness was not.

Williamson and Turi (39) mention some of the reasons for consumption of alcoholic beverages such as the mandatory nature of drinking in some business and social circles, pressures from the big-business aspects of alcohol production, and the lucrative revenues to governments at all levels. These authors consider alcoholism as a medical problem and point out that the individual's attitude toward it is similar to the attitude toward other illnesses, not wanting to accept the responsibility for behavior or treatment, but looking upon alcohol as a socially acceptable drink for relief of stress and anxiety.

Southmayd (35) reported the nutritional and "social aspects of a twenty-one day physical and social rehabilitation program at an alcoholism hospital," emphasizing the need for highly acceptable food served in a pleasant, friendly environment. Two problems that received special attention were providing adequate folic acid and the danger of storage of excessive iron in damaged livers.

Terris suggests environmental control in the form of prohibition of advertising and financial control by much higher taxation to cause a great increase in price, conceding that such measures would encounter great opposition. He further suggests an extensive educational program to change public attitudes and information. (36)

Beauchamp (25) points out that public health leaders, except Terris, have not promoted the establishment of more stringent controls over alcohol in the U.S. He thinks that control may have been confused with prohibition. Beauchamp comments that public health has not challenged the idea of individual responsibility for health protection, which he considers as an unsatisfactory solution. Vladeck and Weiss (37) point out that placing responsibility for action on the individual is currently unpopular, but they question the value of a policy intended to regulate the distribution and consumption of alcohol. They maintain that to some degree there is already control by taxation and distribution constraints and that educational programs show no more promise of success than those for smoking or overeating. Research needs for the future include alcohol control policy and the cause of alcoholism as addictive behavior.

The community nutritionist who works with alcohol programs or alcoholism will need to be informed about both physiological and social aspects of the problem and about resources provided by local groups, agencies and programs. These may be funded by local, state, or federal governments, or by private agencies. Alcoholics Anonymous, which is privately funded, assists individuals by providing companionship and counseling for members to help them refrain from drinking. Local health departments, free clinics, and other agencies may have programs with specially trained staff to work with alcoholics. The nutritionist must also understand the social significance of drinking in the specific community.

The method of providing service for individuals or groups of clients will need to be planned according to the policies of the project or agency so that nutritional care can be integrated with other treatment.

SUMMARY

The causes of the major chronic diseases—atherosclerosis, hypertension, diabetes, and cancer—are unknown, but they develop over a long period of time and evidence is growing that diet is involved in the etiology of each of these diseases. Dietary intakes of animal fats and refined sugars, along with deficiencies of some nutrients are suspect, indirectly by causing obesity, and directly through effects on the body processes. It has been suggested that the best preventive for cancer at the present time is use of the prudent diet that is currently used for prevention of heart disease.

The possible role of salt in the etiology of hypertension has been considered, moderation in salt intake has been defined, and a way has been proposed to achieve it.

Diet affects tooth formation before birth and in early life, and food provides a favorable or unfavorable climate for tooth decay. During regular work with individuals and families, nutritionists can teach a noncariogenic diet of basic foods. Community and nutrition education can both incorporate the value of fluoridated water for prevention of dental decay.

Nutritionists who work with alcoholics or drug addicts should have inservice education in methods to use with these groups. Most of the nutritionist's work will be done in a clinic, home, or halfway house.

REFERENCES CITED

Atherosclerosis, Hypertension, Salt, Cancer, and Diabetes

1. Almy, Thomas, P., The Role of Fiber in the Diet, Ch. 9 in Winick, Myron, ed., *Nutrition and Aging,* John Wiley & Sons, New York, 1976, 155.
2. American Diabetes Association, *Annual Report, 1974.* New York.
3. American Heart Association, *Heart and Blood Vessels,* American Heart Association, Dallas, 1975.

4. American Heart Association, *Heart Facts,* American Heart Association, Dallas, 1975.
5. American Heart Association, Release NR 76-3017 on Statement of the Nutrition Committee, Dallas, March 29, 1976.
6. Dahl, Lewis K., Salt Intake and Hypertension, *Dietetic Currents,* 2 9-10/75 1, Ross Laboratories, Columbus, OH.
7. Gori, Geo. B. The Diet, Nutrition, and Cancer Program of the NCI National Cancer Program, *Cancer Research,* 35 11/75(Part 2) 3545–47.
8. Haughton, James G., The Role of the General Hospital in Community Health, *Am. J. Pub. Health,* 65 1/75 21.
9. Hegsted, D. Mark, Summary of the Conference on Nutrition in the Causation of Cancer, Symposium on Nutrition and Cancer, *Cancer Res.,* 35 11/75(Part 2).
10. Legislative Highlights, *J. Am. Diet Assoc.,* 69 10/76 426.
11. McGandy, Robert B., and Jean Mayer, Atherosclerotic Disease, Diabetes, and Hypertension: Background Considerations, in *U.S. Nutrition Policies In the Seventies,* Jean Mayer, ed., W. H. Freeman and Company, San Francisco, 1973, 42.
12. National Research Council, Food and Nutrition Board, *Recommended Dietary Allowances,* 8th ed., National Academy of Sciences, Washington DC, 1974, 89.
13. Prater, Barbara M., The Diabetic Center: A Self-Care Living-In Program, *J. Am. Diet. Assoc.,* 64 2/74 180.
14. Salt Intake and Eating Patterns of Infants and Children in Relation to Blood Pressure, *Pediatrics,* 53 1/74 115.
15. Smith, Nathan J., *Food for Sport,* Bull Publishing Co., Palo Alto, CA, 1976, 90.
16. Terris, Milton J., The Epidemiological Revolution, National Health Insurance, and the Role of the Health Department, *Am. J. Pub. Health,* 66 12/76, 1157.
17. U. S. Congress, The National Diabetes Research and Education Act, PL 93-354, enacted 7/74.
18. Wynder, Ernst, Nutrition and Cancer, *Fed. Proc.* 35 5/1/76 1309.

Dental Caries

19. Di Orio, L. P., and K. O. Madsen, A Personalized Approach: Discussing Food in Prevention of Dental Caries, *Nutr. News,* 33 2/70 1.
20. Madsen, Kenneth O., Frequency Of Eating and Dental Health, *Food and Nutrition News,* 46 3–4/75, National Livestock and Meat Board.
21. Nizel, Abraham, *Nutrition in Preventive Dentistry: Science and Practice,* W. B. Saunders Co., Philadelphia, 1972, 361.
22. Nizel, Abraham E., and Judith S. Shulman, Interaction of Dietetics and Nutrition With Dentistry, *J. Am. Diet. Assoc.,* 55 11/69 470.
23. Scism, Thomas E., Fluoridation in Local Politics: Study of the Failure of a Proposed Ordinance in One American City, *Am. J. Pub. Health,* 62 10/72 1344.

24. Shaw, James H., New Knowledge of Nutrition and Dental Health, *Med. Clin. North Am.*, 54 11/70 1555.

Substance Abuse

25. Beauchamp, Dan E., Public Health: Alien Ethic In A Strange Land?, *Am. J. Pub. Health*, 65 12/75 1338.
26. Brenner, M. Harvey, Trends in Alcohol Consumption and Associated Illnesses, *Am. J. Pub. Health*, 65 12/75 1279.
27. Carroll, Sheila, What's Being Done About Drug Abuse?, in *Handbook for the Home*, 1973 Yearbook of Agriculture, U.S. Dept. of Agriculture, Government Printing Office, Washing DC, 55.
28. Chafetz, Morris E., New Federal Legislation on Alcoholism—Opportunities and Problems, *Am. J. Pub. Health*, 63 3/73 207.
29. Einstein, Stanley, Drug Abuse Training and Education, *Am. J. Pub. Health*, 64 2/74 101.
30. Frankle, Reva, and Christakis, George, Some Nutritional Aspects of "Hard" Drug Addiction, *Dietetic Currents,* 2 7–8/75 1, Ross Laboratories, Columbus, Ohio.
31. Frankle, Reva T., Betsy McGregor, Judy Wylie, and Mary B. McCann, Nutrition and Life Style: I. The Door, a Center of Alternatives—the Nutritionist in a Free Clinic for Adolescents, *J. Am. Diet. Assoc.*, 63 9/73 269.
32. Holden, Constance, Drug Abuse 1975: The "War" Is Past, the Problem Is as Big as Ever, *Science,* 190 11/14/75 639.
33. Iber, Frank L., In Alcoholism, the Liver Sets the Pace, *Nutrition Today*, 6 1–2/71 2.
34. Johnston, Lloyd D., Drug Use During and After High School, Results of a National Longitudinal Study., *Am. J. Pub. Health*, Supplement, 64 12/74 29.
35. Southmayd, Edna B., The Role of the Dietitian in Team Therapy for Chronic Alcoholism. *J. Am. Diet. Assoc.*, 64 2/75 184.
36. Terris, Milton, The Epidemiologic Revolution, National Health Insurance, and the Role of Health Departments, *Am. J. Pub. Health*, 66 12/76 1156–58.
37. Vladeck, Bruce C., and Robert J. Weiss, Policy Alternatives for Alcohol Control, *Am. J. Pub. Health*, 65 12/75 1340.
38. Washburn, Alice B., Nutrition Counseling for Drug Addicts in Rehabilitation, *J. Nutr. Educ.*, 6 1–3/74 13.
39. Williamson, Deborah E., and Marvin E. Turi, Nutrition in the Treatment of the Alcoholic, *Dietetic Currents,* 2 1–3/75, Ross Laboratories, Columbus, Ohio.
40. Wolman, Walter, and E. M. Steindler, Identifying Drug Users, in *Handbook For the Home*, 1973 Yearbook of Agriculture, U.S Dept. of Agriculture, Government Printing Office, Washington, DC., 57.

25 PROGRAMING FOR SEX-AGE GROUPS

In community nutrition, the family or household and the community are the patients while the primary focus is on the maintenance of good nutritional health and the prevention of disease. The content and direction of a particular community nutrition program will be determined by the nature of the agency or the scope of the program. For example, the public health department is responsible for the nutritional health of the population within its jurisdiction, the Maternity and Infant Care programs focus on high risk pregnant women and infants, the Heart Association is concerned with prevention of heart disease, and Nutrition for the Elderly tries to improve the diet of senior citizens.

It has been the custom for some years to direct community programs toward "vulnerable groups." Frequently statements have designated specific groups as "nutritionally vulnerable," which is defined as those which have greater needs than others (e.g., the pregnant woman) or those which cannot assume full responsibility for their own needs (e.g., the aged person with restricted mobility).

Some lists of groups include only infants and preschool children, pregnant women, and the elderly; others include also school children and adolescents. Sometimes the only groups excluded are adult non-pregnant women and adult men. These adults, burdened with the responsibility for providing the family sustenance, often have little time and energy to consider their own health needs, especially those of a preventive nature.

It is hardly realistic to exclude from the vulnerable group the male adults who are most likely to die of heart attacks when two of the risk factors are currently believed to be related to diet, or to exclude the female adults who are most prone to obesity that predisposes to a number of chronic diseases or makes them more disabling. The community nutritionist needs to be concerned with all sex-age groups. A major thrust in community nutrition as in community medicine and community nursing must be to consider the object of the specific program in the family setting. One of the problems has been the fragmentation of programs.

Fragmentation of attention to nutritional needs occurs because many persons and agencies for whom nutrition is of major concern have limited interests or concerns produced by the method of funding or by the special area of training and work. Physicians are pediatricians or obstetricians or cardiologists. Some nutritionists have had specialized training for maternal health or chronic disease or another field and so have a particular interest in one group. Teachers are primarily interested in the performance and health of children of a specific age. Many programs are for the poor or for one ethnic group. Sometimes funding for special projects has been restricted in such a way as to create a program within a program, isolating the project within the agency where it is conducted, and providing special benefits or privileges for persons who receive care and for project employees.

At the White House Conference, the Panel on Pregnant and Nursing Mothers and Young Infants expressed its concern in this way: "The nutritional needs of mothers and infants should be met only by future programs that meet the nutritional needs of all family members throughout their life cycle." And again: "No one age is more critical than another and family units comprise all ages. The necessary conclusion is that programs consider the entire age spectrum of normal families." This principle was enunciated another time in the same place: ". . . the family is the basic distributive unit. . . . Programs that assume that some family members can eat less well than others while all are seated together at the family table are unrealistic." (16)

Five years later, during the hearings of the Senate Select Committee on Nutrition and Human Needs, Fomon called attention to that recommendation and expressed disappointment that WIC was oriented only toward limited groups of women and children. (3)

Fortunately there is evidence that leaders in the field are aware of the need for specialized programs to be concerned with the whole family. In discussions about a National Nutrition Policy, Jacobson and Mills (6) emphasized the need to deal with mother, family, and total society in an integrated program rather than as separate groups. Fomon and Egan suggested (4) that a program aimed at one specific family member was likely to fail or to have limited success.

The community nutritionist must consider the needs of all family members and plan with them for their nutritional care.

PARENTS AND CHILDREN

The practices that take place in the family generally determine how well the members are nourished and the effects of other health habits. Each member of the family has an impact on these practices. The mother selects and prepares the food and in an increasing number of families is also the breadwinner. The income, working hours, and food preferences of the father affect what is served and when and how. The ages of the children and their food habits affect the costs in both money and energy.

The problems most likely to be encountered in the family setting are inadequate income, lack of information about money management, misinformation about food and nutrition, poor housekeeping practices, and lack of information about child and family development. Parental indifference, neglect or abuse sometimes occur as does abuse of alcohol and drugs. Health personnel concerned about problems of clients due to lack of money must help the family find satisfactory solutions by locating additional resources or make more effective use of those they already have. The problems of poverty were discussed on page 302. The family may be eligible for WIC, food stamps, Social Security benefits, or other means to increase their resources. The single parent, either female or male is in an especially difficult position as one of the groups most vulnerable to malnutrition in large U.S. cities.

The problems of misinformation have already been discussed (page 322) and they are especially acute when they cause a mother to purchase expensive food supplements or foods with money that might better have been spent for oranges, milk, or meat. The family may also need help to realize the social significance of food, especially family meals that provide a time for the members to be together, to talk, and to strengthen the family bonds.

Another phase of education that has an indirect effect on the family is education in nutrition subject matter and methods of nutrition education for teachers and other persons who look after the children such as the day care center staff and health center personnel. Inservice or other education is necessary to keep the nutritionist informed about current problems and how to meet the needs of the clientele. It should cover planning the program, subject matter, tools, and skills.

Many mothers need help with housekeeping practices since they lack the necessary skills to manage the cooking, laundry, child care, and other household tasks. The nutritionist, home economist, community nurse, or nutrition aide can help with practical guidance about management or skills or can advise the family about available community resources where help with such problems can be found. Sometimes the problem is persuading the family to take advantage of the available resources; pride or indifference or lack of understanding may need to be overcome. Angrist gives some practical suggestions for finding help when socioeconomic problems are too big for the family to handle. (1) Many services are available through the Social Security system or public welfare. A community may also have day care for children, family planning services, or protective services, or day care or meal services for the elderly.

The official services differ in different states and each nutritionist should know how to refer a client to make use of them. Once contact has been made with the right resource to meet a particular need, there is usually assurance that the necessary help will follow. The nutritionist should also know about other agencies and nutrition resources in the particular community and be able to recognize which one is best for a specific need. If there is a social worker in the agency, it may only be necessary to refer the client to that office.

Sometimes the prescription of a therapeutic diet for one member of the family may provide an opportunity to suggest changes that will improve the family diet. Examples of such changes would be to modify the kind of fat used for a controlled-fat diet, or to reduce excessive intakes of salt or sugar or calories. Care should be taken, however, not to impose a very different special diet for one member on the whole family, an action likely to be resented by other family members and to get them accustomed to a food pattern that will complicate their adjustment to food served away from home. The individual on the diet needs to recognize the differences in the diet, to know that most people eat differently, and to learn how to make adjustments for the prescribed diet. The dieter will be able to lead a more comfortable food existence by learning to select foods that fit the prescribed diet when eating away from home, in restaurant or cafeteria or another home.

Some heart disease prevention programs also have a family component attempting to change the habits of the whole family, the man and woman to achieve normal blood pressure, blood cholesterol, and weight, and the children as a means of prevention for their adulthood. Other programs that will affect greater numbers should also be used. Television, radio, demonstrations, food fairs, and similar events may be effective. Sometimes these programs may be a part of larger health education programs. The community nutritionist should keep in mind the need to utilize available resources first, and to conduct programs for the persons who cannot be reached by other resources.

Before programs are started, an evaluation method should be developed. Ideally this will be nutritional surveillance, which may show changes in growth rates, anemia, and weight along with other pertinent parameters to be correlated with changes in diet. This may be done by the nutritionist or it may be possible to get help from a university or college nutrition department, or home economics, anthropology, or other department. In the absence of such resources, the nutritionist may need to develop evaluation methods that are practical and possible without outside help. Summarizing 25 food records from the elderly that show the inadequacies, pricing a week's food list, or calculating the fat content of diets in a few households will provide a way to dramatize local problems. In many cases such simple measures would be as effective in demonstrating the value of a program to the administration, local governing bodies, and financing agencies as would a more extensive study, or a report from national surveys. In the absence of local data, that from national surveys may be applied to the local scene, assuming that problems that occurred in a statistical sample will appear in the same proportion in the local population.

Attempts to help the family develop more nutritious and less costly food practices must also be based on the existing cultural, ethnic, religious, or purely personal patterns. Practical methods for determining such patterns have been discussed.

When family food practices need modifications because a family member has hypertension, diabetes, high blood cholesterol, anemia, obesity, or other nutritional problems, the family may need extra counseling and help. Poor families who have multiple problems will need much help to place on the family table minimum cost meals that meet the nutritional needs of all family members.

PREGNANT AND LACTATING WOMEN

The community nutritionist should be acquainted with the Recommendations of the Committee on Maternal Nutrition of the National Research Council for "a single standard of high quality maternity care, including nutrition, for all pregnant women and adolescents." (9) This standard includes:

Average weight gain of 20 to 25 pounds during the pregnancy.

Monitoring of the pattern of weight gain.

Special attention to the high nutrient needs of the pregnant girl under 17, with a food pattern developed for the group.

Special attention to the nutrient needs and food habits of all females who enter pregnancy in a poor nutritional state.

No routine use of salt restriction, and use of diuretics only on specific clinical indications.

No routine use of vitamin and mineral supplementation for the correction of a poor diet.

Iron supplement of 30 to 60 milligrams per day during the last six months of pregnancy and a daily supplement of 0.2 to 0.4 milligram of folate.

Use of iodized salt where soil is deficient in the element.

Generally, Maternity and Infant Care Projects (page 102) are concerned with poverty families; however, it must be remembered that even well-educated women with plenty of money may eat a poor diet because of limited food likes or of misinformation about what constitutes a good diet. Some physicians and other professionals are not aware of the changes in practices about weight gain and sodium restriction, so the nutritionist may need to find ways to educate both professionals and publics about such changes.

The effects of diet counseling during pregnancy may be measured by comparing the diet record made at the first visit with records taken near the delivery date and at a postpartum visit. The nutritional effects as shown by weight and hemoglobin (or hematocrit) between the first prenatal visit and the postpartum visit should be matched with changes in food intake to evaluate the changes.

The influence of the diet and nutritional status of the female at the time of conception is of much importance in determining the health of the infant at birth and its growth and development in early life. The increase in number of infants born to young girls makes attention to nutrition of this age group especially important.

Pregnant teenagers present particular problems and services are often inadequate to meet their needs. This is one of the times when girls may be motivated toward good nutrition, as many have an interest at this time in their own health and that of the coming baby. However, many teenage girls do not have control over their food because of living in the family home. Often the attitude of the girl's mother must be changed and she must be motivated to provide the necessary food and emotional support for the girl.

In many areas there is a lack of educational and financial resources for this group. A study of services for pregnant teenage girls in 130 cities conducted in 1970–71 by Wallace and coworkers indicated that more nutrition services were needed for both the mothers and their babies. The services needed were education about infant feeding and provision of nutritious foods. (14)

Miller has proposed a National Health Service for Mothers and Children and emphasized the need for national standards and governmental services rather than state services. (8) This is one of the subjects for continuing debate between local, state, and federal governments.

In many prenatal care programs, there was for some years much emphasis on formula feeding and little on breast feeding. Sometimes breast feeding has been practiced more in poor families, but currently poorer mothers are using formula and higher income mothers are nursing their babies. This is related to early return to work as many mothers are employed. The only way these mothers could nurse their babies would be on the basis of a widespread commitment as to its importance with development of government subsidized day care centers at or near the place of work.

The renewed emphasis on the value of breast feeding recognizes that the woman must prepare for it during pregnancy. In some health agencies and hospitals, the benefits and advantages of breast feeding are explained to every pregnant woman although care is taken not to create guilt feelings among women who do not wish to breast feed or are unable to do so.

The benefits and advantages are that (1) human milk is easier for the infant to digest, (2) there is less likelihood of allergic reactions, (3) the antibodies in human milk help the infant resist infection, and (4) breast feeding reduces the probability of overfeeding because the mother is inclined to let the infant decide when enough food has been ingested but apt to urge the formula-fed infant to finish the bottle.

The nutritionist, nurse, and others who are in frequent contact with the pregnant woman can emphasize practical points about the problems of breast feeding that will give the mother confidence to prepare for it.

The community nutritionist should participate in the agency policy setting about the amount and kind of emphasis to be placed on breast feeding and in planning the education program to encourage its use. Agency programs to encourage breast feeding must include commitment of funds for personnel to conduct the educational program.

INFANTS AND PRESCHOOL CHILDREN

It appears logical that all child-citizens of the U.S. should have access to the same quality of care. This should not be denied because of the conservatism of local government, which sometimes does not provide good programs. Members of the community must be informed of standards and available programs so they can elect politicians who will provide the services desired by the community.

Health personnel should promote the development of good food habits in early life as the basis for lifelong good food practices. The anxious or competitive mother who urges the infant to finish the bottle or to eat a wide variety of solid foods at an earlier age than other babies sets the stage for obesity at a later date. Perhaps health workers should promote compliments for slender babies to replace those about the "fine big baby" that are frequently heard. The nurse or nutritionist who counsels the parents should help them recognize the wisdom of letting the child stop eating when ready rather than encourage cleaning the plate and drinking large amounts of milk, and rewarding the child with dessert for having eaten all of the food.

Undernutrition is a problem with some population groups, and some of the effects are irreversible. Dobbing believes that these "diffuse deficits of growth attainment" may cause a lower level of intellectual well-being. (2)

EPSDT, which is now operative in most states, needs the help of nutritionists to develop the nutrition component. The nutritional assessment of this program should be done carefully and accurately from four parameters—height, weight, hemoglobin or hematocrit, and dietary record. The assessment should be followed by counseling for correction of inadequate diet even when the growth data and blood iron are normal, because the effects of the poor diet may not be seen until sometime after the nutritional deficit has occurred. Nutritionists should be included on the staff that supervise and conduct these programs. The community nutritionist must know about these programs and work for nutritional assessment and follow-up.

Nutrition education should incorporate desirable patterns of physical activity that should be established during childhood by developing attitudes and teaching skills. The former involves the acceptance of the importance of activity and exercise in maintaining physical fitness and the need to make time for it in the adult schedule. Lack of time is the most common reason given by adults for not following good health practices in activity and a frequent reason for not eating properly. The preschool period is a good time to set the example and begin to instill the attitudes that will be followed by good practices in children, youths, and adults.

SCHOOL CHILDREN

School nutrition programs are usually restricted in scope. Fomon and Egan (4) suggest that in addition to nutritional assessment, they include proper food, nutrition education for children and parents, and education for school personnel. The latter should include subject matter and methods of nutrition education.

There are two points of view about food provided at school and in other child-feeding locations. One is that the program should make up for the deficiencies in diet caused by the home situation, giving breakfast, snacks, and a noon meal when needed. The other holds that the parents should be responsible for the child's nutrition, and the program should provide only the foods normally indicated by the hour. Teachers who have to cope with problems caused by hunger usually advocate breakfast programs.

It has been estimated that about 30 percent of children under 18 live in families in which both parents work. Many of these children eat one or more meals a day in camps, schools, Head Start centers, day care centers, or other places. Many additional children eat in residential institutions. The community nutritionist may work with these organizations in a variety of ways. Group care centers should consider not only the provision of proper food and development of good food habits, but also the social needs of the individuals. Such programs should include nutrition education for children and parents.

Day care should be more than a custodial service. It should include nutrition services, health services, social services, education for children and parents, and special services for handicapped children and for those who have a language problem. Nutritionists should participate in efforts to develop good day care. One of their special contributions is providing the nutrition component of the inservice education for staff.

Smith (11) urges teachers to become aware of the effects of malnutrition on ability to learn, and reports some of the studies that have shown the effects of nutrition on school achievement.

Mentally and physically handicapped children need special attention to help them reach their full potential. The method is the same as for other children except when a therapeutic diet is required as when there is an inborn error of metabolism. The nutritionist, nurse, occupational therapist, and others should work with the parents to resolve the problems of the child and family. Sometimes this care is given in special programs and sometimes it is provided by the regular health team. In either case, there is need for the special skills of the nutritionist in planning the services needed and in providing the services. (13)

YOUTH

The nutrition problems of young people are due to obesity, food misinformation, adherence to fad diets or diets of the counterculture, abuse of alcohol and drugs, and indifference about the importance of food and nutrition.

There are great differences among adolescents, some being still emotionally dependent on their parents, others emotionally emancipated and very sure of themselves and their ideas. The nutritionist must learn to assess the emotional state of the adolescent and to adapt approach and methods accordingly. Above all, the nutritionist must adjust teaching to each individual according to the characteristics of that individual.

Those who would work with youth must be able to establish rapport. This has been done by some workers by dressing and talking like them. Others have achieved it by persuading the youths of their interest and concern while retaining their own identity, for example, a long-haired, mini-skirted nurse and a gray-haired, motherly nutritionist both worked successfully in the same youth clinic.

One investigation of factors affecting teen-age food habits showed that the occupational level of parents, educational level of the mother, social activity, and employment affected the complexity of the diet but that age, sex, family size, and number of nutrition information channels did not. (10)

A realistic goal for the obese early adolescent when motivation is limited is to stabilize weight, and for the older adolescent to achieve a slow, constant loss. Motivation for teenagers usually is not related to health but is for appearance, for dates, for ease in finding clothes, or for greater prowess in athletics. Efforts to increase the activity of the obese teenager are of much importance and may center on social activities built around hiking, biking, or swimming.

A study of 75 transient youths (32 females, 43 males) in Hawaii, most between the ages of 16 and 25, revealed that the choice of foods depended on having money and access to food. The diets of both sexes were considered deficient in calories while the girls' diets were also deficient in protein. There were many misconceptions about food, especially in the list of those considered to be "unhealthy and bad for the body." (7)

Frankle and Heussenstamm (5) reviewed the three diets most common among youths in the counterculture, namely vegetarian, organically grown and health foods, and the Zen macrobiotic regimen. They point out the sharp contrast between these overconcerned youths and the soda-and-candy-bar crowd. They suggest as a preliminary step to starting programs that an agency organize a board of teenage advisors and make sure in nutrition education of youth groups to teach them what they want to know.

OLDER AMERICANS

One of the recommendations of the White House Conference on Aging was that health care be considered as a basic right of the elderly, that it should be comprehensive and systematic and should provide:

1. Assessment of health.
2. Education to preserve health.
3. Appropriate preventive and outreach services.
4. All physical, mental, social, and supportive services necessary to maintain or restore health.
5. Rehabilitation.
6. Maintenance and long term care when disability occurs. (20)

Having a large aged population is a characteristic of this century. There are now more than 22 million persons over 65 in the U.S. and it is estimated that by the year 2000 there will be 29 million. (18) Moreover, a major medical advance such as eliminating over-65 deaths from cardiovascular-renal disease would change the present life expectancy of the 65-year-old from 15 years to 25 years, resulting in a marked increase in the number of older persons. In 1972 the median age for the elderly (i.e., persons 65 or older) was 73 years.

The need for the community nutritionist to work on problems of the elderly depends largely on the locale. Most of the elderly and the large concentrations are in a few states; ten states (California, New York, Pennsylvania, Illinois, Ohio, Texas, Florida, Michigan, New Jersey, and Massachusetts) account for 55 percent of them. However, the elderly are often clustered in certain areas so there may be a high concentration in one part of a state even when the total number for that state is small.

There are several stereotypes about older persons. One stereotype is that they live in institutions, but in fact in 1972 over 95 percent lived in the community and only 4 percent in institutions. Sixteen percent of the men lived alone and 80 percent in a family setting, 70 percent being with their wives. In contrast, 35 percent of the women lived alone or with nonrelatives, 34 percent with husband and 61 percent in a family setting. However, because women have a greater life expectancy, most older women are widows and most older men are married. Another stereotype is that most older persons have physical handicaps; in fact, 81 percent had no limitations on their mobility. It has been estimated that 80 to 90 percent of persons over 65 can manage on their own in the community if essential services such as health care and transportation are provided. (18, 20)

Encouraging as these figures are, there is still a sizable problem among the aged. Some who live in their own homes are bedfast or housebound, while others find it hard to get outdoors.

Food intakes of the aged need to be improved. Pao reported (21) information from the 1965 food consumption studies about the food intakes of the elderly in the North Central Region. Fifty-four percent had three meals a day and 42 percent had more than three meals, but many of the meal patterns did not meet the recommendations for older people for vegetables, citrus fruits, and milk although intakes of protein-rich foods and cereals were adequate.

Another problem is low income. In 1971 one-fourth of all Americans over 65 had incomes below the poverty level. Of these, 65 percent were women, and 85 percent were white. The spending practices of those who had money were similar to the spending practices of younger persons, most of it going for necessities (food, housing and medical care), which took a large part of the income. (18)

Though the above statistics are encouraging, the fact remains that for most aged life is a struggle for economic survival and is marked by the need for a great effort to stay in the mainstream. The major problems are concerned with shopping, getting medical care, and attending social, cultural or recreational events because of both limited physical ability and lack of suitable transportation. A disturbing phenomenon of the 1970's, which further contributes to these problems, is the increase in crime and violence against older persons, especially women, and mainly in large cities.

Unfortunately, bringing the benefits of a better diet to older persons is difficult. Organizations for the aged do not usually stress the benefits of good nutrition because it is not a popular subject. Older people in good health think they know what to eat. (22)

Aging takes place from conception to death but its course is determined in early life by genetic patterning, especially during the fetal period and up to age 2. Properly managed environmental factors and nutrition will help prevent obesity, atherosclerosis, osteoporosis, and dental caries. Few other things contribute as much to the comfort and life enjoyment of the older person as good food served in a pleasant way. Many older persons need help in knowing how to market or cook or serve for one; they tend to eat inadequate meals while standing in the kitchen. The nutrition counselor needs to check carefully into the nutrient intakes of older persons and, when indicated, help them find other resources so they can purchase an adequate diet.

Many older persons, especially those who have lost their spouses, lose interest in life and health. The nutritionist and others who work with them need to point out the significance of their new single existence and the importance of maintaining their physical and mental health. Participation in feeding programs for the elderly, trying new recipes, having a guest, using pleasing appointments or eating outdoors, are possible ways to add zest and interest to mealtime and improve the food intake.

Another health problem in older people is their lack of activity which leads to obesity and restricted mobility. Several studies have demonstrated that older persons can be physically benefited by exercise retraining programs. Adams and DeVries have demonstrated this with groups of older men and women. (17, 19) Some senior citizens' groups are now conducting exercise programs for members. The problem of obesity in older persons is actually one of substitution of fatty tissue for lean tissue during adulthood. Body conditioning and vigorous activity will prevent the loss of lean tissue.

Older persons must be recognized as individuals rather than put into rigid categories, and each should be considered according to specific needs. A problem in dealing with their health needs is that the elderly poor make less use of health services than those with more money. Well-chosen methods of motivation with attention to individual needs will help the nutritionist get the elderly to attend special meal programs or to improve their eating and exercise practices.

Screening programs of multiphasic type or those for detection of specific conditions such as diabetes offer a way to identify problems and to get the elderly into the health care system. Nutritionists will find frequent opportunities to participate in these programs.

The nutritionist might find opportunity to talk with adult groups about the need for child nutrition services in the community and how they could promote better nutrition for children. The community nutritionist or other professionals might be able to interest seniors as volunteers in child nutrition services to promote better nutrition. Many older adults do not know the relationship of nutrition to brain development and ability to learn, and feel no responsibility for education and welfare of children. Perhaps motivation might result if they were shown they could help prevent in others the disabilities they suffer. Watkin has made the point that good nutrition in the first two years of life can have a favorable influence on the aging process. (22)

Research is needed to fill some of the gaps in information about aging and the aged. The natural process of aging must be distinguished from disease, with a description of the aging process for all cell and organ systems. Research is also needed on how nutritional requirements change with age and how the impairments of age become permanent disabilities.

SUMMARY

Some members of the family group need special attention because of physical or mental problems or because they are unable to look after themselves. The policies that govern specially financed programs for some family members have resulted in fragmentation of programs. Such fragmentation should be avoided.

A family group may consist of two parents and children or a single parent with children, or children with parent-substitute. Any group may have the problem of inadequate diet due to lack of money, information, or interest. The Committee on Maternal Nutrition has recommended that there be a single standard for high quality maternal care of all pregnant females.

Parents should be taught how to instill good nutrition habits in children and why good habits acquired in early life are a lifelong asset. Pregnancy and obesity are the two greatest problems of teen-age girls. Sometimes changes in the girl's lifestyle can be accomplished only by making changes in the mother's attitudes and practices.

The proportion of aged in the population is increasing. Most of the aged live in a few states, many women live alone, and most aged have no limitations on their mobility. However, a sizable number of aged are unable to care for their own needs because of inadequate funds, decreased mobility, or illness. Some older persons need many kinds of help. Many older persons need to improve their diets, but do not recognize the need or are not interested in changing.

REFERENCES CITED

Parents and Children

1. Angrist, Walter J., Special Problems of Families: How To Obtain Help, in *Handbook for the Home,* 1973 Yearbook of Agriculture, U.S. Department of Agriculture, Government Printing Office, Washington DC, 32.
2. Dobbing, J., Undernutrition and the Developing Brain, *Am. J. Dis. Child,* 120 11/70 411.
3. Fomon, Samuel J., Nutrition and Health of Infants and Children, in *National Nutrition Policy Study,* Part 6—Nutrition and Health, Hearings Before the U.S. Senate Select Committee on Nutrition and Human Needs, June 21, 1974, Government Printing Office, Washington DC, 2577.
4. Fomon, Samuel J., and Mary C. Egan, Infants, Children and Adolescents, in *U.S. Nutrition Policies In the Seventies,* Jean Mayer, ed., 1973, 4.
5. Frankle, Reva T., and F. K. Heussenstamm, Food Zealotry and Youth, *Am. J. Pub. Health,* 64 1/74 11.
6. Jacobson, Howard N., and Susan H. Mills, Pregnant and Lactating Women, Ch. 2 in *U.S. National Nutrition Policies In the Seventies,* Jean Mayer, ed., W. H. Freeman and Co., San Francisco, 1973, 20.
7. Jane, Diane E., Jean E. Hankin, Setsu Furuno, and Neal E. Winn, Nutri-

tion in Action for Young Transients in Hawaii, *Am. J. Pub. Health,* 62 9/72 1202.

8. Miller, C. Arden, Health Care of Children and Youth In America, *Am. J. Pub. Health,* 65 4/75 353.

9. National Research Council, Food and Nutrition Board, *Maternal Nutrition and the Course of Pregnancy: Summary Report,* Reprinted by U.S. Dept. of Health, Education, and Welfare, Public Health Service, Pub. No. 2114, 1970, 16.

10. Schorr, Bernice C., Diva Sanjur, and Eugene C. Erickson, Teen-Age Food Habits, *J. Am. Diet. Assoc.,* 61 10/72 419.

11. Smith, Nila Banton, Child Nutrition In a Changing World, *Childhood Education,* 51 1/75 142.

12. United States Department of Health, Education, and Welfare, Bureau of Community Health Service, *Promoting Community Health,* DHEW Pub. No. (HSA) 75-5016, 1975, 33.

13. United States Department of Health, Education, and Welfare, Public Health Service, Nutrition Section, *Nutrition Services for Children Who Are Mentally or Physically Retarded,* leaflet.

14. Wallace, Helen M., Edwin M. Gold, Hyman Goldstein, and Allan C. Oglesby, A Study of Services and Needs of Teenage Pregnant Girls in the Large Cities Of the United States, *Am. J. Pub. Health,* 63 1/73 5.

15. Watkin, Donald M., A Year of Developments in Nutrition and Aging, *Med. Clin. North Am.,* 54 11/70 1589.

16. *White House Conference On Food, Nutrition, and Health, Final Report,* Government Printing Office, Washington DC, 1970, 38.

Older Americans

17. Adams, Gene M., and Herbert A. DeVries, Physiological Effects of an Exercise Training Regimen upon Women Aged 52 to 79, *J. Geront.,* 28 1973 50.

18. Brotman, Herman B., The Fastest Growing Minority: The Aging, *Am. J. Pub. Health,* 64 3/74 249.

19. DeVries, Herbert A., *Physiology of Exercise for Physical Education and Athletics,* W. C. Brown Co., Dubuque, Iowa, 1974, 261.

20. Hammerman, Jerome, Health Services: Their Success and Failure in Reaching Older Adults, *Am. J. Pub. Health,* 64 3/74 253.

21. Pao, Eleanor, Food Patterns of the Elderly, *Fam. Econ. Rev.,* ARS 62-5, U.S. Dept of Agriculture, Agricultural Research Service, Hyattsville MD, 16.

22. Watkin, Donald M., A Year of Developments in Nutrition and Aging, *Med. Clin. North Am.,* 54 11/70 1589.

CHAPTER 26

QUALITY STANDARDS FOR COMMUNITY NUTRITION

Community nutrition programs must be evaluated to determine whether the standards on which they are based will assure high quality nutritional care. Nutritionists need to maintain an ongoing assessment of their own standards, which are first acquired during their academic preparation for the profession. These standards will be modified to meet the exigencies of the job and the changes that take place in scientific knowledge and practice.

Because many community nutritionists work independently, they need to engage in continual self-assessment to maintain high standards. The current emphasis on review by professional peers may result in review by another community nutritionist. Such review is more desirable than review by a professional from another field whose orientation, viewpoint, and standards of practice are different.

Community nutritionists should develop quality standards for the practice of community nutrition. Since none have been established, the author is proposing a number for use in evaluating some of the activities of practice. These standards should be based on nutritional status rather than on food. However, the effects of nutrition education must be measured by change in food practices.

1. *Nationally accepted standards are used.* The nutritionist should try to establish the acceptance of such standards in the agency and the community. They include the NRC Recommended Dietary Allowances, the NRC recommended percentage of calories from fat, the NRC policies on enrichment and fortification of foods, the

growth tables of the National Center for Health Statistics, and similar standards. These standards should be used for the purposes intended. Sometimes a problem arises when the nutritionist teaches accepted national standards to nurses but a physician accepts standards established by a professional association. This kind of situation may occur frequently unless national standards are adopted. Standards should be based on an unbiased, professional concensus.

2. *Legal or program standards are met for nutrition programs for which they have been established.* This includes standards for Head Start, WIC, Child Nutrition Programs, and other programs. They should be monitored to be sure the standards are met. If it appears that the standards are unrealistic or too difficult to meet, changes should be requested.

3. *Programs are conducted to meet identified needs.* The problems of the specific community should be identified rather than assumed to exist. Local figures should be used if available. If there are none, the figures from HANES should be used and projected to the local area. Frequent review of existing programs will indicate when one is no longer needed and may be eliminated. Review also shows how an existing program may be modified to make it more efficient, thus freeing resources to meet current program needs.

4. *Program plans include the naming of broad goals and specific objectives.* A goal is based on concrete data that show a need. Specific measurable objectives for meeting the goal are then established, with method and target dates.

5. *Large-scale efforts are used to attack nutrition problems that affect large numbers of people.* Investigation is conducted to identify the problems. Then intervention is planned to attack the most serious problems. A community with a higher than average incidence of hypertension might organize an educational program by press, radio, and television to urge people to have blood pressure taken and to seek regular medical care for high blood pressure. If the problem is a high number of obese teenagers, a task force from that group might be encouraged to develop a program of weight control. A high incidence of retarded growth as shown by EPSDT indicates a need for intervention on this problem.

6. *Nutritional status is monitored by a surveillance system.* A system may start with convenience samples established by utilizing data from records taken in regular programs (e.g., WIC, EPSDT) or by establishing a special data collection (e.g., regular

taking of height and weight at school). These data identify needs and indicate the kind of intervention that is needed.

7. *Children with growth problems are identified by regular weighing and measuring.*   This may be accomplished in a health center, HMO, private physician's office, school, or other place where children receive care. Height and weight are recorded on a growth chart and monitored to identify growth problems at an early stage. Action is then taken to correct the retarded growth or obesity.

8. *Attempts to change food practices are based on a food record and success is measured by change in food practices.*   The food record shows dietary inadequacies which form the basis for nutrition counseling. A second food record taken after counseling shows the changes that have been made. The success of a program should be measured by change in nutrition practices rather than by number of persons exposed to nutrition education.

9. *Client is referred for biochemical tests when food record indicates a continued low nutrient intake.*   A continued low nutrient intake is a danger signal even in the absence of clinical signs of malnutrition, because low biochemical values reflect past intake and precede the appearance of clinical signs.

10. *Nutrients are supplied with food rather than with supplements.*   Adequate nutrients can be supplied by a good diet of basic foods, with choices of the best foods from each Food Group except iron during the prenatal period. Money is better spent for basic foods than for supplements so that meals will be more appealing and nutritious.

11. *Nutrition education is regularly initiated when indicated.*   This includes counseling for individual problems and counseling of parent about food served in the home. It includes attention to problems of food money management, home management, and child development. Nutritionists should also participate in developing policies and practices for others responsible for food service as in school, institution, and elderly meal programs.

12. *Weight control is incorporated into all materials used for nutrition education.*   This is accomplished by limiting sugar, fat, and alcohol. Materials might also be adjusted to conform to the current recommendation that the same diet is indicated as a preventive measure against cancer, heart disease, diabetes, and obesity. Changes should be incorporated into both teaching materials and resource materials. Though there is no conclusive evidence that this diet will prevent these diseases, it is the best preventive measure currently known.

13. *Nutrition education encompasses related health habits.*   Activity and sleep affect appetite, food consumption, and weight. Several factors affect dental health, including the effect of food during the prenatal period, and in early life, and regular use of noncariogenic and detersive foods. The value of fluoride obtained in the water supply or by other means can also be included as part of nutrition education.

14. *Professional education is evaluated by increase in services as well as increase in knowledge.*   Increase in knowledge is important, but change must also occur in attitudes and willingness to provide nutrition services not previously provided, or to keep records, or to make a greater effort to motivate changes in the patient.

15. *An ongoing review of information sources is maintained.*   The nutritionist always keeps materials to provide information about current scientific data and recommended practices. The community nutritionist may take leadership for preparation of an unbiased joint statement about an issue. Sometimes it is helpful to prepare a position statement on a specific topic based on national standards when available, or on one's own judgment of current research and other evidence. One example is the author's statement about use of salt on page 395. The nutritionist should modify such statements when the need is indicated by new evidence or by other circumstances. Sometimes different judgments make it necessary to compromise with medical personnel in the agency or with nutrition personnel in the community.

16. *A permanent official record is kept of each client and each activity.*   The patient's record shows the problems and action taken to handle them. It includes all significant information. Each team member records nutrition contacts with the patient. Records should likewise be kept of each activity to show the action that has been taken and serve as a basis for evaluating change that indicates progress. This helps the nutritionist to decide whether a program or activity is productive.

Evaluation of nutrition education and other programs should be conducted by use of the most effective means available. The methds should answer three specific questions: (1) Is this activity needed for good nutrition? (2) Does this activity conform to standards generally recognized by the profession? (3) Is this activity provided in the most appropriate way? Often it is useful to make program changes or to initiate new programs in accordance with nationwide emphasis, such as the program mentioned in the yearly USDHEW *Forward Plan for Health.* Recently these have included improving food consumption practices, integrating nutrition into health care systems, training health personnel so they can work for better nutrition, and determining the nutritional status of people in the nation.

Community nutrition programs do not just happen. New ideas are not just luck. The community nutritionist must innovate and develop new programs or new ways to make old programs more effective at less cost. The community nutritionist who depends on others to carry much of the nutrition message must develop in those persons a confidence that they can do the task, and must take leadership to establish an environment in which they can teach nutrition effectively.

Health policy is often made by administrative personnel who are business school graduates without experience in the health field. The community nutritionist should find ways to participate in this policy-making and to develop in administrators a knowledge of the requirements for successful nutrition programs.

SUMMARY

The author has suggested 16 points for use in assessing quality in community nutrition. They may be used by an experienced nutritionist working alone or in cooperation with administrative personnel, or by the individual nutritionist as an ongoing program check.

GLOSSARY

activist one who makes judgments and acts on a professional appraisal of community needs.

activity (1) a specialized action that is characteristic of community nutrition; (2) state of action.

additive a substance that is added to a food to produce a specific desired effect, improving nutritional value or the quality of the finished product. "Food additive" has a specific legal meaning in the U.S.

adviser one who suggests possible resources or activities for handling a problem.

advocate one who promotes nutrition activities for the solution of problems; to speak out in favor of something or to recommend publicly.

alcoholism regular excessive drinking of alcoholic beverages.

ambulatory care care given to the noninstitutionalized patient, including home care, primary, secondary, and emergency care.

anemia the final stage in development of iron deficiency after body iron stores are depleted.

anomie lack of purpose, identity or ethical values in a person or a society; disorganization, rootlessness, and so forth.

anthropometry the science dealing with measurement of the human body to determine differences in individuals, groups, and so forth.

atherosclerosis a disease in which the linings of the arteries are thickened and partly blocked by a build-up of fatty deposits narrowing the inside channel.

behavior modification a method of changing eating behavior by changing the circumstances that precede and follow eating.

birth defect an abnormality of structure, function, or metabolism existing at birth and resulting from a genetic or an environmental cause.

429

cancer a group of diseases characterized by uncontrolled growth and invasion of other body systems.

cariogenic favoring the development of dental caries.

carrier private insurance organization that handles claims from doctors and others who supply services under the medical insurance part of Medicare.

cholelithiasis gallstones.

client the recipient of nutrition service.

clinical dietetics the part of medical care concerned with the nutritional care of sick persons.

clinical nutrition treatment of disease through attention to nutritional care of the individual.

community a social group of any size whose members have a common bond such as the same city, same culture, or same language.

community education activities planned to change the knowledge, attitudes, or actions of the publics who influence the making of policies and decisions that affect nutrition.

community medicine scientific study of the health problems of the community and application of the knowledge to the solution of those problems.

community nursing the field of nursing that functions in home and community with family and community as patients.

community nutrition the branch of nutrition that works with the entire range of health and illness of the individual and family as a part of the community, but that focusses primarily on prevention of disease and maintenance of health by interaction of nutrition personnel and community.

community nutritionist a nutritionist who applies the subject matter of nutrition in the community setting.

community organization a process by which individuals, groups, or organizations find solutions to social problems by planned action in which forces, people, and resources are organized and used to meet needs.

conference a formal meeting in which members of the audience discuss a particular topic; may be between two persons or include a large group.

consult to ask for advice or information to help solve a problem.

consultation a process by which a specialist makes professional knowledge and skill available to help other professionals with problems.

consultee person who requests help by consultation.

consumerism the practices and policies of protecting the consumer by developing awareness of defective and unsafe products, misleading business practices, and so forth.

convenience food a food that has been partially prepared by a food manufacturer to reduce work and ingredients to be added at home.

coordinate to combine in harmonious action.

coronary heart disease blockage of the coronary artery that causes a heart attack.

counsel to provide individualized guidance for the purpose of helping adjust daily food consumption to meet health needs.

decision choice of a course of action.

decision-making deciding among alternatives to determine policy.

detersive exerting a cleansing action.

diabetes a disease that occurs when the metabolism of carbohydrate is incomplete due to insufficient production of insulin.

dietitian a specialist educated for a profession responsible for the nutritional care of individuals and groups. . . . participation may be in . . . foodservice systems management; in extending knowledge of food and nutrition principles; in teaching these principles . . . ; or in dietary counseling. (*J. Am. Diet. Assoc., 64:* 661, June 1974.)

drug a substance that, by its chemical activity, alters body function or structure.

elderly age 65 or older.

enabler person who acts as a catalytic agent to help a community state its problems.

enrichment increasing the amount of nutrients in a food to a higher level than they naturally occur.

evaluation to ascertain the worth of a program or activity by measuring the results.

exercise test (stress test)—a medical test used by physician or exercise physiologist to determine how the heart responds to stress or exertion.

existing nutrition problem a problem based on conditions that are already present.

external poverty a temporary form of poverty as when one is out of work.

faddism excessive emphasis on a topic over a period of time, usually as a result of fashion.

failure-to-thrive a condition of young infants characterized by failure to grow at a normal rate.

food contact taking food or drink.

food recall a list from the client's memory of food eaten in the preceding 24 hours.

food record (1) a form for recording food intake, (2) a list of food eaten by an individual in a specified period of time.

fortification adding nutrients that do not naturally occur in a food.

foundation a nongovernmental, nonprofit organization that makes grants for purposes serving the common welfare.

habit an acquired pattern of action that has become automatic.

health maintenance organization (HMO) an organization that provides prepaid comprehensive health services with emphasis on primary care and preventive services.

high blood pressure common term for hypertension, used in public education.

Hispanic native to or descended from a native of any country in the Western Hemisphere south of the United States where Spanish or Portuguese is the official language; including Mexico and all countries of Central America, the West Indies, and South America.

home economist person with a college major in home economics; for work in a nutrition program, one should have a good background in foods and nutrition, food economics, and home management.

hunger   discomfort, pain, or weakness caused by inadequate intake of food.

hypertension   medical term for abnormally high blood pressure; normal range for systolic pressure is 100 to 140 millimeters (mm) of mercury; for diastolic, 70 to 90 mm.

income maintenance   a plan to provide a guaranteed annual income for each individual and family.

institute   a short teaching program for people in the same field of work.

instruct   to furnish information in a systematic manner.

instructional medium   any medium (plural, *media*) used for teaching, as printed matter, films, charts, posters, field trips, role-playing, chalkboard, projector, and so forth.

intermediary   private insurance organization that handles hospital, nursing home, and home health care for Medicare.

internal poverty   the culture of poverty.

intervention   any action to stop the cause or progress of a nutrition problem.

interview   a directed conversation for the purpose of gathering information.

iron deficiency   low body iron as shown by transferrin saturation level.

lecture   an informative talk presented to an audience.

legislation   the making of laws.

lobby   persuasive activity that tries to influence the passage of a bill.

logrolling   the process by which politicians give mutual aid by supporting each other's bills.

malnutrition   a state of disease caused by sustained deficiency, excess, or imbalance of the supplies of calories, nutrients, or both, that are available for use in the body.

malnutrition control   the prevention and treatment of malnutrition by identification of nutrition problems and action to prevent or control them.

management   the control of time, energy, money, and other resources to achieve goals.

mediator   one who acts as a link between two groups, as public and officials.

Medicaid   the program under federal law, administered by the individual state, that provides payment for medical care for eligible needy persons.

Medicare   the federal health insurance program for persons over 65 financed and administered by the Social Security Administration.

migrant worker   a farm worker who moves from place to place to work with seasonal crops.

misinformation   incorrect information based on inaccurate facts, misinterpretation of facts, or ignoring of facts.

mutagenic   causing a sudden variation in inherited characteristics.

national health insurance   a federal system of health care financing to cover individuals with basic benefits and reimburse for the costs of catastrophic illness.

negotiator   one who helps two groups reach agreement.

nutrition   series of processes by which an organism ingests and assimilates the nutrients necessary for body function.

nutrition aide   a person trained by the nutritionist for a helping role in the nutrition program; the aide is often from the neighborhood in which the work is to be done.

nutrition (or nutritional) care   application of the science and art of nutrition to help individuals and groups achieve good nutrition through proper diet and attention to related health habits.

nutrition counselor   nutritionist, dietitian, nurse, or other person who teaches nutrition to individuals or small groups.

nutrition education   the process of applying a knowledge of nutrition, related scientific information, and the social and behavioral sciences in ways designed to influence individuals and groups to eat the kinds and amounts of foods that will make a maximum contribution to health and social satisfaction.

nutrition educator   a person who conducts nutrition education.

nutrition problem   any situation that adversely affects nutrition and therefore needs to be changed to improve nutrition.

nutrition program manager   person responsible for a program with staff; any nutritionist who works alone and is responsible for planning and carrying out a program.

nutrition (nutritional) surveillance   continuous collection of data for evaluating nutritional status and showing points of intervention.

nutrition technician   a technically skilled person who has completed the specified two-year college program for the position of dietetic technician and has had courses and experience to qualify for work in a community setting.

nutritional status   the physical health of a person as it results from consumption and utilization of food in the body.

nutritionist   a person whose primary discipline is nutrition and whose major work is in the field of nutrition, especially in activities designed to promote health, or prevent, or control disease.

obesity   any body weight in excess of 20 percent above normal; lesser degrees may be termed *overweight.*

official agency   one established by government and financed with public moneys.

overnutrition   malnutrition resulting from excessive intake of calories or nutrients, or both.

panel discussion   a discussion carried on among a selected group of speakers before an audience, sometimes in response to questions posed by a panel leader.

paraprofessional   a worker trained to perform certain functions but not prepared to practice as a professional.

partisan   one who takes sides in a social conflict.

planner   a person who has a special background for helping the community plan ways to deal with its problems.

ponderal index   a method of assessing weight based on the ratio of height in inches to the cube root of weight in pounds.

potential nutrition problem   problem likely to develop because of existing factors.

poverty   lacking resources for reasonably comfortable living compared with the standard of living for the community.

practice   (1) the doing of something in the same way repeatedly; (2) the exercise of a profession.

prevention   action or intervention designed to prevent disease. See also *primary prevention, secondary prevention,* and *tertiary prevention.*

primary prevention   an early attack on the cause of disease, before disease has developed.

problem-solving   using decisions to determine a course of action on everyday operations.

process   a series of loosely connected changes taking place in a definite manner or pattern.

professional education   education for professionals to enhance their skills and abilities.

program   a plan of activities that combines personnel, money, equipment, supplies, and other resources to accomplish goals.

public   the people who constitute a community.

public education   education of the people as a whole, or a part of the people; includes community education and nutrition education.

public health   all aspects of the health of all of the people. The classic definition of C.E.A. Winslow is "the Science and Art of preventing disease, prolonging life and promoting health and efficiency through organized community effort."

public health agency   the government agency that is responsible for the health of the people within its geographic area.

public health nutrition   the nutrition program conducted by a state, county, city, or other governmental agency that has the responsibility for the health of persons living in the area over which it has jurisdiction.

public health nutritionist   a nutritionist with advanced study in nutrition, public health, and educational methods, whose function is to assess nutrition needs in the area served, and to plan and direct a public health nutrition program to meet the needs. (Adapted from definition in *Personnel in Public Health Nutrition,* American Dietetic Association, 1976, pp. 4–5.)

quackery   professing to have qualifications or knowledge one does not actually have.

quasi-governmental agency   a nongovernmental agency which, because of the nature of its work and charter, appears to be a governmental agency.

rapport   development of mutual trust and understanding, confidence, and respect as a basis for continued communication.

regimen   a regulated course or manner of living intended to preserve or restore health.

research   scholarly, carefully controlled, exhaustive, critical investigation or experimentation for the purpose of discovering and interpreting new facts of wide significance. Sometimes used to refer to surveys, studies or literature review for the purpose of obtaining information for use in program planning.

retarded growth   failure to reach the expected growth potential.

secondary prevention   early detection of disease before individual shows symptoms.

skill   the ability to do something well because of knowledge, training, and practice, with proficiency resulting from many repetitions.

staff nutritionist   a nutritionist who works under direction in an agency where there is more than one nutritionist.

standard of identity   a statement of the required and permissible ingredients in a food that bears a particular name, for example, mayonnaise. Any food that bears the name must conform to the standard, and thus the label does not have to show a list of ingredients.

stress test   exercise test.

substance abuse   excessive use of alcohol or drugs.

symposium   a program in which a particular subject is discussed, usually with a number of speakers.

technique   systematic employment of basic skills to carry out an operation.

teratogenic   causing malformation of a fetus.

tertiary prevention   treatment of disease to prevent damage to future health.

tool   any implement or object used in carrying on an occupation.

trade association   a nonprofit, voluntary association of business competitors in the same trade or industrial operation, formed to provide services to the members.

training   making proficient by practice.

undernutrition   malnutrition that results from an inadequate amount of calories, or nutrients, or both.

vegetarian diet   a meatless diet composed of vegetables, fruits, grains and nuts, sometimes with animal products such as milk, cheese and eggs.

voluntary health agency   a private, nonprofit organization that conducts activities designed to mitigate a specific health problem and that is supported by voluntary contributions.

weight control   a regimen for achieving and maintaining normal weight with correction to the normal range when necessary.

workshop   an action-oriented meeting to help the participant acquire specific skills.

INDEX